Taenzer/Zeitler
Contrast Media

Überreicht
von Schering

# Fortschritte auf dem Gebiete der Röntgenstrahlen und der Nuklearmedizin

Diagnostik, Physik, Biologie, Therapie

Supplement Volume 118

Edited by W. Frommhold and P. Thurn

In Collaboration with G. Breitling, E. Vogler and K. zum Winkel

1983
Georg Thieme Verlag
Stuttgart · New York

Thieme-Stratton Inc.
New York

# Contrast Media
in Urography, Angiography
and Computerized Tomography

Edited by
Volker Taenzer and Eberhard Zeitler

With Contributions by

| | | | |
|---|---|---|---|
| P. Anger | B. Hagen | X. Papacaralampous | A. Thron |
| T. Baitsch | H. G. Hartmann | W. R. Press | K. Tremmel |
| D. Baller | P. Hartwig | M. Ratzka | H. Tschakert |
| D. Banzer | H. Heep | W.-D. Reinbold | S. Tuengerthal |
| V. Barth | G. Hellige | E.-I. Richter | U. Uthmann |
| D. Beduhn | A. Hoeft | J. E. Scherberich | K. Voigt |
| H. K. Beyer | R. Keysser | D. Schlürmann | H.-J. Weinmann |
| K. Böhnlein | G. Klink | R. Schräder | W. Wenz |
| U. Borst | J. Kollath | B. Schulze | V. Wiebe |
| W. Clauss | H. Korb | W. Seyferth | K. Wiemers |
| N. Freudenberg | T. Kröpelin | H. M. Siefert | K. Wink |
| H. Gailer | R. Lindner | U. Speck | J. Wissert |
| H. P. Geisen | P. Meiisel | B. Steidle | K.-J. Wolf |
| E. Glück | W. Mützel | H. Straub | H. G. Wolpers |
| Ch. Gospos | M. Nadjmi | V. Taenzer | E. Zeitler |

106 Figures, 86 Tables

1983
Georg Thieme Verlag   Thieme-Stratton Inc.
Stuttgart · New York   New York

**Deutsche Bibliothek Cataloguing in Publication Data**

**Contrast media in urography, angiography and computerized tomography** /
ed by Volker Taenzer and Eberhard Zeitler. With contributions by P. Anger . . . –
Stuttgart ; New York : Thieme ; New York : Thieme-Stratton, 1983.

(Fortschritte auf dem Gebiete der Röntgenstrahlen und der Nuklearmedizin : Suppl. ; Vol. 118)

NE: Taenzer, Volker [Hrsg.]; Anger, P. [Mitverf.]; Fortschritte auf dem Gebiete der Röntgenstrahlen und der Nuklearmedizin / Ergänzungsband

**Important Note:**
Medicine is an ever-changing science. Research and clinical experience are continually broadening our knowledge, in particular our knowledge of proper treatment and drug therapy. Insofar as this book mentions any dosage or application, readers may rest assured that the authors, editors and publishers have made every effort to ensure that such references are strictly in accordance with the state of knowledge at the time of production of the book. Nevertheless, every user is requested to carefully examine the manufacturers' leaflets accompanying each drug to check on his own responsibility whether the dosage schedules recommended therein or the contraindications stated by the manufacturers differ from the statements made in the present book. Such examination is particularly important with drugs which are either rarely used or have been newly released on the market.

Some of the product names, patents and registered designs referred to in this book are in fact registered trademarks or proprietary names even though specific reference to this fact is not always made in the text. Therefore, the appearance of a name without designation as proprietary is not to be construed as a representation by the publishers that it is in the public domain.

All rights, including the rights of publication, distribution and sales, as well as the right to translation, are reserved. No part of this work covered by the copyrights hereon may be reproduced or copied in any form or by any means – graphic, electronic or mechanical including photocopying, recording, taping, or information and retrieval systems – without written permission of the publisher.

© 1983 Georg Thieme Verlag, Rüdigerstrasse 14, D-7000 Stuttgart 30
Printed in Germany
Typesetting by Druckhaus Dörr, Ludwigsburg (Linotron 202). Printing by Gutmann + Co., Heilbronn

| ISBN 3-13-645501-0 | Georg Thieme Verlag | ISBN 0-86577-104-9 | Thieme-Stratton | |
|---|---|---|---|---|
| ISSN 0342-6114 | Stuttgart · New York | LC 83-050145 | Inc., New York | 1 2 3 4 5 6 |

# Adresses

*Anger, P., Dr.*
Abteilung Röntgendiagnostik am Zentrum Radiologie der Albert-Ludwigs-Universität Freiburg
Hugstetter Straße 55, D-7800 Freiburg

*Baitsch, T., Dr.*
Radiologische Abteilung des Kreiskrankenhauses Lahr
Klostenstraße 19, D-7630 Lahr

*Baller, D., Dr.*
Abteilung für experimentelle Kardiologie am Zentrum Physiologie und Pathophysiologie der Universität Göttingen
Humboldtallee 7, D-3400 Göttingen

*Banzer, D., Priv.-Doz. Dr.*
Klinik für Radiologie und Nuklearmedizin der Freien Universität Berlin, Klinikum Charlottenburg
Spandauer Damm 130, D-1000 Berlin 19

*Barth, V., Prof. Dr.*
Radiologisches Zentralinstitut der Städtischen Krankenanstalten Esslingen
Hirschlandstraße 97, D-7300 Esslingen

*Beduhn, D., Prof. Dr.*
Radiologische Klinik des Kreis- und Stadtkrankenhauses Wetzlar
Forsthausstraße 1, D-6330 Wetzlar

*Beyer, H. K., Prof. Dr.*
Radiologisches Institut des Marienhospitals der Universität Bochum
Hölkeskampring 40, D-4690 Herne 1

*Böhnlein, K.*
Klinikum Nürnberg, Radiologisches Zentrum, Abteilung Diagnostik
Flurstraße 17, D-8500 Nürnberg 91

*Borst, U., Dr.*
Radiologisches Zentralinstitut der Städtischen Krankenanstalten Esslingen
Hirschlandstraße 97, D-7300 Esslingen

*Clauss, W., Dr.*
Schering AG
Müllerstraße 170–172, D-1000 Berlin 65

*Freudenberg, N., Priv.-Doz. Dr.*
Pathologisches Institut
der Albert-Ludwigs-Universität Freiburg
Hugstetter Straße 55, D-7800 Freiburg

*Gailer, H.*
Klinikum Nürnberg, Radiologisches Zentrum, Abteilung Diagnostik
Flurstraße 17, D-8500 Nürnberg 91

*Geisen, H. P., Priv.-Doz. Dr.*
Klinisches Labor und Blutbank der Chirurgischen Universitätsklinik Heidelberg
Im Neuenheimer Feld 110, D-6900 Heidelberg

*Glück, Elvira, Dr.*
Abteilung für Röntgendiagnostik der Chirurgischen Universitätsklinik Heidelberg
Im Neuenheimer Feld 110, D-6900 Heidelberg

*Gospos, Ch., Dr.*
Sektion Medizinische Klinik,
Abteilung Röntgendiagnostik
am Zentrum Radiologie
der Albert-Ludwigs-Universität Freiburg
Hugstetter Straße 55, D-7800 Freiburg

*Hagen, B., Dr.*
Röntgenabteilung am Martin-Luther-Krankenhaus
Caspar-Theyß-Straße 27, D-1000 Berlin 33

*Hartmann, H. G., Dr.*
Abteilung für Nephrologie der Medizinischen Klinik und Poliklinik der Universität Homburg
D-6650 Homburg/Saar

*Hartwig, P.*
Abteilung Röntgendiagnostik des Krankenhauses Moabit, Berlin-Tiergarten
Turmstraße 21, D-1000 Berlin 21

*Heep, H., Dr.*
Radiologische Abteilung des Städtischen Krankenhauses Frankfurt-Höchst
Gotenstraße 6–8, D-6230 Frankfurt 80

*Hellige, G., Prof. Dr.*
Abteilung für experimentelle Kardiologie am Zentrum Physiologie und Pathophysiologie der Universität Göttingen
Humboldtallee 7, D-3400 Göttingen

*Hoeft, A., Dr.*
Abteilung für experimentelle Kardiologie am Zentrum Physiologie und Pathophysiologie der Universität Göttingen
Humboldtallee 7, D-3400 Göttingen

*Keysser, R., Dr.*
Schering AG
Müllerstraße 170–172, D-1000 Berlin 65

*Klink, G., Dr.*
Schering AG
Müllerstraße 170–172, D-1000 Berlin 65

*Kollath, J., Prof. Dr.*
Abteilung Allgemeine Röntgendiagnostik II
am Klinikum der Johann Wolfgang Goethe-
Universität Frankfurt
Theodor-Stern-Kai 7, D-6000 Frankfurt 70

*Korb, H., Dr.*
Abteilung für experimentelle Kardiologie am
Zentrum Physiologie und Pathophysiologie der
Universität Göttingen
Humboldtallee 7, D-3400 Göttingen

*Kröpelin, Traute, Prof. Dr.*
Sektion Medizinische Klinik, Abteilung
Röntgendiagnostik, am Zentrum Radiologie der
Albert-Ludwigs-Universität Freiburg
Hugstetter Straße 55, D-7800 Freiburg

*Lindner, R.*
Klinikum Nürnberg, Radiologisches Zentrum,
Abteilung Diagnostik
Flurstraße 17, D-8500 Nürnberg 91

*Meiisel, P., Dr.*
Radiologische Abteilung des
Wenckebach-Krankenhauses
Wenckebachstraße 23, D-1000 Berlin 42

*Mützel, W., Dr.*
Schering AG
Müllerstraße 170–172, D-1000 Berlin 65

*Nadjmi, M., Prof. Dr.*
Abteilung Neuroradiologie,
Neurologische Klinik und Poliklinik
im Kopfklinikum der Universität Würzburg
Josef-Schneider-Straße 11, D-8700 Würzburg

*Papacaralampous, X., Dr.*
Sektion Medizinische Klinik,
Abteilung Röntgendiagnostik,
am Zentrum Radiologie
der Albert-Ludwigs-Universität Freiburg
Hugstetter Straße 55, D-7800 Freiburg

*Press, W. R., Dr.*
Schering AG
Müllerstraße 170–172, D-1000 Berlin 65

*Ratzka, M., Dr.*
Abteilung Neuroradiologie, Neurologische Klinik
und Poliklinik im Kopfklinikum der Universität
Würzburg
Josef-Schneider-Straße 11, D-8700 Würzburg

*Reinbold, W.-D., Dr.*
Abteilung Röntgendiagnostik am Zentrum
Radiologie der Albert-Ludwigs-Universität Freiburg
Hugstetter Straße 55, D-7800 Freiburg

*Richter, E.-I.,*
Klinikum Nürnberg, Radiologisches Zentrum,
Abteilung Diagnostik
Flurstraße 17, D-8500 Nürnberg 91

*Scherberich, J. E., Priv.-Doz. Dr.*
Abteilung für Nephrologie am Zentrum der Inneren
Medizin, Klinikum der Johann Wolfgang Goethe-
Universität Frankfurt
Theodor-Stern-Kai 7, D-6000 Frankfurt 70

*Schlürmann, D., Dr.*
Abteilung Anästhesiologie und Intensivtherapie,
Anästhesiologisches Institut
der Albert-Ludwigs-Universität Freiburg
Hugstetter Straße 55, D-7800 Freiburg

*Schräder, R., Dr.*
Abteilung für experimentelle Kardiologie am
Zentrum Physiologie und Pathophysiologie der
Universität Göttingen
Humboldtallee 7, D-3400 Göttingen

*Schulze, B., Dr.*
Radiologisches Zentralinstitut der Städtischen
Krankenanstalten Esslingen
Hirschlandstraße 97, D-7300 Esslingen

*Seyferth, W., Dr.*
Klinikum Nürnberg, Radiologisches Zentrum,
Diagnostische Abteilung
Flurstraße 17, D-8500 Nürnberg 91

*Siefert, H. M.,*
Bayer AG
Postfach 10 17 09, D-5600 Wuppertal

*Speck, U., Dr.*
Schering AG
Müllerstraße 170–172, D-1000 Berlin 65

*Steidle, B., Dr.*
Medizinisches Strahleninstitut der
Universität Tübingen
Röntgenweg 11, D-7400 Tübingen

*Straub, H., Dr.*
Abteilung für Kardiologie und Angiologie der
Berufsgenossenschaftlichen Krankenanstalten „Berg-
mannsheil" Bochum, Universitätsklinik
Hunscheidtstraße 1, D-4630 Bochum

*Taenzer, V., Prof. Dr.*
Abteilung Röntgendiagnostik des Krankenhauses
Moabit, Berlin-Tiergarten
Turmstraße 21, D-1000 Berlin 21

*Thron, A., Dr.*
Abteilung Neuroradiologie des Medizinischen
Strahleninstituts der Universitätsklinik Tübingen
Röntgenweg 11, D-7400 Tübingen

*Tremmel, K., Dr.*
Radiologisches Zentralinstitut der Städtischen
Krankenanstalten Esslingen
Hirschlandstraße 97, D-7300 Esslingen

*Tschakert, H., Dr.*
Radiologische Abteilung des Knappschaftskrankenhauses Recklinghausen
Westerholter Weg 82, D-4350 Recklinghausen

*Tuengerthal, S., Dr.*
Abteilung Allgemeine Röntgendiagnostik I am
Klinikum der Johann Wolfgang Goethe-Universität
Frankfurt
Theodor-Stern-Kai 7, D-6000 Frankfurt 70

*Uthmann, U., Dr.*
Abteilung für Urologie
der Chirurgischen Universitätsklinik Heidelberg
Im Neuenheimer Feld 110, D-6900 Heidelberg

*Voigt, K., Prof. Dr.*
Abteilung Neuroradiologie des
Medizinischen Strahleninstituts
der Universitätsklinik
Tübingen
Röntgenweg 11, D-7400 Tübingen

*Weinmann, H.-J., Dr.*
Schering AG
Müllerstraße 170–172, D-1000 Berlin 65

*Wenz, W., Prof. Dr.*
Abteilung für Röntgendiagnostik am Zentrum
Radiologie der Albert-Ludwigs-Universität Freiburg
Hugstetter Straße 55, D-7800 Freiburg

*Wiebe, V., Dr.*
Radiologische Abteilung
der Berufsgenossenschaftlichen Krankenanstalten
„Bergmannsheil" Bochum, Universitätsklinik
Hunscheidtstraße 1, D-4630 Bochum

*Wiemers, K., Prof. Dr.*
Institut für Anästhesiologie
der Albert-Ludwigs-Universität Freiburg
Hugstetter Straße 55 , D-7800 Freiburg

*Wink, K., Prof. Dr.*
Abteilung Kardiologie
der Albert-Ludwigs-Universität Freiburg
Hugstetter Straße 55, D-7800 Freiburg

*Wissert, J., Dr.*
Abteilung Kardiologie
der Albert-Ludwigs-Universität Freiburg
Hugstetter Straße 55, D-7800 Freiburg

*Wolf, K.-J., Prof. Dr.*
Medizinisches Strahleninstitut
der Universität Tübingen
Röntgenweg 11, D-7400 Tübingen

*Wolpers, H. G., Dr.*
Abteilung für experimentelle Kardiologie am
Zentrum Physiologie und Pathophysiologie der
Universität Göttingen
Humboldtallee 7, D-3400 Göttingen

*Zeitler, E., Prof. Dr.*
Klinikum Nürnberg, Radiologisches Zentrum,
Diagnostische Abteilung
Flurstraße 17, D-8500 Nürnberg

# Preface

A new era in contrast media began with the introduction of the first water-soluble, non-ionic x-ray contrast medium, Metrizamide (1973). Initially only the low neurotoxicity of this substance on administration in the subarachnoid area was utilized. The instability of the solution and its extremely high cost prevented use of the substance in other indications or at least limited it to a few high-risk patients.

The general good tolerance of Metrizamide and, in particular, the almost complete absence of pain during intra-arterial injection, which consequently obviated the need for anaesthesia, encouraged the development of other, more stable and less expensive contrast media with similar properties.

The fact that new contrast media have been introduced in Germany or are currently undergoing clinical trials prompted us to assemble available experiences in a special edition of "Röntgen-Fortschritte". Particular prominence is given in the publication to preclinical and clinical experiences with another new non-ionic contrast medium, Iopromide.

Experimental and clinical studies both indicate changes in certain clinically pertinent properties of the new contrast media:

- a reduction in general reactions (nausea, vomiting, allergic reactions)
- a diminution of cardiovascular reactions
- decreased painful reactions
- renal tolerance

The reasons for this are to be found in the absence of any electrical charge in the non-ionic contrast media, in the lowering of the osmotic pressure and in the very low chemical toxicity.

The renal tolerance of contrast media with reduced osmotic pressure in the excretory phase after a fairly high total dose cannot yet – on the basis of the material available – be unequivocally distinguished from that of the hypertonic ionic contrast media.

The reduction in the osmotic pressure of the ionic contrast media is a decisive factor in the reduction in painfulness and for the circulatory effect. The non-ionic contrast media have, in addition, much better general and neural tolerance. The superior general tolerance of the non-ionic contrast media is beneficial both to intravenous urography and computed tomography and to peripheral, cerebral and cardioangiography.

A wide range of application in catheter arteriography is envisaged for the non-ionic contrast media, whereas their significance for intravenous administration is dependent on whether

1. the incidence of serious general reactions can also be decisively reduced in more protracted series of examinations, and
2. these non-ionic, ready-for-injection substances can be made available at a reasonable price.

The current state of contrast medium development shows considerable promise in this direction.

We would like to thank the publishers of "Röntgen-Fortschritte", Mr Frommhold and Mr Thurn, for giving us this exceptional opportunity to present this subject in a comprehensive manner. Our thanks are also due to "Thieme-Verlag", especially to Mr Hauff, for their generous support.

October 1982     *V. Taenzer*     *E. Zeitler*

# Vorwort

Mit der Einführung des ersten wasserlöslichen nicht-ionischen Röntgenkontrastmittels Metrizamid (1973) begann ein neues Kontrastmittelzeitalter. Ursprünglich wurde bei dieser Substanz lediglich die geringere Neurotoxizität bei der Kontrastmittel-Applikation für den Subarachnoidalraum genutzt. Instabilität der Kontrastmittellösung und extrem hohe Kosten erlaubten eine Anwendung in anderen Indikationsgebieten nicht oder beschränken diese auf einige Risikopatienten.

Die generell gute Verträglichkeit des nicht-ionischen Metrizamid und insbesondere dessen nahezu vollständige Schmerzlosigkeit bei intraarterieller Injektion mit daraus resultierendem Verzicht auf Anästhesie waren Anlaß für die Entwicklung anderer, stabilerer und preisgünstigerer Kontrastmittel mit ähnlichen Qualitäten.

Die Tatsache, daß in Deutschland neue Röntgenkontrastmittel eingeführt sind oder sich in klinischer Prüfung befinden, veranlaßt uns, die Erfahrungen in einem Sonderband der Röntgen-Fortschritte zusammenzufassen. Einen Schwerpunkt des Heftes bilden darüber hinaus vorklinische und klinische Erfahrungen mit einem weiteren neuen nicht-ionischen Röntgenkontrastmittel, dem Iopromid.

Experimentelle und klinische Arbeiten weisen übereinstimmend auf Änderungen der für die klinische Anwendung entscheidenden Eigenschaften der neuen Röntgenkontrastmittel hin:

- die Reduzierung von Allgemeinreaktionen (Übelkeit, Erbrechen, allergieartige Reaktionen)
- die Minderung von Herz-Kreislaufreaktionen
- verminderte Schmerzreaktionen
- die Nierenverträglichkeit

Die Ursachen dafür liegen in der fehlenden elektrischen Ladung der nicht-ionischen Kontrastmittel, in der Senkung des osmotischen Druckes und der sehr geringen chemischen Toxizität.

Die Nierenverträglichkeit der Kontrastmittel mit vermindertem osmotischen Druck in der Ausscheidungsphase nach hoher Gesamtdosis ist bisher anhand des vorliegenden Materials nicht sicher gegen die der ionischen hypertonen Kontrastmittel abzugrenzen.

Die Reduktion des osmotischen Druckes der ionischen Kontrastmittel ist entscheidend für die Verminderung der Schmerzhaftigkeit und der Kreislaufwirkung. Die nicht-ionischen Kontrastmittel haben darüber hinaus eine deutlich bessere allgemeine und neurale Verträglichkeit. Die bessere Allgemeinverträglichkeit der nicht-ionischen Kontrastmittel kommt sowohl bei der intravenösen Urographie und Computer-Tomographie, als auch bei der Angiographie im peripheren, cerebralen und cardangiographischen Bereich zum Tragen.

In der Katheterarteriographie ist mit einem umfangreichen Einsatz der nicht-ionischen Röntgenkontrastmittel zu rechnen, während die Bedeutung bei intravenöser Applikation davon abhängt ob

1. die Häufigkeit ernsterer Allgemeinreaktionen auch bei größeren Untersuchungsserien entscheidend zu reduzieren ist und
2. diese nicht-ionischen, injektionsfertigen Substanzen zu einem günstigen Preis angeboten werden können.

Die derzeitigen Kontrastmittelentwicklungen sind in diesem Bezug vielversprechend.

Den Herausgebern der Röntgen-Fortschritte, den Herren Frommhold und Thurn danken wir für die außergewöhnliche Möglichkeit, dieses spezielle Thema im Zusammenhang darstellen zu können. Dem Thieme-Verlag, insbesondere Herrn Hauff danken wir für die großzügige Unterstützung des Vorhabens.

Oktober 1982  *V. Taenzer*  *E. Zeitler*

# Contents

## Animal and Clinical Pharmacology

**Chemistry, Toxicity and Biochemical Basis of Allergy-like Reactions**    2

Chemistry, Physicochemistry and Pharmacology of Known and New Contrast Media for Angiography, Urography and CT Enhancement . . . . . . . .    2
*U. Speck, W. Mützel and H.-J. Weinmann*

Tolerance and Biochemical Pharmacology of Iopromide . . . . . . . . . . . .    11
*W. Mützel and U. Speck*

The Action of Iohexol on Clotting, Fibrinolysis, Complement and Kallikrein System . . . . . . . . . . . . . . . . . . . . . . . . . . . . . . . . . . . . . . . . . . . . . . . . .    18
*B. Schulze, H. K. Beyer, V. Barth, K. Tremmel and U. Borst*

**Renal Tolerance** . . . . . . . . . . . . . . . . . . . . . . . . . . . . . . . . . . . . . . . . . . .    25

Albuminuria Following Renal Arteriography with Various Ionic and Non-ionic Contrast Agents in the Rat . . . . . . . . . . . . . . . . . . . . . . . . . . . . . . .    25
*U. Speck, W. R. Press and W. Mützel*

Enzymuria after Administration of Water-soluble X-ray Contrast Media . . .    30
*H. G. Hartmann*

Monitoring of Contrast Media Nephrotoxicity by Specific Kidney Tissue Proteinuria of Membrane Antigens . . . . . . . . . . . . . . . . . . . . . . . . . . . . . .    37
*J. E. Scherberich, S. Tuengerthal and J. Kollath*

Urinary β-2-Microglobulin Determinations in Assessment of Tubular Dysfunction after X-ray Contrast Media Application . . . . . . . . . . . . . . . . . . . .    43
*U. Uthmann, H. P. Geisen and E. Glück*

**Vascular Tolerance** . . . . . . . . . . . . . . . . . . . . . . . . . . . . . . . . . . . . . . . .    50

Contrast Media and Pain: Hypotheses on the Genesis of Pain Occurring on Intra-arterial Administration of Contrast Media . . . . . . . . . . . . . . . . . . .    50
*B. Hagen and G. Klink*

Increased Pain Reactions as Hang-over Phenomena after Intra-arterial Injections of Contrast Media in Rats . . . . . . . . . . . . . . . . . . . . . . . . . . . . . . . .    57
*B. Hagen, H. M. Siefert, W. Mützel and U. Speck*

Effects of Ionic and Non-ionic Contrast Media after Selective Peripheral and Cerebral Arterial Injections in Rats . . . . . . . . . . . . . . . . . . . . . . . . . . . . .    62
*W. Mützel and U. Speck*

**Haemodynamics** . . . . . . . . . . . . . . . . . . . . . . . . . . . . . . . . . . . . . . . . . .    67

Reduced Side Effects of Low Osmolality Non-ionic Contrast Media in Coronary Arteriography – Comparative Experimental Study in Dogs . . . . . . .    67
*R. Schräder, D. Baller, A. Hoeft, H. Korb, H. G. Wolpers and G. Hellige*

Haemodynamic Side Effects of Meglumine Ioglicate, Meglumine Sodium Ioxaglate and Iohexol in Aortofemoral Angiography: Comparison of a High-osmolar and Two Low-osmolar Radiological Contrast Media ........... 78
V. Wiebe and H. Straub

**Pharmacokinetics** .................................. 85

Pharmacokinetics of Iopromide in Rat and Dog .................. 85
W. Mützel, U. Speck and H.-J. Weinmann

# Clinical Application

**Angiography** .................................... 92

Anaesthesia Problems in Angiography with Special Reference to Modern Contrast Media ................................... 92
W. Wenz, K. Wiemers, D. Schlürmann, W.-D. Reinbold and P. Anger

Comparative Evaluation of Low Osmolar Contrast Media in (Femoral) Arteriography ..................................... 102
K.-J. Wolf, B. Steidle, D. Banzer, W. Seyferth and R. Keysser

Iohexol and Iopromide – Two New Non-ionic Water-soluble Radiographic Contrast Media: Randomized, Intraindividual Double-blind Study Versus Ioxaglate in Peripheral Angiography ...................... 107
B. Hagen

Iohexol and Ioxaglate in Cerebral Angiography ................. 115
A. Thron, M. Ratzka, K. Voigt and M. Nadjmi

Cardiovascular Side Effects of Various Conventional, Low-osmolar and Non-ionic Contrast Media ............................ 120
K. Wink and J. Wissert

Contrast Media in Intravenous Digital Subtraction Angiography (Initial Experience) ..................................... 125
W. Seyferth and E. Zeitler

**Urography** ..................................... 129

The Risk Liability of Nephrotropic Contrast Media: Clinical and Experimental Results ..................................... 129
T. Kröpelin, Ch. Gospos, X. Papacaralampous and N. Freudenberg

Double Blind Comparison of Ioglicate and Iothalamate in Intravenous Urography ...................................... 143
T. Baitsch, D. Beduhn and G. Klink

Urography with Non-ionic Contrast Media:
I. Diagnostic Quality and Tolerance of Iohexol in Comparison with Meglumine Amidotrizoate ............................... 148
V. Taenzer, H. Heep and W. Clauss

Urography with Non-ionic Contrast Media:
II. Diagnostic Quality and Tolerance of Iopromide in Comparison with Ioxaglate ..................................... 153
V. Taenzer, P. Meiisel and P. Hartwig

**Computerized Tomography** . . . . . . . . . . . . . . . . . . . . . . . . . . . . 156
Contrast Medium Tolerance in Computed Tomography . . . . . . . . . . . 156
*H. Tschakert*

Experiences with Rayvist and Iopromide in Head and Body CT . . . . . . . . 162
*E. Zeitler, K. Böhnlein, H. Gailer, R. Lindner and E.-I. Richter*

**Index** . . . . . . . . . . . . . . . . . . . . . . . . . . . . . . . . . . . . . . . . 173

# Synopsis of Contrast Media for Uro-angiography and the Trade Names Assigned to them in Various Countries

| Generic name<br>Patent holder | Trade name |
|---|---|
| | **Salts of tri-iodinated benzoic acids** (high osmolality)<br>**Salze trijodierter Benzoesäuren** (hoher osm. Druck) |
| Amidotrizoate<br>(previous name: diatrizoate)<br>Schering AG and Winthrop | Angiografin, Hypaque, Kardiografin, Peritrast, Pielografin, Radioselectan urinaire, Renografin, Renovist, Selectografin, Triombrast, Triombrin, Tryosom, Urografin, Urovison, Urovist, Verografin, Visotrast |
| Iodamide<br>Bracco | Angiomiro(n), Conraxin, Odiston, Ryomiro, Renovue, Triomiro, Uromiro(n) |
| Ioglicate<br>Schering AG | Rayvist |
| Iothalamate<br>Mallinckrodt | Angio-Conray, Conray, Sombril, Vascoray |
| Ioxithalamate<br>Guerbet | Telebrix, Vasobrix |
| Metrizoate<br>Nyegaard | Isopaque, Ronpacon, Triosil |
| | **Salt of a hexaiodinated acid** (low osmolality)<br>**Salz einer hexajodierten Säure** (niedriger osm. Druck) |
| Ioxaglate<br>Guerbet | Hexabrix |
| | **Nonionic tri-iodinated compounds** (low osmolality)<br>**Nichtionische Trijodverbindungen** (niedriger osm. Druck) |
| Iohexol<br>Nyegaard | Omnipaque |
| Iopamidol<br>Bracco | Iopamiro(n), Solutrast |
| Iopromide<br>Schering AG | – |
| Metrizamide<br>Nyegaard | Amipaque |

# Animal and Clinical Pharmacology

# Chemistry, Toxicity and Biochemical Basis of Allergy-like Reactions

## Chemistry, Physicochemistry and Pharmacology of Known and New Contrast Media for Angiography, Urography and CT Enhancement

U. Speck, W. Mützel, and H.-J. Weinmann

### Summary

The chemistry of water-soluble x-ray contrast media is based on triiodobenzene. 30 years of development led to diaminobenzoic acid, monoaminoisophthalic acid and only recently to trimesic acid derivatives. Nonionic and hexaiodinated compounds as well as triiodocations which can be used instead of sodium or meglumine were synthesized to lower the osmotic activity of contrast materials. The physicochemical properties relevant to the clinical application of contrast media are outlined. Examples are given how electrical charge, osmotic pressure and chemotoxicity due to lipophilicity or electron density of the benzene ring influence tolerance. From this, recommendations for the clinical application of new and conventional contrast materials are derived.

### Zusammenfassung

Die Chemie wasserlöslicher Kontrastmittel basiert auf dem Trijodbenzol. Die 30jährige Entwicklung dieses Grundkörpers führt von der Diaminobenzoesäure zur Monoaminoisophthalsäure und erst kürzlich zur Trimesinsäure. Es wurden nichtionische und hexajodierte Verbindungen sowie Trijodkationen, die anstelle von Natrium oder Meglumin genutzt werden können, synthetisiert, um den osmotischen Druck der Kontrastmittel zu senken. Die für die klinische Anwendung bedeutsamen physikochemischen Eigenschaften der Kontrastmittel werden dargestellt. An Beispielen wird gezeigt, welchen Einfluß die elektrische Ladung, der osmotische Druck und die durch Lipophilie oder höhere Elektronendichte im Benzolring bedingte Chemotoxizität auf die Verträglichkeit haben. Daraus werden Empfehlungen für die klinische Anwendung der neuen und der konventionellen Kontrastmittel abgeleitet.

### Introduction

X-ray contrast media for angiography, urography and related applications should not exhibit any pharmacological action. Their radiological efficacy in angiography does not require any activity on the part of the organism with the exception of a minimum blood flow. Even the filling of the urinary tract with the iodinated contrast medium as a prerequisite for excretion urography occurs without any specific action directed toward the contrast material: The fact that contrast media do not pass through cell membrane preserves them from too much dilution after intravenous injection. Low molecular weight and the lack of protein binding guarantees effective glomerular filtration, which does not require additional effort. Tubular reabsorption of water leading to a sufficient iodine concentration in urine occurs to an extent which is mainly controlled by the actual water demand of the individual undergoing the urographic examination and the concentration of non-absorbable solutes in the urine.

CT enhancement is achieved either by the passive transport of the contrast medium with the blood or by its diffusion through the capillary wall in the interstice, which in cerebral blood vessels is dependent on the disruption of the blood-brain barrier.

Thus, chemists are free to modify chemical structures of contrast media without too much concern about their efficacy.

The known toxic effects of X-ray contrast media cannot be related to specific actions of the iodinated molecules on receptor sites of proteins or membranes but to a rather unspecific binding. Moreover, a great number of side effects caused by

---

*Acknowledgement:* Thanks are due to Dr. C. Herrmann of the Department of Quantum Chemistry, for the calculation of the electron densities of various benzoic acid derivatives.

contrast injections are explained by the physicochemical properties of contrast media and are at least partly independent of the exact chemical structure of the particular product.

Therefore, it may be concluded that improvement of contrast tolerance can be achieved simply by modifying the physicochemical properties of iodinated molecules in the direction towards biological inertness. The development of x-ray contrast media has been successfully proceeding in this direction.

## Chemistry

### Improving the Basic Triiodinated Ring

All modern water-soluble contrast media are based on the triiodinated benzene ring. The first clinically used derivative was acetrizoate (Fig 2). Due to the lack of one side chain acetrizoate was rather lipophilic and toxic. The introduction of a second side chain led to diatrizoate, the still most widely used contrast agent for urography, angiography and CT enhancement, which became well known as Urografin, Angiografin, Urovison, Urovist, Renografin and Hypaque. Even today diatrizoate is unique among the conventional ionic contrast media because of its cardiovascular tolerance. It contains two side chains in addition to the carboxylic group, both bonded to the benzene ring by nitrogen atoms (Fig 1). Ten years later Hoey and coworkers (6) succeeded in synthesizing an analogous chemical structure called iothalamate having two carboxy groups and only one nitrogen as substituents of triiodobenzene (Fig 1). In spite of the fact that the cardiovascular toxicity of iothalamate was slightly increased, it became famous due to its improved neural tolerance. From this time it was clear that a molecule bearing no nitrogen on the benzene ring would be worth synthesizing and investigating for pharmacological properties. Nevertheless, it took about 20 years until Gries and coworkers (5) presented triiodotrimesic acid, which might be the chemical basis of a new series of ionic and non-ionic contrast media in the future, as triiodoisophthalamic acid has been during the last 20 years.

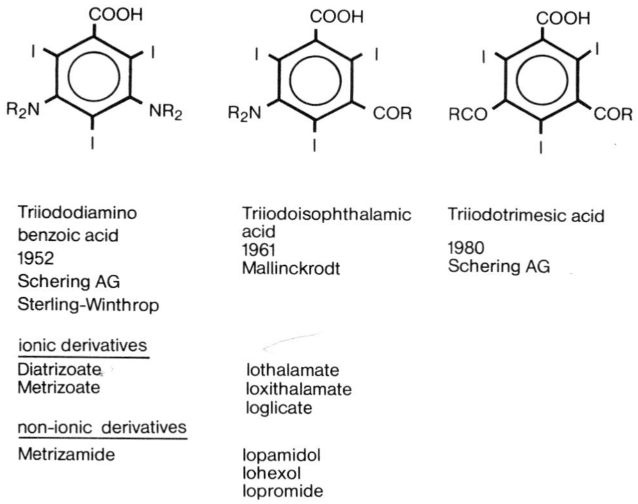

### Increasing Hydrophilicity of Ionic Contrast Media

The correlation between lipophilicity and toxicity of contrast material was recognized very early (7). Whereas diatrizoate and iothalamate contain only short side chains in positions 3 and 5 on the benzene ring, a better tolerance especially of the iothalamate derivatives ioxithalamate and ioglicate (3, 13) was achieved by the introduction of larger, more hydrophilic substituents. On the other hand, increasing viscosity of the larger molecules limits the use of even more hydrophilic side chains.

Fig 1  Three different basic structures used in the synthesis of ionic and non-ionic contrast media

Triiododiamino benzoic acid
1952
Schering AG
Sterling-Winthrop

ionic derivatives
Diatrizoate
Metrizoate

non-ionic derivatives
Metrizamide

Triiodoisophthalamic acid
1961
Mallinckrodt

Iothalamate
Ioxithalamate
Ioglicate

Iopamidol
Iohexol
Iopromide

Triiodotrimesic acid
1980
Schering AG

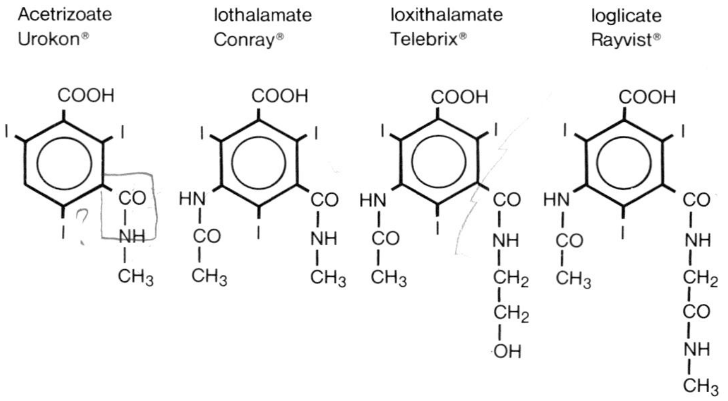

Fig 2  Increasing hydrophilicity by the introduction of hydrophilic side chains

Acetrizoate — Urokon®
Iothalamate — Conray®
Ioxithalamate — Telebrix®
Ioglicate — Rayvist®

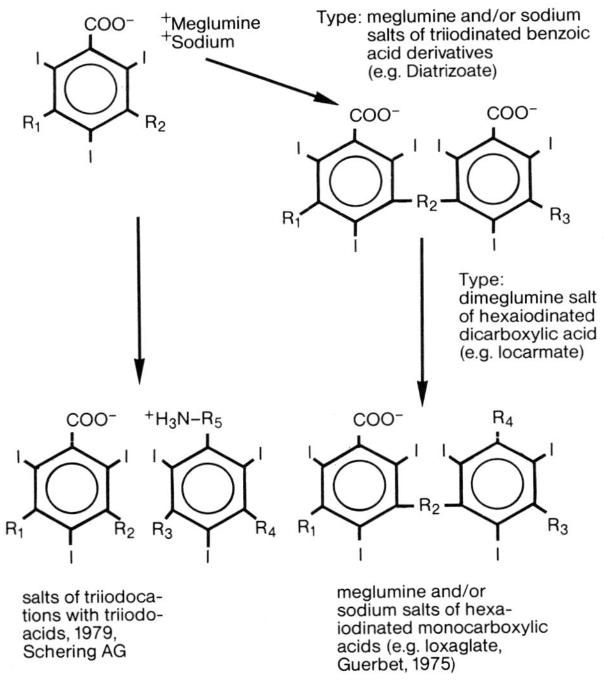

# 4 Chemistry, Toxicity and Biochemical Basis of Allergy-like Reactions

Fig 3 Decreasing osmotic pressure of ionic contrast media

## Reduction of Osmotic Pressure

Almen (1) proposed several ways to reduce the osmotic pressure of contrast media while maintaining the iodine concentrations within the demands of angiographic examinations. A reduction of osmotic activity can be realized either with ionic or with non-ionic molecules.

Dimerization of two carboxy acids led to iocarmic acid (Fig 3), a myelographic agent with only very slightly reduced osmotic pressure. A definite reduction of osmotic activity was obtained by the connection of one benzene ring with a free carboxy group to another benzene without free carboxy group, resulting in a monocarboxy dimer (20). One candidate from this work became known as ioxaglate. In the meantime, ioxaglate is used in several countries, preferably in peripheral angiography. The lipophilic properties of non-ionic triiodobenzene in the molecule and the increased viscosity of dimers are the principal drawbacks of this class of compounds.

Both of them can be avoided if triiodinated cations are used instead of sodium or meglumine in connection with conventional triiodinated benzoic acid derivatives. First examples of such low osmotic contrast media were characterized by Sovak and cowirkers (17) and Speck and coworkers (18).

## Nonionic Contrast Media

The most promising approach to well-tolerated contrast media is the synthesis of nonionic compounds (Fig 4). The first clinically useful product was metrizamide, whose chemical structure still

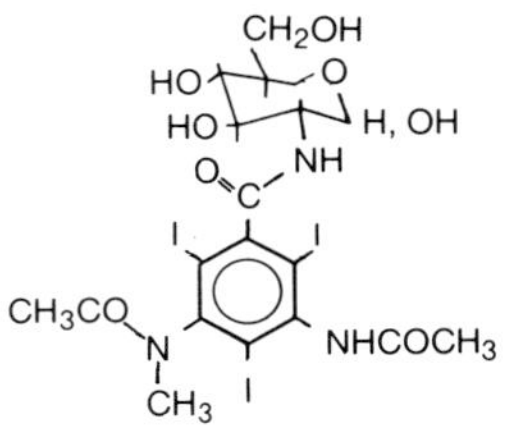

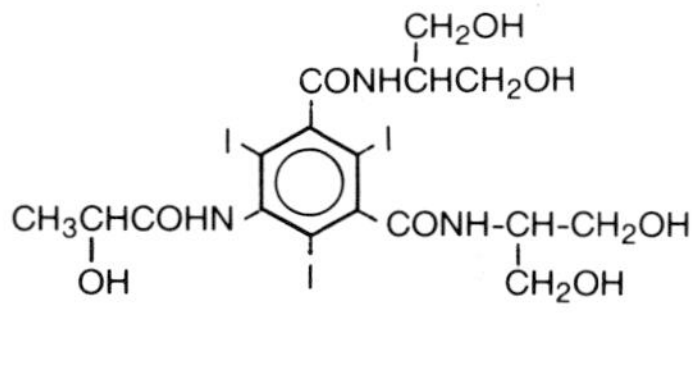

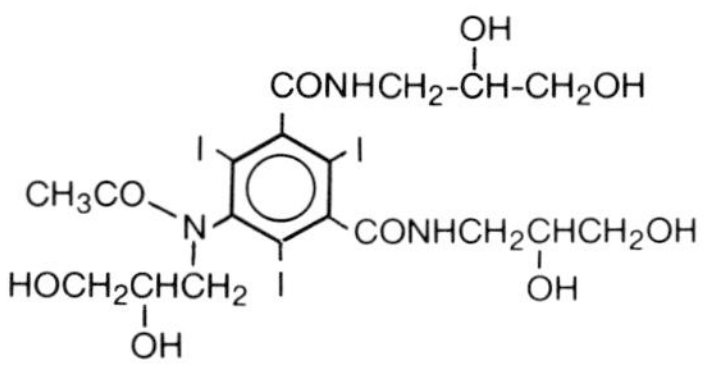

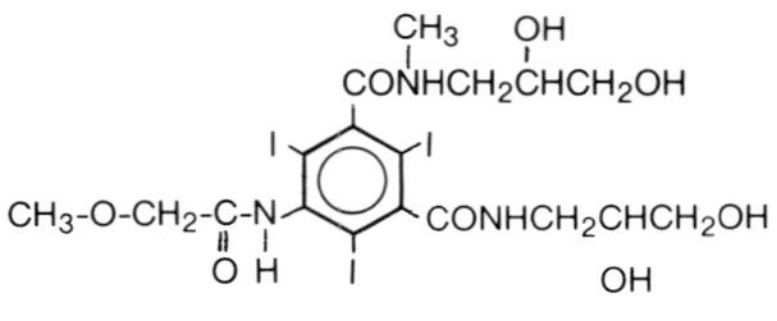

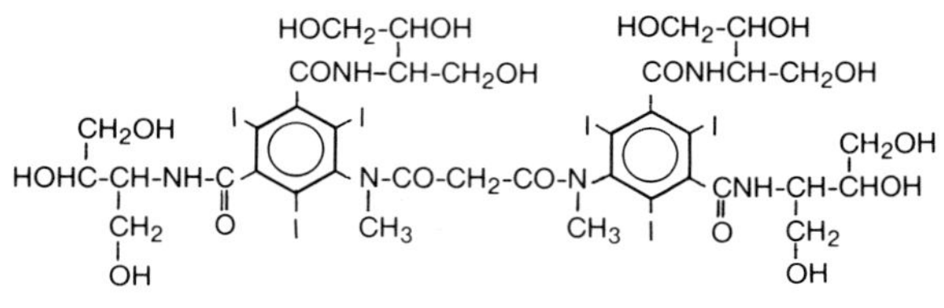

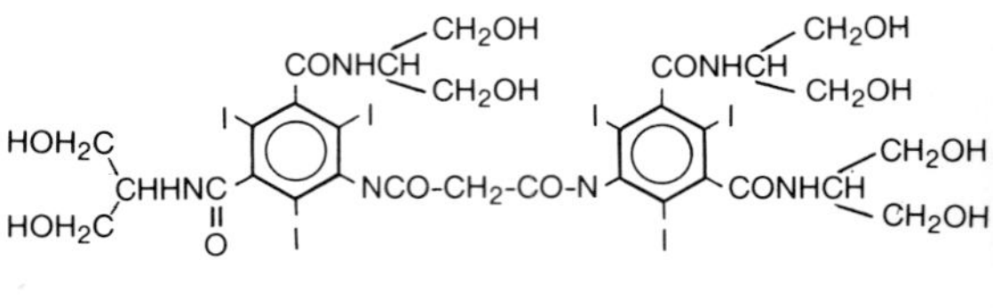

Fig 4 Non-ionic contrast media

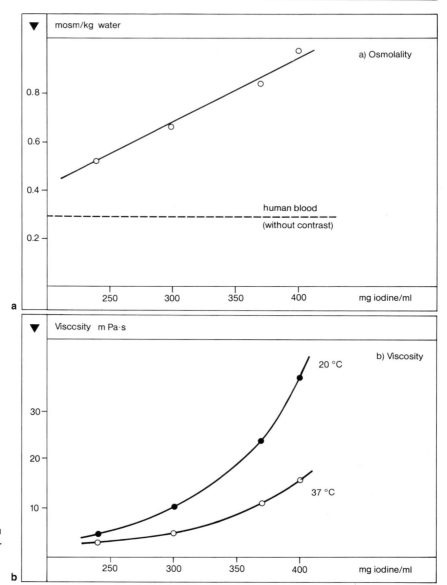

Fig 5 Osmolality and viscosity of Iopromide, a typical nonionic monomer, within the concentration range suitable for angiographic examinations
a) Osmolality
b) Viscosity

resembles the conventional ionic agents insofar as it contains two short side chains which do not contribute to the solubility to a great extent and only one highly hydrophilic substituent, the amino sugar. Metrizamide cannot be sterilized by heating and long-term storage in solution is not possible because of its degradation.

The new nonionic triiodinated monomers iopamidol, iohexol and iopromide were synthesized according to somewhat different principles: the hydrophilic side chains are more or less equally distributed around the iodinated benzene ring. All the products are sufficiently stable to be delivered as solution ready for injection. Neither the above-mentioned ionic contrast media nor the triiodinated nonionic monomers are actually isotonic with blood or cerebrospinal fluid at concentrations above 140–180 mg iodine per ml (Fig 5a). Therefore, attempts were undertaken to synthesize nonionic hexaiodinated dimers to further decrease osmolality and molarity of contrast solutions (19). Two candidates from this group of compounds have been identified until now: Iotrol (16) as a myelographic agent and Iodecol (18) for intravascular use.

# Physicochemical Properties of Contrast Media Relevant to Their Application

Contrast media are believed to act on the organism almost exclusively in an unspecific way due their physicochemical properties. Three different categories of such interactions have been described

a) electrical charge,
b) hyperosmolality,
c) chemotoxicity.

With regard to these parameters the above-mentioned contrast agents differ very significantly from each other.

## Electrical Charge and Solubility

Ionic contrast media are soluble in water due to the fact that they form ions bearing either a positive (cation) or negative (anion) electrical charge. The solubility of nonionic contrast media is mainly achieved by the introduction of a sufficient number of (nonionic) hydroxylic groups. Independently of the solubility of the amorphous material in water and their hydrophilicity, ionic and nonionic contrast media may crystallize.

a) if the energy level of the molecules within the crystal is lower than the energy level of dissolved and hydrated molecules and

b) if a first crystal appears spontaneously in the solution or has been added to the solution.

## Osmotic Pressure

Osmotic pressure of solutions depends on the number of dissolved and freely mobile molecules or ions within a given amount of solute. The chemical structures given in Figs 1, 3 and 4 indicate distinct differences between the various contrast media with regard to the osmotic pressure of solutions with equal iodine concentration. In addition to the effects which can be derived directly from the chemical structure the association of molecules within the solution influences the osmotic pressure in a significant but hardly predictable way (4, 11). Therefore, the measured osmolality of contrast media is lower than it should be from the theoretical point of view and differences are measured between compounds of the same class (e.g. nonionic monomers). Data for representative contrast media are given in Table 1.

## Chemotoxicity

Chemotoxicity is believed to be the reason for toxic effects which otherwise cannot be explained. At least two properties of contrast media should be mentioned, which seem to correlate with known side effects of contrast material:

Table 1 Osmolality of various contrast media with a concentration of 300 mg iodine/ml at 37° C in comparison to human blood

| Compound | mosm/kg $H_2O$ |
|---|---|
| Blood | 290 |
| *Conventional ionic media* | |
| Diatrizoate, meglumine | 1500 |
| Diatrizoate, sodium | 1570 |
| Ioglicate, meglumine | 1790 |
| *Ionic media with reduced osmotic pressure* | |
| Ioxaglate, meglumine | 560 |
| Diatrizoate/Triiodocation | 500 |
| *Nonionic monomers* | |
| Metrizamide | 480 |
| Iopamidol | 616 |
| Iohexol | 690 |
| Iopromide | 630 |
| *Nonionic dimers* | |
| Iotrol | 360 |
| Iodecol | 280 |

Table 2 Partition coefficient of various contrast agents between butanol and buffer, contrast medium concentration 0.01 mg iodine/ml. The distinct difference between partition coefficents at pH 7.6 (anions) and pH 1 (no electrical charge) in the case of ionic contrast media indicates the contribution of the electrical charge to the hydrophilicity of these compounds

| Contrast agents | Partition coefficient | |
|---|---|---|
| | pH 7.6 | pH 1 |
| *Ionic* | | |
| Diatrizoate | 0.045 | |
| Iothalamate | 0.054 | |
| Ioxithalamate | 0.039 | 0.62 |
| Ioglicate | 0.034 | 0.89 |
| Ioxaglate | 0.104 | |
| Triiodocation | 0.001 | |
| *Nonionic* | | 0.39 |
| Metrizamide | 0.37 | |
| Iopamidol | 0.11 | |
| Iohexol | 0.07 | |
| Iopromide | 0.14 | |
| Iotrol | 0.005 | 0.021 |
| Iodecol | 0.019 | |

- Lipophilicity/Hydrophilicity
Lipophilicity means the preference of a molecule for lipid-like organic solvents or fats whereas hydrophilicity means the opposite quality, the preference for water and aqueous solvents. To measure the lipophilic/hydrophilic qualities of contrast media, the compounds were dissolved in water or in a buffer. A known amount of a lipophilic solvent like n-butanol is added which is not well soluble in water. After shaking this mixture for a while, the solvents are allowed to separate again and the concentration of the iodinated molecules within the aqueous and the organic phase is measured. The partition coefficient is calculated by dividing the concentration of the contrast material in the organic solvent by the concentration in water (Table 2).

The electrical charge of triiodobenzoic acid derivatives contributes to an extremely high extent to the hydrophilicity of contrast medium acids. Biological investigations do not clearly indicate that the portion of hydrophilicity which is caused by the electrical charge is reflected completely in the expected tolerance. At this time, it is our impression that a comparison of partition coefficients of ionic and nonionic contrast media does not allow conclusions on the toxicity of products of these different classes of compounds, whereas a convincing correlation seems to exist within each of the separate groups of contrast media.

- Distribution of ring electrons
Sovak (15) suggested to explain the difference in the pharmacological quality of diatrizoate and iothalamate by the different distribution of ring electrons in both molecules. Whereas the acylamido group (nitrogen on the ring, diatrizoate) donates electrons to the benzene ring, the carbamoyl group (carboxy group on the ring, triiodotrimesic acid) withdraws ring electrons (Fig 1). According to Sovak's hypothesis triiodotrimesic acid derivatives should be less toxic than triiododiaminobenzoic acid derivatives (e.g. diatrizoate) and triiodoisophthalamic acid derivatives (e.g. iothalamate).

## Viscosity

The viscosity of contrast media is primarily important for the application process, e.g. the rate of infusion or the pressure necessary for rapid injection. Viscosity of contrast media increases as the water content of the aqueous solutions decreases. This means that more concentrated solutions and solutions of molecules with lower iodine content (low percentage iodine of the molecular weight) are more viscous. In fact the demand for molecules with a high iodine content is a severe limitation for

| Structure | Partition coefficient[1] | Protein-binding[2] |
|---|---|---|
| ionic: iodipamide 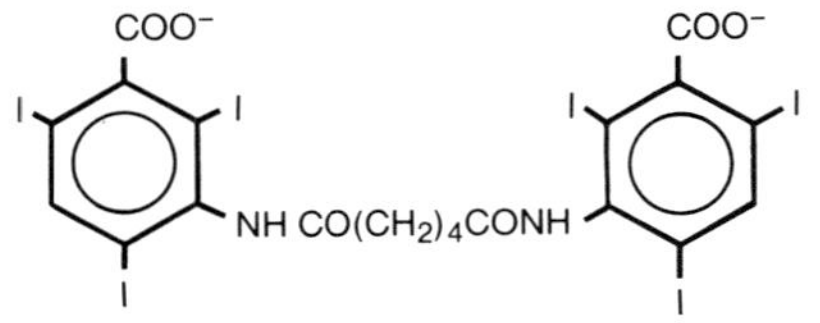 $COO^-$ ... $NH\,CO(CH_2)_4\,CONH$ ... $COO^-$ | 0.20 | 73 % |
| nonionic 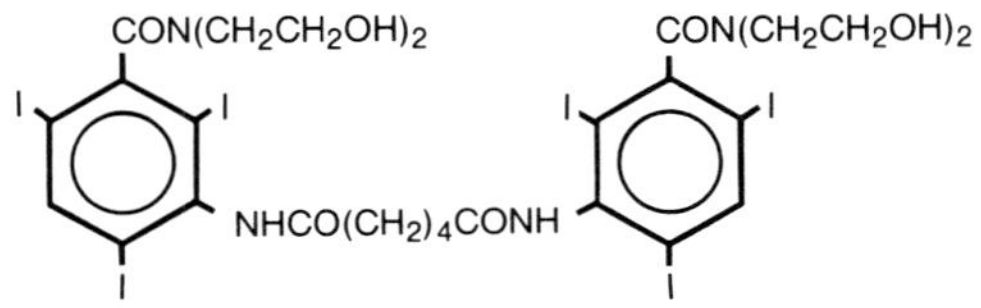 $CON(CH_2CH_2OH)_2$ ... $NHCO(CH_2)_4CONH$ ... $CON(CH_2CH_2OH)_2$ | 0.54 | < 10 % |

1) n-butanol/buffer pH 7.6
2) equilibrium dialysis at 1.2 mg iodine/ml for iodipamide and 0.01 mg iodine/ml for the nonionic compound

Fig 6  Protein-binding of ionic and nonionic contrast media

the synthesis of well-tolerated water-soluble contrast media. Furthermore, dimers (hexaiodinated) and polymers are more viscous than monomers (triiodinated). The individual chemical structure has an additional influence on the viscosity. All contrast medium solutions become less viscous at increasing temperature. The last effect is very pronounced (Fig 5b) and can help to overcome viscosity problems in clinical practice.

## Physicochemistry and Pharmacology

### Biological Effects Due to Ions

First of all, the electrical charge of ionic contrast molecules contributes to a large extent to their hydrophilicity and tolerance after i.v. injection. Electrical charge is at least one factor limiting the distribution of ionic contrast media almost exclusively to the extracellular space and by this means excludes toxic actions of contrast material within most compartments of the organism.

On the other hand contrast ions are known to cause several side effects, primarily

- epileptogenic activity after subarachnoidal injection (2) and
- reactions induced by the binding of calcium ions (21).

A comparison of the protein-binding of iodipamide and its nonionic derivative indicates a significant contribution of free carboxy groups to this kind of interaction (Fig 6). Nevertheless, Speck and coworkers (18) demonstrated that ionic contrast media (e.g. salt of triiodocations with triiodoacids) were as well tolerated after intravenous injection in rats as nonionic monomers.

Table 3  Side effects of contrast media at least partly attributed to their osmotic activity

hypervolaemia
vasodilatation
increase in pulmonary arterial pressure
endothelial injury
blood-brain barrier breakdown
pain
thrombogenesis
bradycardia in cardioangiography
diuresis
disturbance of osmotic balance in newborn

### Side Effects Due to Hypertonicity

Extensive literature is available with regard to this topic. However, it is not always certain to what extent side effects are caused by the hypertonicity of contrast material and if all of the osmotic effects are already known. Table 3 summarizes what side effects have been assigned to the osmotic activity of contrast media.

### Side Effects Caused by Chemotoxicity

Chemotoxicity is an inherent property of ionic and nonionic, hypertonic and isotonic contrast media solutions. Whereas the correlation between the lipophilicity of contrast molecules, their affinity to proteins and toxicity is well established (7, 8, 9, 13) no other explanations of chemotoxicity were available. In 1978 Sovak (15) proposed his electron density hypothesis, drawing attention to the way by which side chains are fixed to the benzene ring. In the meantime, the synthesis of triiodotrimesic acid derivatives by Gries and coworkers (5) allowed further testing of this correlation. According to our experience the electron density hypothesis applies preferably to neural tolerance, as it is observed after subarachnoidal injection. A convincing example is shown in Fig 7 since the investigated compounds differ only with regard to the relevant substituents of the benzene ring.

Another observation may support the electron density hypothesis too: from a very large number of non-ionic monomers tested with regard to acute intravenous tolerance in rats one triiodotrimesic acid derivative achieved a significantly higher $LD_{50}$ (18.7 g iodine/kg body weight) than all other contrast media based on aminobenzenes (10.3 to 12.9 g iodine/kg, see 12).

## Discussion and Conclusions

A great number of iodinated water-soluble contrast media are already available and further promising products are under development. Therefore, it might be useful to find out whether the decision what product is suitable for what examination and what patient can be made on the basis of a few principles equally true for all the different compounds. Provided the obvious demand is followed to use the minimum concentration and amount of contrast material that gives unequivocal diagnostic information, the following rules may help:

- A lower incidence of common side effects like nausea, vomiting and allergy-like reactions

| Contrast media meglumine salts | Structure | number of ring π-electrons in addition to the 6 benzene electrons | neural tolerance mg iodine/kg body weight |
|---|---|---|---|
| Diatrizoate 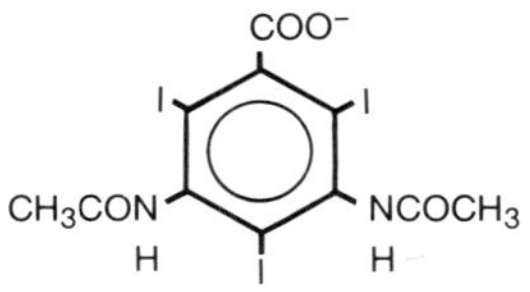 | COO⁻ substituted benzene with I, I, I and CH₃CONH–, –NHCOCH₃ | 0.1077 | 4.2 (3.0-5.4) |
| Iothalamate 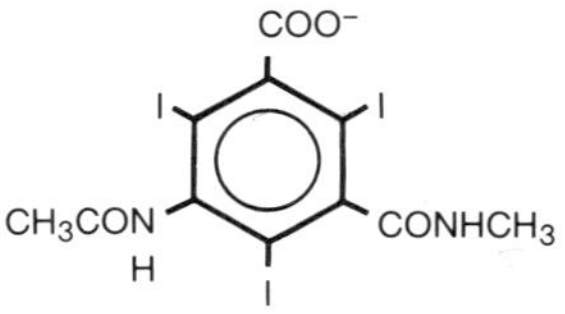 | COO⁻ substituted benzene with I, I, I and CH₃CONH–, –CONHCH₃ | 0.0947 | 11.4 (9.0-15.2) |
| Triiodotrimesic acid derivative 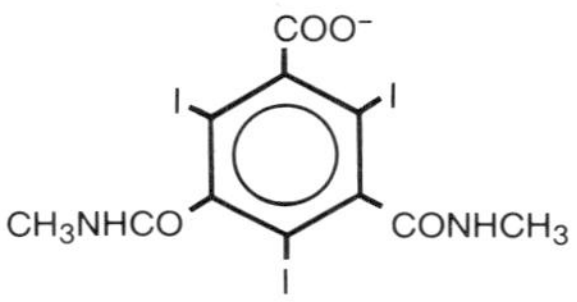 | COO⁻ substituted benzene with I, I, I and CH₃NHCO–, –CONHCH₃ | 0.0815 | 22.7 (16.3-31.0) |

Fig 7 Neural tolerance of contrast media distinguished by different substituents of the benzene ring which influence its electron density. Neural tolerance is given as dosage necessary to produce signs of neurotoxicity in 50% of rats after intracisternal injection and 95% confidence limits[1])

1) Experimental method as described by Siefert and coworkers (1980)

should be achieved by more hydrophilic contrast media (sodium salts should be avoided).
- Local side effects like endothelial damage, pain, etc. are mainly dependent on the osmotic pressure. Low-osmotic ionic and nonionic contrast media are equally well tolerated.
- Diuresis is an osmotic effect and can be reduced by the use of any low osmotic contrast medium (and sodium salts).
- Sodium-meglumine salts of diatrizoate (Urografin 76 and 60, Renografin 76, Hypaque 76) are superior to other conventional ionic agents with regard to cardiovascular tolerance. Since nonionic contrast media do not bind calcium ions and have reduced osmotic pressure, they produce hardly any cardiovascular effect and no disturbance of the osmotic or ionic balance.
- From the theoretical point of view nonionic contrast media should be substantially safer than ionic products (least possibility of interaction) with the exception of renal tolerance, where the higher concentration of nonionic contrast media in renal tubules during excretion might offset better tolerance.

## Development of New Contrast Materials

New contrast media are synthesized and developed up to the stage of clinical trials on the basis of the hypothesis as discussed above. From time to time, these hypotheses need confirmation by clinical experience. This is especially true if new principles are introduced. At the present time, clinical trials, introduction and first experience in practice with nonionic contrast agents better suitable for intravascular application than metrizamide are under way. It depends very much on the outcome of this process in what direction further development of contrast media should be pursued.

Further improvement of the typical nonionic monomers iopamidol, iohexol and iopromide seems to be possible, both by dimerization to a new class of isotonic contrast media which have shown extremely low acute toxicity in animal experiments and by the introduction of triiodotrimesic acid derivatives to further decrease toxicity of the basic iodinated benzene ring.

The fate of ionic contrast agents in radiology should depend

a) on the incidence of severe and fatal reactions due to the new nonionic agents and

b) on the cost of non-ionic compounds.

Although in the meantime low-osmotic ionic contrast media have been synthesized which were found to be well tolerated in animal experiments, it is doubtful whether they would be as safe as the nonionics in clinical practice. In myelography, at least, water-soluble nonionic contrast media only will be used in the future, probably as dimers.

## References

1 Almén, T.: Contrast agent design. J. theoret. Biol. 24: 216–226, 1969
2 Almén, T.: Experience from 10 years of development of water-soluble nonionic contrast media. Invest. Radiol. 15, 6: 283–288, 1980
3 Baitsch, T., D. Beduhn, G. Klink: This volume, p. 143
4 Felder, E., D. Pitre, P. Tirone: Radiopaque contrast media. Farmaco, Ed. sci. 32, 11: 835–844, 1977
5 Gries, H., H. Pfeiffer, U. Speck, W. Mützel: Ionische 5-C-substituierte 2, 4, 6-Trijod-Isophthalsäure-Derviate, deren Herstellung und diese enthaltende Röntgenkontrastmittel. Europäische Patentanmeldung No. 0032 388, 1980
6 Hoey, G. B., R. D. Rands, G. Dela Mater, D. W. Chapman, P. E. Wiegert: Synthesis of derivatives of isophthalamic acid as X-ray contrast agents. J. med. Chem. 6: 24–26, 1963
7 Knoefel, P. K., K. C. Huang: The biochemorphology of renal tubular transport: Iodinated benzoic acids. J. Pharmacol. exp. Ther. 117: 307–316, 1956
8 Lang, J. H., E. C. Lasser: Binding of roentgenographic contrast media to serum albumin. Invest. Radiol. 2: 396–400, 1967
9 Lasser, E. C., J. H. Lang: Contrast-protein interactions. Invest. Radiol. 5: 446–451, 1970
10 Melartin, E., P. J. Tuohimaa, R. Dabb: Neutrotoxicity of iothalamates and diatrizoates. I. Significance of concentration and cation. Invest. Radiol. 5: 13–21, 1970
11 Miklautz, H., J. Riemann: Über das Assoziationsverhalten von Methylglukaminsalzen der Dicarbonsäure-bis-(3-carboxy-2,4,6-trijod-anilide) in wäßrigen Lösungen. Arch. Pharm. 308: 760–768, 1974
12 Mützel, W., U. Speck: This volume, p. 11
13 Rapoport, S. I., H. Levitan: Neurotoxicity of X-ray contrast media. Amer. J. Roentgenol. 122: 186–193, 1974
14 Siefert, H.-M., W.-R. Press, U. Speck: Tolerance to iohexol after intracisternal, intracerebral and intraarterial injection in the rat. Acta radiol. (Stockh.) Suppl. 362: 77–81, 1980
15 Sovak, M., R. Ranganathan, J. H. Lang, E. C. Lasser: Concepts in design of improved intravascular contrast agents. Ann. Radiol. 21 (4–5): 283–289, 1978
16 Sovak, M., R. Ranganathan, U. Speck: Nonionic dimer: Development and initial testing of an intrathecal contrast agent. Radiology 142: 115–118, 1982
17 Sovak, M., F. L. Weitl, J. H. Lang, C. B. Higgins: Development of a radiopaque cation: Toxicity of the benzylammonium group. Europ. J. Med. Chem. 14: 257–260, 1979
18 Speck, U., W. Mützel: Two New Classes of Low-Osmotic Contrast Agents: Triiodinated Cations and Nonionic dimers. Contrast Media in Radiology. Springer, Berlin 1982
19 Speck, U., W. Mützel, G. Mannesmann, H. Pfeiffer, H. M. Siefert: Pharmacology of nonionic dimers. Invest. Radiol. 15: 317–322, 1980
20 Tilly, G., M. J.-C. Hardouin, J. Lautrou: Kontrastmittel für Röntgenaufnahmen. Offenlegungsschrift des Deutschen Patentamtes No. 2523567, 1974
21 Wolpers, H. G., D. H. Hunneman, M. Stellwaag, G. Hellige: Calcium binding by arteriographic contrast media. J. pharm. Sci. 70: 231–232, 1981

# Tolerance and Biochemical Pharmacology of Iopromide

W. Mützel and U. Speck

## Summary

The new nonionic, monomeric, triiodinated contrast agent iopromide has been shown to have a remarkably low intravenous toxicity in mice and rats. Neural tolerance of iopromide was found to be equal to or better than that of metrizamide, when injected into rats intracisternally and intracerebrally, respectively. The interaction of iopromide with proteins was demonstrated in several in-vitro test models to be considerably low. On the basis of these preclinical studies iopromide is a very promising intravascular contrast agent being most suitable for angiography, urography and computed tomography.

## Zusammenfassung

Das neue nichtionische monomere trijodierte Kontrastmittel Iopromid zeigte nach intravenöser Injektion an Maus und Ratte eine bemerkenswert geringe Toxizität. Nach zisternaler bzw. intrazerebraler Injektion an Ratten wurde Iopromid gleich gut bzw. besser vertragen als Metrizamid. Die außerordentlich geringe Interaktion von Iopromid mit Proteinen konnte anhand einiger In-vitro-Versuche nachgewiesen werden. Aufgrund der vorliegenden vorklinischen Untersuchungen dürfte Iopromid ein vielversprechendes intravasales Kontrastmittel sein, das besonders gut in der Angiographie, Urographie und in der Computertomographie eingesetzt werden kann.

## Introduction

Iopromide is a nonionic, water-soluble triiodinated aromatic compound being developed for use in angiography, urography and computed tomography (17).

In order to define the margins of safety afforded by the new contrast agent when employed in human clinical use, the compound was subjected to a number of pharmacological experiments as well as to several biochemical tests. The experiments were designed to reveal qualitative and quantitative aspects of toxic effects by comparing iopromide with metrizamide and iopamidol, which have been shown to be very well tolerated (1, 4).

## Material and Methods

### Contrast Media

Iopromide was used as a sterile, aqueous solution containing 300 mg I/ml (Schering, Berlin). Metrizamide was in the form of the lyophilized substance (Nyegaard & Co., Oslo), which was dissolved in the required concentration with 5 mg sodium bicarbonate/100 ml solution immediately before the experiments. Iopamidol, too, was in the form of a sterile, aqueous solution containing 300 mg I/ml (Bracco, Milan).

## Acute Tolerance after a Single i.v. Injection in the Mouse

The acute tolerance of iopromide, metrizamide and iopamidol after a single intravenous injection was investigated on 6 mice per dose in each case. The animals were Schering AG SPF-outbred animals from the Naval Medical Research Institute strain, weighing 18–22 g; male and female animals were used in a 50 : 50 ratio.

The aqueous contrast medium solutions, which contained 300 mg I/ml in each case, were injected once in varying volumes at a rate of 2.0 ml/min into a lateral tail vein. The mortality of the animals was observed over a period of 7 days.

## Acute Tolerance after Single i.v. Injection in the Rat

The acute general tolerance of iopromide, metrizamide and iopamidol after a single intravenous injection was investigated on 6 (or 4) rats per dose in each case. The animals were Schering AG SPF-outbred animals of the Wistar strain weighing 90–110 g; male and female animals were used in each case in a 50 : 50 ratio.

The aqueous contrast medium solutions, which contained 300 mg I/ml in each case, were injected once in varying volumes at the rate of 2.0 ml/min into a lateral tail vein. The mortality of the animals was observed over a period of 7 days.

## Tolerance after Intracerebral Administration in the Rat

A comparative investigation was carried out into the neural tolerance of iopromide, metrizamide and iopamidol in rats after intracerebral administration.

The substances to be tested were administered once as aqueous solutions in 5 dosages in the range of 10–240 mg iodine/kg in a constant volume (0.4 ml/kg) and varying concentrations to 10 animals for each dose (SPF-outbred animals of Wistar strain, 90–110 g, ♀ : ♂ = 50 : 50, bred by: Schering AG) intracerebrally according to the method of Valzelli (19). The investigations were carried out on one day. The animals were allocated to the substances and dosages completely at random. The criteria of action were: unequivocal postural abnormalities, excitation states and mortality. The animals were observed over a period of 24 hours in each case.

## Tolerance after Intracisternal Administration in the Rat

A comparative investigation was carried out into the (neural) tolerance of iopromide, metrizamide and iopamidol in rats after administration into the cisterna cerebello-medullaris.

The contrast medium solutions (300 mg I/ml) to be tested were diluted with 0.9% NaCl solution for each test dose, in such a way that the administration volume amounted to 40 µl/animal.

Five female and five male rats (SPF-outbred animals of a Wistar strain, bred by: Schering AG) weighing 140–160 g, received the substances once in 6 dosages in the range of 32–152 mg iodine/kg injected into the cisterna cerebello-medullaris, after the cisternal position of the injection cannula (injection depth 5 mm) had been checked through puncture with clear CSF (approx. 20 µl). 0.9% NaCl solution were used as the volume control, this being administered to another 10 rats in the same way. The animals were allocated to the substances purely at random.

The criteria of action (= "findings") were: unequivocal postural abnormalities, states of excitation and mortality within 24 hours after injection.

Statistical evaluation of all experiments mentioned hitherto was performed using a computer program for probit analysis.

## Protein Binding

Protein binding was determined by equilibrium dialysis according to Scholtan (14) using a Dianorm dialysis apparatus (Diachema AG, Zürich, Switzerland) according to Weder and Bickel (20). Human plasma (protein content: 6 g/100 ml) was dialysed at room temperature for 4 hours with contrast medium solution (final concentration in the total mixture: 1.2 mg I/ml) against buffered physiological saline (pH 7.0). The contrast medium concentrations were determined by spectrophotometry at 238 nm (6-fold determination).

## Lysozyme Inhibition

Lysozyme (EC 3.2.17; Boehringer, Mannheim, Germany) hydrolyzes β-1,4-bonds between N-acetylmuramic acids and 2-acetyl-amino-2-deoxy-D-glucose in monopeptides and polysaccharides. The enzyme activity was observed according to Shugar (15), i.e. dissolution of the cell wall of Micrococcus luteus, since a yellow dye is liberated during this process. The time course of dye liberation was followed with a spectrophotometer, and is proportional to the enzyme activity.

For observation of lysozyme inhibition by iopromide, metrizamide and iopamidol, 2 ml of contrast medium solution containing increasing concentrations of the media were incubated with 1 ml of a fresh suspension of 0.6 mg lyophilized Micrococcus luteus (Boehringer) in phosphate buffer according to Sörensen (16) for 2 min at 34 °C in a measuring cuvette, then mixed with 5 µg lysozyme (ex chicken protein, Boehringer) dissolved in 0.1 ml re-distilled water, and incubated for a further 3 min at 34 °C. Liberation was observed during the last 1.5 min of incubation with the aid of a recording spectrophotometer at 450 nm.

Relative inhibition of lysozyme was yielded by the slope of the reaction curve obtained from a mixture not containing contrast medium and the slopes of the curves obtained on addition of the contrast media.

## Histamine Liberation

For observation of histamine liberation from mast cells by iopromide, metrizamide and iopamidol, 0.5 ml of contrast media solutions containing 200, 250 and 300 mg I/ml was mixed with 0.5 ml of a fresh mast cell suspension of heparinized peritoneal fluid from rats (250–350 g, male : female = 1 : 1, Schering SPF breed), and incubated for 10 min at 37 °C. The liberated histamine found in the cell-free supernatant was isolated by ion-exchange chromatography on Dowex 50-W-X-9, $H^+$, and condensed in an alkaline medium with o-pthaldialdehyde according to Lorenz et al. (10). Fluorescence intensity of the complex was determined by fluorometry in a phosphoric acid medium; it is directly proportional to the amount of histamine in the sample for the range 0.1 ng to 10 µg. In order to ascertain the total content of histamine in the mast cell suspensions used, preparations of the latter were mixed with a solution of the Wellcome histamine liberator Compound 48/80 instead of the contrast media solutions (= 100 per cent value). The values measured in mixtures containing contrast media were calculated as percentages of the former 100 per cent value.

## Erythrocyte Morphology

Iopromide, metrizamide and iopamidol, in each case 6 parts by volume of fresh, heparinized whole blood (4 subjects, male : female = 2 : 2) were mixed with one part by volume of test solution, and immediately examined under a light microscope. The morphologic changes of the erythrocytes were scored (degree of damage 0–6) according to Speck et al. (18). The controls used were saline solution or distilled water (= diluent for the hypertonic contrast media solutions), which were added to the blood instead of contrast medium solutions. For the experiments, the sequence of the substances and their concentrations were randomized. The injury indices were calculated by probit analysis, and the potencies of iopromide and iopamidol compared with one another in relation to metrizamide as reference substance (= 1.00).

## Complement Activation

For determination of serum complement activation by iopromide, metrizamide and iopamidol, 0.3 ml of contrast medium solution in gelatin-veronal-buffer (GVB) was incubated in increasing concentration with 0.1 ml of fresh human serum for 1 h at 37 °C. The mixtures were then diluted with 10 ml of GVB. In each case 0.8, 1.2, 1.6, 2.0 and 2.6 ml of the dilutions were mixed with 0.4 ml of a suspension of antibody-coated sheep erythrocytes ($5 \times 10^8$ cells/ml), and made up to 3.0 ml with GVB. This mixture was again incubated for 1 h at 37 °C. The amount of haemoglobin liberated was determined by spectrophotometry at 541 nm, and the $CH_{50}$ values according to Mayer (11) calculated from this. Finally, the dose-effect relationship yielded the relative activity of the contrast media on the untreated complement system: the relative activity 1.0 signifies that the complement system was not activated, and the relative activity 0.0 that the complement system was activated to the highest extent possible under the experimental conditions.

## Results

The intravenous toxicity of iopromide in male and female mice (Table 1) is statistically significantly ($p \leq 0.05$) lower than that of metrizamide. The $LD_{50}$ at 16.5 g iodine/kg is comparable to that of iopamidol determined concurrently.

The intravenous toxicity of iopromide in male and female rats (Table 2) was found to be 11.4 g iodine/kg, which is very close to that of metrizamide (10.3 g I/kg) and iopamidol (11.3 g I/kg).

The tolerance of iopromide after intracerebral injection in rats (Table 3) was found to be significantly ($p \leq 0.05$) higher than that of metrizamide. Iopamidol was tolerated better ($p \leq 0.05$) than iopromide and metrizamide.

Intracisternal administration of saline caused no changes of the behaviour in any animal. After administration of iopromide, metrizamide and iopamidol, disturbances in physiological coordination and occasionally spasm were observed, but no lethal effects (Table 4). The effective doses of iopromide and metrizamide were very similar, while iopamidol was tolerated better ($p \leq 0.05$) than the other two agents.

In the concentration of 1.2 mg I/ml binding of iopromide to the proteins of human plasma was $0.9 \pm 0.2$ per cent, that of metrizamide $4.3 \pm 0.3$ per cent and that of iopamidol $2.9 \pm 0.2$ per cent.

Table 1 Acute tolerance after a single i.v. injection of iopromide, metrizamide and iopamidol in the mouse

| Compound | dose g I/kg | mortality up to 7 d p. appl.* | lethal dosages with 95 per cent confidence intervals (g I/kg) |
|---|---|---|---|
| iopromide | 12.0 | 1/6 | $LD_{50}$ 16.5 (13.8–18.9) |
| | 15.0 | 1/6 | |
| | 18.0 | 4/6 | $LD_5$ 11.4 ( 6.1–13.7) |
| | 21.0 | 5/6 | |
| | 24.0 | 6/6 | $LD_{95}$ 23.9 (20.4–40.3) |
| metrizamide | 8.25 | 0/6 | $LD_{50}$ 12.1 (10.6–13.6) |
| | 10.5 | 2/6 | |
| | 12.0 | 2/6 | $LD_5$ 9.2 ( 5.8–10. 5.) |
| | 14.25 | 5/6 | |
| | 16.5 | 6/6 | $LD_{95}$ 15.8 (13.9–24.4) |
| iopamidol | 12.0 | 0/6 | $LD_{50}$ 16.4 (14.8–17.6) |
| | 14.25 | 1/6 | |
| | 16.5 | 2/6 | $LD_5$ 13.8 ( 9.7–15.1) |
| | 18.0 | 5/6 | |
| | 19.5 | 6/6 | $LD_{95}$ 19.5 (18.0–25.8) |

* The quotient from the number of animals which died and the number of animals used is given in the table.

Table 2  Acute tolerance after a single i.v. injection of iopromide, metrizamide and iopamidol in the rat

| Compound | dose g I/kg | mortality up to 7 d p. appl.* | lethal dosages with 95 per cent confidence intervals (g I/kg) |
|---|---|---|---|
| iopromide | 9.0 | 1/6 | $LD_{50}$ 11.4 ( 9.1–13.1) |
|  | 10.5 | 3/6 |  |
|  | 12.0 | 3/6 | $LD_5$ 7.3 ( 2.6– 9.6) |
|  | 13.5 | 4/6 |  |
|  | 15.0 | 5/6 | $LD_{95}$ 17.7 (14.7–40.8) |
|  | 16.8 | 4/4 |  |
| metrizamide | 7.5 | 1/6 | $LD_{50}$ 10.3 ( 8.1–11.9) |
|  | 9.0 | 0/6 |  |
|  | 10.0 | 3/6 | $LD_5$ 6.8 ( 3.0– 8.2) |
|  | 10.5 | 5/6 |  |
|  | 12.0 | 4/6 | $LD_{95}$ 15.4 (12.8–35.3) |
|  | 13.5 | 5/6 |  |
| iopamidol | 7.5 | 1/6 | $LD_{50}$ 11.3 ( 9.4–13.8) |
|  | 9.0 | 1/6 |  |
|  | 10.5 | 3/6 | $LD_5$ 6.8 ( 2.7– 8.5) |
|  | 12.0 | 2/6 |  |
|  | 13.5 | 4/6 | $LD_{95}$ 18.6 (14.8–48.9) |
|  | 15.0 | 6/6 |  |

* The quotient from the number of animals which died and the number of animals used is given in the table.

Table 3  Tolerance to iopromide, metrizamide and iopamidol after intracerebral administration in rats. Effective doses (lack of motor coordination, epileptoid fits) with 95 per cent confidence intervals

| iopromide ($n = 50$) | $ED_{50}$ | 85.9 ( 69.4–113.0) mg I/kg |
|---|---|---|
|  | $ED_5$ | 37.4 ( 12.3– 51.7) mg I/kg |
|  | $ED_{95}$ | 197.6 (137.2–711) mg I/Kg |
| metrizamide ($n = 50$) | $ED_{50}$ | 52.2 ( 39.3– 79.0) mg I/kg |
|  | $ED_5$ | 18.3 ( 4.7– 27.8) mg I/kg |
|  | $ED_{95}$ | 155.1 ( 96.0–766) mg I/kg |
| iopamidol ($n = 50$) | $ED_{50}$ | 154.1 (122.7–215.8) mg I/kg |
|  | $ED_5$ | 62.6 ( 26.0– 86.1) mg I/kg |
|  | $ED_{95}$ | 379.7 (253.7–1237) mg I/kg |

Table 4  Tolerance to iopromide, metrizamide and iopamidol after intracerebral administration in rats. Effective doses (lack of motor coordination, epileptoid fits) with 95 per cent confidence intervals

| iopromide ($n = 50$) | $ED_{50}$ | 53.2 ( 47.5– 61.5) mg I/kg |
|---|---|---|
|  | $ED_5$ | 27.4 ( 12.7– 36.5) mg I/kg |
|  | $ED_{95}$ | 103.0 ( 83.1–178.3) mg I/Kg |
| metrizamide ($n = 50$) | $ED_{50}$ | 52.8 ( 45.4– 60.7) mg I/kg |
|  | $ED_5$ | 29.7 (18.6– 36.6) mg I/kg |
|  | $ED_{95}$ | 93.7 ( 79.9–144.6) mg I/kg |
| iopamidol ($n = 50$) | $ED_{50}$ | 127.1 (109.9–161.9) mg I/kg |
|  | $ED_5$ | 72.7 ( 42.4– 88.3) mg I/kg |
|  | $ED_{95}$ | 222.2 (170.6–495.6) mg I/kg |

The 50 per cent inhibition of lysozyme was observed from iopromide at 142 mg I/ml ($\triangleq 0.37$ mol/l), that for metrizamide at 132 mg I/ml ($\triangleq 0.35$ mol/l) and that for iopamidol at 157 mg I/ml ($\triangleq 0.41$ mol/l; Fig 1).

At the final concentration of 150 mg I/ml of the incubation mixture iopromide liberated about 7 per cent of the maximum amount of histamine possible from the mast cells of rats, metrizamide about 25 per cent and iopamidol 17 per cent (Fig 2). After incubation of human blood with metrizamide the shape of erythrocytes changed markedly even

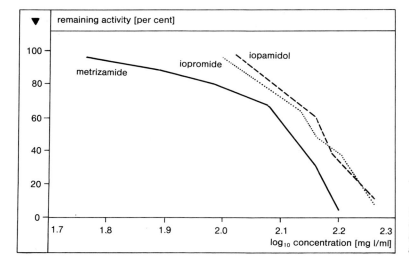

Fig 1  Dependence of remaining activity (per cent) of lysozyme on concentration ($\log_{10}$ mg I/ml) of metrizamide, iopromide and iopamidol in vitro

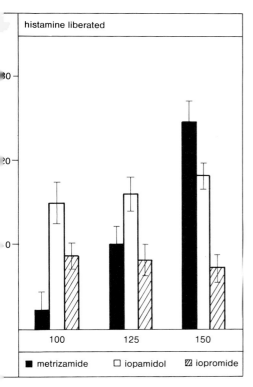

Fig 2 Liberation of histamine (per cent) from mast cells after incubation with contrast media with 3 different concentrations (mg I/ml)

Fig 3 Mean damage index of erythrocytes when exposed to contrast media in vitro

Fig 4 Complement activation (per cent) as a function of contrast media concentration ($\log_{10}$ mg I/ml) in vitro

at low concentrations. The occurrence of, e.g., echinocytes and spherocytes, was significantly ($p < 0.01$) more frequent than in the mixture with iopromide and iopamidol. Taking the dose-dependent effects of metrizamide as 1, the relative effects of iopromide and iopamidol were 0.15 in each case (Fig 3).

The activation of the complement system in human serum by iopromide, metrizamide and iopamidol is given in Fig 4. Under experimental conditions at an iopromide concentration of 176 mg I/ml, a metrizamide concentration of 101 mg I/ml and an iopamidol concentration of 190 mg I/ml, 50 per cent of the activity of the complement employed remained.

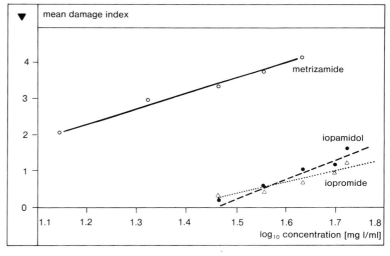

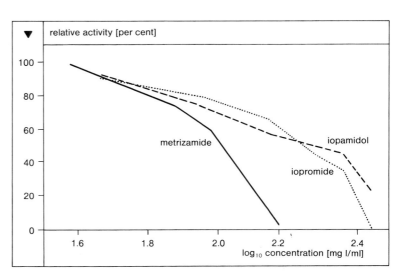

## Discussion

The systemic tolerance of iopromide, which was explored in tests of acute intravenous toxicity in two rodent species, was found to be remarkably good. In rats tolerance was found to be equal to that of metrizamide and iopamidol. In mice iopromide was tolerated as well as iopamidol and better than metrizamide.

The substantial improvement in general tolerance achieved by contrast agents of the nonionic type compared to ionic urographic agents is very well reflected by the median lethal dose in test animals. For meglumine-sodium ioglicate and for meglumine-sodium ioxaglate we reported median lethal doses ($LD_{50}$) of about 8.5 g iodine per kg of rat (12), which is considerably lower than the $LD_{50}$ reported here of about 11 g I/kg of three nonionic monomeric agents.

The absolute values for the lethal doses of metrizamide and iopamidol resulting from this study appear to be different from data published by other groups (5, 13). Typically, the strain of test animals and other experimental conditions may cause such differences. The ranking of values from a comparative study is best suited best to give reliable information.

If the low toxicity of iopromide in test animals is related to nonidiosyncratic pathophysiologic dose-depending reactions in man, the new contrast agent should induce fewer adverse reactions than conventional agents.

Neural tolerance of iopromide was found to be equal to or higher than that of metrizamide and somewhat lower than that of iopamidol when injected into rats intracisternally and intracerebrally, respectively. Even for a contrast agent designed predominantly to be used for intravascular use, good neural tolerance appears to be gratifying. Although it is unlikely that a very hydrophilic contrast agent like iopromide could penetrate into neural tissues, in some diseased states penetration may occur. Our results with iopromide may indicate that this compound will not provoke any major reactions in patients with specific neuropathophysiological dispositions, as is the case in clinical experience with metrizamide.

Iopromide has very low binding affinity to serum albumin at a concentration of 1.2 ml I/ml which was observed 5–10 minutes after bolus injection of 15 g iodine intravenously to patients (21). Moreover, the low affinity of iopromide to proteins was demonstrated by the fact that the compound is unable to inhibit lysozyme in concentrations lower than 100 mg iodine per ml. From these observations and against the background of the experiences of Lasser and his collaborators (6, 7) iopromide is considered to be a contrast agent with an extremely low capacity to displace physiologic, highly effective compounds by competition for the binding sites or to alter the configuration of enzymes and thus inactivate them.

The observations of Lasser et al. (7) that protein binding capacity is correlated also to crenation and agglutination of red blood cells was reconfirmed in our studies: Iopromide and iopamidol induced only minor changes in erythrocyte morphology, while metrizamide, which is more lipophilic, induced significantly more echinocytes and spherocytes. In order to minimize disturbances in the microcirculation caused by the rigidification of the erythrocytes, the use of contrast agents producing only minor changes in red cell morphology is favourable.

The property of the contrast media tested of liberating histamine from rat peritoneal mast cells might have a direct relationship to their affinity to proteins also; iopromide exhibited less influence than iopamidol and metrizamide, in particular at high concentrations of the contrast agents. On the basis of clinical investigations it may be assumed that the property of iodinated contrast media of liberating histamine from basophilic cells and mast cells in vivo is directly related to the idiosyncratic (anaphylactoid) reactions developing in 5 to 8 per cent of patients (2, 3). On the basis of the low liberation of histamine by iopromide observed in vitro, a markedly lower rate of side-effects can be expected compared with currently known contrast media.

Activation systems, i.e., the complement, fibrinolytic and coagulation systems, have been shown to be involved in severe reactions to contrast media (8, 9). Our results indicate iopromide can also activate the complement system in principle. Again, iopromide and iopamidol exhibited less activity than metrizamide. Iopromide may accordingly have even fewer side-effects clinically than metrizamide, which is tolerated very well in man when applied intravascularly.

It is concluded from our preclinical studies with iopromide reported here that the new contrast agent shows properties predicting a broad margin of safety when employed in human clinical use. Chemotoxic reactions following the intravascular injection of high concentrations of iopromide as well as systemic anaphylactoid reactions may occur less frequently than with conventional contrast agents and metrizamide.

# References

1. Almén, T.: Experience from 10 years of development of water-soluble nonionic contrast media. Invest. Radiol. 15: 282–283, 1980
2. Bhat, K. N., C. M. Arroyave, R. Crown: Reaction to radiographic contrast agents. New developments in etiology. Ann. Allergy 37: 169, 1976
3. Cogen, F. C., M. E. Norman, E. Dunsky, J. Hirschfeld, B. Zweiman: Histamine release and complement changes following injection of contrast media in humans. J. Allergy Clin. Immunol. 64 (1979) 299
4. Felder, E., J. Dossnini: Water soluble contrast media for urography, angiography and myelography: a review. Rays 6: 3–10, 1981
5. Felder, E., D. Pitrè, P. Tirone: Radiopaque contrast media. XLIV. Preclinical studies with a new nonionic contrast agent. Farmaco Ed. sci. 32: 835–844, 1977
6. Lasser, E. C., J. W. Lang: Contrast-protein interactions. Invest. Radiol. 5: 446, 1970
7. Lasser, E. C., R. S. Farr, T. Fujimagari, W. M. Tripp: The significance of protein binding of contrast media in roentgen diagnosis. Amer. J. Roentgenol. 87: 338–360, 1962
8. Lasser, E. C., J. H. Lang, S. G. Lyon, A. E. Hamblin: Complement and contrast material reactors. J. Allergy clin. Immunol. 64: 105–112, 1979
9. Lasser, E. C., J. H. Lang, A. E. Hamblin, S. G. Lyon, M. Howard: Activation systems in contrast idiosyncrasy. Invest. Radiol. 14: 52–55, 1980
10. Lorenz W., L. Benesch, H. Barth, E. Matejky, R. Meyer, J. Kusche, M. Hutzel, E. Weile: Fluorometric assay of histamine in tissues and body fluids. Choice of the purification procedure and identification in the nanogram range. Z. anal. Chem. 252: 94, 1970
11. Mayer, M. M.: Complement and complement fixation. In Kabat, E. A., M. M. Mayer: Experimental Immunochemistry. Thomas, Springfield/Ill. 1971 (p. 133)
12. Mützel, W.: Properties of conventional contrast media. In Felix, R., E. Kazner, O. H. Wegener: Contrast Media in Computed Tomography. Excerpta Medica, Amsterdam 1981 (pp. 19–30)
13. Salvesen, S.: Acute toxicity test of metrizamide. Acta radiol. Suppl. 335: 5–13, 1973
14. Scholtan, W.: Über die Bindung der Langzeit-Sulfonamide an die Serumeiweißkörper. Makromol. Chem. 54: 24, 1962
15. Shugar, D.: The measurement of lysozyme activity and ultraviolet inactivation of lysozyme. Biochim. biophys. Acta 8: 302, 1952
16. Sörensen, S. P. L.: Enzymstudien II. Mitteilung. Über die Messung und die Bedeutung der Wasserstoffionenkonzentration bei enzymatischen Prozessen. Biochem. Z. 21: 131, 1909
17. Speck, U., W. Mützel, H.-J. Weinmann: This volume, p. 2
18. Speck, U., B. Düsterberg, G. Mannesmann, H. M. Siefert: Pharmakologie der Iotroxinsäure, eines neuen Cholegraficums. II. Tierexperimentelle Untersuchungen zur Verträglichkeit. Arzneimittel-Forsch. 28: 2290, 1978
19. Valzelli, L.: A simple method to inject drugs intracerebrally. Med. exp. (Basel) 11: 23, 1964
20. Weder, H. G., M. H. Bickel: Verbessertes Gerät zur Gleichgewichtsdialyse. Z. anal. Chem. 252: 253, 1970
21. Wolf, K. J., B. Steidle, T. Skutta, W. Mützel: Iopromide – first clinical experience with a new non-ionic, renally excreted X-ray contrast medium. Acta radiol. (Stockh.) (in press)

# The Action of Iohexol on Clotting, Fibrinolysis, Complement and Kallikrein System

B. Schulze, H. K. Beyer, V. Barth, K. Tremmel and U. Borst

## Summary

Iohexol, a new non-ionic, low osmolar radiographic contrast medium, causes a dose dependent lengthening of global coagulation tests (thrombin time, calciumthromboplastin time, partial thromboplastin time, thrombin coagulase time). Plasminogen levels and thrombin activity are not affected by iohexol. Iohexol triggers activation of complement system by the alternative pathway. The complement activation is enhanced by EACA. It is not due to inhibition of C 3 b – inactivator.

In comparison to ioxaglate, iohexol affects coagulation far less. Both substances do not interfere with fibrinolysis. Activation of properdin pathway by iohexol and other non-ionic contrast media is probably due to macromolecular aggregates formed at high RCM concentrations.

In vivo, an acceptable contrast and only occasional minor osmotic pain reactions were recorded during extensive angiographic routine examinations using iohexol. Poor contrast was noted for translumbar aortography and imaging of the aortic arch using iohexol at a concentration of 300 mg iodine/ml. Phlebography by iohexol rendered excellent contrast.

The application of iohexol is highly recommended for arterial and venous angiography.

## Zusammenfassung

*Iohexol* bewirkt eine dosisabhängige Verlängerung der Thrombinzeit, Thrombincoagulase-Zeit, Calcium,Thromboplastin-Zeit und partiellen Thromboplastinzeit. Die Thrombinaktivität und Plasminogenkonzentration werden durch Iohexol nicht beeinflußt. Iohexol führt zu einer Nebenschlußaktivierung des Komplementsystems, die nicht durch eine Hemmung des C3b-Inaktivators bedingt ist, und die durch EACA dosisabhängig verstärkt wird.

Ein Vergleich mit *Ioxaglat* zeigt, daß Iohexol die Gerinnung wesentlich weniger beeinflußt. Hinsichtlich der Fibrinolyse verhalten sich beide Substanzen gleich.

Die Komplementaktivierung ist wahrscheinlich durch Micellenbildung von Iohexol bei hohen Konzentrationen bedingt. Angiographische In-vivo-Untersuchungen aller Gefäßprovinzen unter Routinebedingungen zeigen eine gute Verträglichkeit von Iohexol im Konzentrationsbereich 300–350 mg Jod/ml bei zufriedenstellendem Kontrast. Bei Darstellungen des Aortenbogens und translumbalen Aortographien wird allerdings die höhere Konzentration (350 mg Jod/ml) empfohlen. Phlebographien zeigen einen sehr guten Kontrast. Zur Vermeidung zusätzlicher osmotisch bedingter Gefäßschäden wird der Einsatz von Iohexol 300 zur Shunt-Darstellung bei Dialysepatienten sowie bei akuten tiefen Pflebothrombosen empfohlen.

## Introduction

The following pathogenesis appears to underlie the anaphylactoid intolerance reactions of iodinated water-soluble x-ray contrast media:

The activation threshold of clotting, fibrinolysis, complement and kallikrein systems is lowered by a diminution of C1-esterase inhibitor serum level.

The contrast media (RCM) directly or indirectly trigger off contact activation of Hageman-Factor-XII thus initiating fibrinolysis and the complement system. In addition, the conversion of pre-kallikrein to kallikrein is set in motion. As a consequence to activation of these systems, biological cleavage products are formed, such as histamine and bradykinin, which underlie the clinical symptomatology of the RCM-intolerance reactions.

Therefore, it seems reasonable to investigate the effect of iohexol on essential parameters of the above-mentioned systems under in vitro conditions, and to compare them with the results using other contrast media.

The following parameters were included in the investigation:

– Clotting assays for the terminal clotting phase: thrombin time, thrombin-coagulase time and thrombin activity; for the endogenous clotting system: the partial thromboplastin time, and for the exogenous clotting system: the calcium thromboplastin time.

In addition, because of its importance, the RCM-induced activation of Factor XII was measured.

– Fibrinolysis: the plasminogen consumption of RCM-incubated plasma was measured.
– Complement systems: Factor B cleavage by iohexol was demonstrated by means of two-dimensional immuno-electrophoresis. In addition, the extent to which Factor B conversion is influenced by EACA was investigated.
– Kallikrein system: we examined the question of a RCM-induced kallikrein formation. In addi-

tion, the rate of conversion of pre-kallikrein to kallikrein after RCM-incubation of citrated plasma was measured.

## Materials and Methods Obtained

from Behring: Standard human plasma, test thrombin, calcium thromboplastin, pathromtin, plasminogen assay kit including plasminogen standard plasma, agarose and anti-serum against Factor B.
from Boehringer Mannheim: Thrombin-coagulase reagent, PK test, Chromozym-TH.
from Merck: Tris, TRA, barbital and sodium barbital, sodium chloride.
from Roche: EACA (400 mg/ml).
The contrast medium iohexol from Schering AG/Berlin (350 mg iodine/ml: batch No. 111027) was kindly supplied by Dr. Clauss.

## Conditions of Incubation

Standard human plasma was mixed with increasing amounts of iohexol (1000 µl plasma − 0–300 µl iohexol 350) and all mixtures were made up with isotonic saline solution to the same final volume of 1.300 µl. After that the mixtures were incubated in the water bath at 37° for 30 minutes. The duration of incubation for plasminogen, Factor B conversion and kallikrein amounted to 60 minutes. The coagulation times for thrombin time, thrombin-coagulase time, PTT, calcium-thromboplastin time and plasminogen were measured using Schnitger and Gros coagulometer. 10 determinations were carried out for each concentration range.
The determination of thrombin and kallikrein activities was carried out photometrically in plastic cuvettes at 37° and 405 nm. In testing the thrombin activity, an increasing amount of iohexol was added to the incubation mixture in the cuvette, so as to avoid diluting of contrast medium by buffer and substrate.
The details of the determinations respectively were carried out according to the test instructions.

## Statistics

For graphical representation of the results the mean, standard deviation and variance were ascertained. The concentrations of contrast medium were given in mg iodine/ml.

## Results

Fig 1–3 show the results of the investigations of the terminal sequence of the clotting system. These show a calcium-independent, dose-dependent prolongation of clotting times, and a slight reduction in thrombin activity.
In particular a doubling of the thrombin time by iohexol was found at a concentration of about 45 mg iodine/ml. At this concentration ioxaglate causes a 6-fold prolongation of thrombin time.
At the highest iohexol concentrations (80 mg iodine/ml) investigated by us, an almost 6-fold prolongation of the thrombin time is found, whereas at the same concentration ioxaglate causes incoagulability.
The thrombin-coagulase time shows a doubling of the initial value with iohexol at barely 30 mg iodine/ml. In the same concentration range ioxaglate effects a 5 to 6-fold prolongation of the initial value. Similary for this parameter it is noteworthy that up to 80 mg iodine/ml of iohexol a 5 to 6-fold prolongation of clotting time occurs, whereas ioxa-

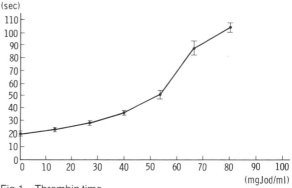

Fig 1  Thrombin time

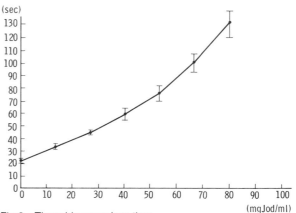

Fig 2  Thrombin coagulase time

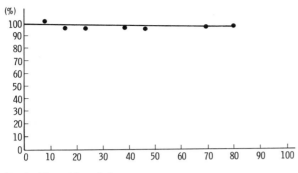

Fig 3 Thrombin activity

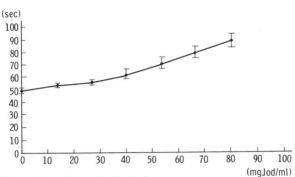

Fig 4 Partial thromboplastin time

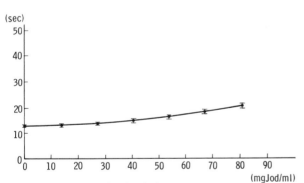

Fig 5 Calcium thromboplastin time

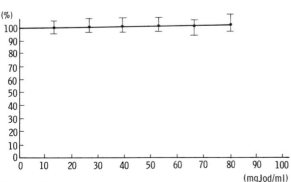

Fig 6 Plasminogen

glate already displays incoagulability below 40 mg iodine/ml.

Assays of thrombin activity (Fig 3) showed no depressing effect in the concentration range between 0–80 mg iodine/ml of iohexol. Of course it must be borne in mind that for the enzyme determination the serum used in the test mixture is diluted to 1:200 with buffer and substrate. Since the binding affinity of iohexol to protein is very slight, a corresponding dilution of contrast medium can arise by dissociation. We therefore changed the experimental procedure in such a way that we added iohexol directly to fresh thrombin-containing serum in the assay mixture. The actual thrombin activity was measured beforehand. After addition of contrast medium (1–300 μl) the thrombin activity was once more determined over several minutes thereafter. The dilution caused by addition of contrast medium was taken into account in the evaluation. The results show in the highest concentration ranges (45 mg iodine/ml) a reduction of thrombin activity by 12%.

Fig 4 shows the changes of the PTT with increasing concentrations of iohexol. Even at the highest concentrations investigated by us (80 mg iodine/ml) there is only a 1.8-fold increase in coagulation time. For ioxaglate incoagulability occurs from 60 mg iodine/ml onward or a doubling of the initial clotting time at around 25 mg iodine/ml.

Fig 5 shows the dose-dependent prolongation of the calcium-thromboplastin time by iohexol. There occurs only a minimal increase of coagulation time of 13 to 20 seconds in the concentration range of 0–80 mg iodine/ml. Expressed as percentage of the value for the RCM-free plasma sample this corresponds to a reduction from 100 to 40%. For ioxaglate a diminution of the quick value to 10% was calculated at a concentration of 50 mg iodine/ml.

Fig 6 shows the dose-dependent behaviour of plasminogen with increasing concentrations of iohexol. Identical with the behaviour of ioxaglate, no changes in plasminogen concentrations for all tested concentrations were found. These findings are of special importance, since according to several authors, in contrast to our results, a RCM-induced activation of fibrinolysis is believed to be responsible for triggering off RCM adverse reactions.

Fig 7 summarizes the results of activation of complement Factor B by iohexol.

In particular the figures on the electropherogram illustrations signify the following:

1 = complement factor B in fresh serum with minimal spontaneous activation after 60 minutes incubation at 37 °C.
2 = zymosane-activated serum with clearly detectable cathodic cleavage product Bb.
3 = behaviour of Factor B with EACA (concentration: 120 mg/1.3 ml mixture). Behaviour identical to 1 is apparent.
4 & 5 = serum incubated with iohexol (70 mg or 88 mg iodine/ml). A clear precipitate of the Bb cleavage product is visible.
6 = serum incubated with iohexol (80 mg iodine/ml) + 40 mg EACA/1.400 ml mixture. The activation of B is clearly evident, being demonstrable more extensive than that under (4) and (5). This finding clearly proves that EACA neither suppresses nor diminishes complement activation induced by RCM.

Table 1 shows the results of Factor XIIa formation at increasing concentrations of iohexol. Under conditions of excess prekallikrein, after incubation with citrated pooled plasma at 37 °C for 60 minutes in the concentration range 0–80 mg iodine/ml, there is no increase of kallikrein activity suggestive of factor XIIa generation.

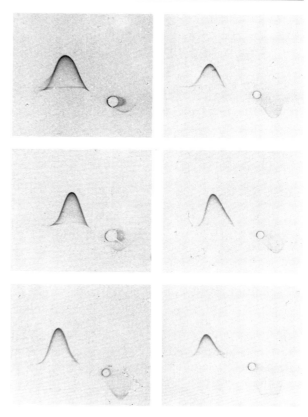

Fig 7   Immuno-electrophoresis Complement factor B

Table 1   XIIa Activity in Iohexol-incubated citrat plasma

| Iohexolconcentration (mg iodine/ml) | ΔE/min | Substrate (µl) | Sample (µl) | Chromozyme PK (µl) | Buffer (µl) | EACA (µl) |
|---|---|---|---|---|---|---|
| 0 | 0.009 | 20 | 20 | 300 | 500 | 25 |
| 0 | 0.019 | 50 | 50 | 300 | 500 | 25 |
| 0 | 0.019 | 50 | 50 | 300 | 500 | 25 |
| 40.4 | 0.009 | 20 | 20 | 300 | 500 | 25 |
| 40.4 | 0.004 | 10 | 10 | 300 | 500 | 25 |
| 40.4 | 0.021 | 50 | 50 | 300 | 500 | 25 |
| 80.3 | 0.009 | 20 | 20 | 300 | 500 | 25 |
| 80.3 | 0.020 | 50 | 50 | 300 | 500 | 25 |
| 80.3 | 0.019 | 50 | 50 | 300 | 500 | 25 |

Substrate = inactive pooled citrated plasma (prekallikrein)

Table 2   Conversion inhibition of prekallikrein to kallikrein by iohexol

| Buffer (µl) | Chromozyme PK (µl) | Iohexol (µl) | Citrated Plasma (µl) | Dextran Sulphate (µl) | ΔE/10 min. (µl) |
|---|---|---|---|---|---|
| 1.500 | 500 | 0 | 10 | 10 | 0.013 |
| 1.500 | 500 | 8.45 | 10 | 10 | 0.005 |
| 1.500 | 500 | 0 | 50 | 50 | 0.022 |
| 1.500 | 500 | 8.14 | 50 | 50 | 0.016 |
| 1.500 | 500 | 0 | 100 | 100 | 0.072 |
| 1.500 | 500 | 7.77 | 100 | 100 | 0.051 |

Table 2 shows that on addition of iohexol to Factor XIIa-activated citrated pooled plasma an inhibition of kallikrein activity results. This effect can also be detected for other enzyme activities with all contrast media so far investigated by us. The concentrations of contrast media necessary for inhibition of enzyme activity exist under in vivo conditions for only a few seconds, and are in general completely reversible.

## Discussion

In order to obtain comparable and reproducible results, we carried out the investigations described above using pooled plasma. For reason of comparison we referred to our earlier investigations on ioxaglate. This appears to be reasonable, since ioxaglate is a RCM with low osmolarity and identical spectrum of clinical application and similar iodine concentrations.

With regard to the effects on coagulation, iohexol exerts considerably less anticoagulant activity than ioxaglate. The inhibitory effect on coagulation is, as with ioxaglate, not brought about by EDTA or an inactivation of thrombin induced by RCM.

The minimal effect of iohexol on calcium thromboplastin time or PTT requires special mention. These latter findings argue strongly against contact activation by iohexol. In the case of ioxaglate, both parameters show considerable prolongations of clotting time right up to incoagulability.

A decline of plasminogen as an indication of an activation of fibrinolysis could neither be found for iohexol nor for ioxaglate.

Further, the results are interesting as regards the question of complement activation by RCM. A shunt activation, measured by Factor B conversion, indeed occurs for iohexol at a concentration of 70 mg iodine/ml. For ioxaglate no C-3 conversion was found.

Thus iohexol behaves similarly to the two other non-ionic RCM metrizamide and iopamidol. With the latter, we verified complement activation both by Factor B as well as Factor C-3 conversion. According to our interpretation, the complement activation is released by non-ionic RCM by the formation of micelles at high concentrations of conctrast medium. This also explains why we found no complement activation with ionised contrast media despite a similar chemical structure and comparable concentrations, even with EDTA-free preparations.

In practice this means that no correlation exists between the capability for complement activation and the toxicity of a contrast medium. The correlation between $LD_{50}$ and reduction in complement activity (CH-50 method) is, in our opinion, no evidence for a complement activation, but much more the demonstration of a contrast medium mediated inactivation of the complement cascade.

Under conditions of excess prekallikrein, we investigated in vitro the possiblity of a contrast medium activation of Factor XII (Hageman Factor). In the range of concentrations investigated by us, no elevation of kallikrein activity was found as an expression of Factur XIIa formation.

Kallikrein activity released in citrated plasma by dextran sulphate could be suppressed dose-dependently by addition of iohexol.

For in vivo conditions our model is too simple. Here it would be desirable to allow for corpuscular blood elements and endothelial cells as a source of partial thromboplastin during incubation by RCM. In vivo we investigated in 28 patients during routine arterial angiographies the pain reactions elicited by injection of RCM, as well as the contrast after intra-arterial administration of iohexol, 300, 350 and ioxaglate. Anaphylactoid side effects did not appear, and blood pressure changes and vomiting were not observed. Immediately following administration of contrast medium, the patients were questioned about the occurrence of feelings of heat or of pains. After the first injection of contrast medium there followed, if necessary, a second injection of the competitive preparation, so that an immediate comparison of pain reactions between both preparations (iohexol/ioxaglate) by the patient was possible.

Iohexol 300 and ioxaglate behaved identically in respect of feelings of heat and painful reactions. There occurred only a slight feeling of warmth, and arm and leg angiographies were possible without sedation. Iohexol 350 caused in 3 of 12 patients to some extent considerable osmotic pain reactions on peripheral angiography.

With regard to contrast, iohexol 300 was graded inferior to ioxaglate as evaluated by examining radiologists. On the other hand, contrast with iohexol 350 was rated as good to very good. The poorest contrasts were obtained with iohexol 300 on translumbar aortography and for contrasting the aortic arch.

Summing up our in vivo and in vitro investigations, we confirm that iohexol proved to be a suitable substance for angiography.

# References

1 Hasselbacher, P., J. Hahn: In vitro effects of radiographic contrast media on the complement system. J. Allergy clin. Immunol. 66: 217–222, 1980
2 Lasser, E. C. et al: Complement and contrast material reactors. J. Allergy clin. Immunol. 64: 105–112, 1979
3 Lasser, E. C., J. H. Lang, A. E. Hamblin, S. G. Lyon, M. Howard: Activation systems in contrast idiosyncrasy. Invest. Radiol. 15, 6 Suppl.: 3–5, 1980
4 Lasser, E. C. et al.: Changes in complement and coagulation factors in a patient suffering a severe anaphylactoid reaction to injected contrast material: Some considerations of pathogenesis. Invest. Radiol. 15, 6 Suppl.: 6–12, 1980
5 Lasser, E. C. et al: Prekallikrein,Kallikrein conversion rate as a predictor of contrast material catastrophies. Radiology 140: 11–5, 1981
6 Neoh, S. H. et al.: The in vitro activation of complement by radiological contrast materials and its inhibition with ε-amino caproic acid. Invest. Radiol. 16: 152–158, 1981
7 Roth, F. J.: Ergebnisse der klinischen Prüfung der Testsubstanz AG 6227 bei der Extremitäten-Angiographie. In: Zukunft der Angiographie – Schmerzfreiheit. Byk Gulden Symposium, Juli 1979 (pp. 127–130)
8 Schulze, B.: In vitro Wirkung von Ioxaglat (Hexabrix®) auf Gerinnung, Fibrinolyse und Komplementsystem. Fortschr. Röntgenstr. 134: 566–570, 1981
9 Schulze, B., H. K. Beyer: The effect of radiographic iodized contrast media on coagulation, fibrinolysis and complement system. In Amiel, M.: Contrast Media in Radiology. Bergmann, München 1982 (pp. 31–39)
10 Till, G., U. Rother, D. Gemsa: Activation of complement by radiographic contrast media: Generation of chemotactic and anaphylatoxin activities. Int. Arch. Allergy 56: 543–550, 1978
11 Vinazzer, H.: Assay of Total Factor XII and of Activated Factor XII in Plasma with a chromogenic Substrate. Haematologica 65: 636–643, 1980
12 Zeitler, E. et al.: Angiography in Lower Extremities with new Contrast Media: Review of Double Blind Studies. In: First European Workshop: Contrast Media in Radiology, Lyon 1981. Springer, Berlin (pp. 57)

# Renal Tolerance

## Albuminuria Following Renal Arteriography with Various Ionic and Nonionic Contrast Agents in the Rat

U. Speck, W. R. Press and W. Mützel

### Summary

Albuminuria was measured up to 2 hours p. inj. following bilateral selective renal arteriography in anaesthetized rats using meglumine salts of conventional ionic contrast media, sodium diatrizoate, sodium-meglumine ioxaglate and various nonionic agents at about 300 mg iodine/ml. The nonionic contrast media were also employed with 370 mg iodine/ml. A comparison with 0.9% sodium chloride and two hypertonic controls was performed. Metrizamide and all ionic contrast media revealed the same degree of albuminuria as a hypertonic (1.8 osm/kg) sorbitol solution. The nonionic contrast agent iopromide did not cause albuminuria at all at 300 mg iodine/ml but did so slightly at 370 mg iodine/ml. The properties of contrast media which might cause kidney toxicity in nephroangiography are discussed.

### Zusammenfassung

An narkotisierten Ratten wurde die Albuminausscheidung bis 2 Stunden nach beidseitiger selektiver Nierenarteriographie mit Megluminsalzen gebräuchlicher ionischer Kontrastmittel, dem Natriumamidotrizoat, dem Natrium-Meglumin Ioxaglat und verschiedenen nicht ionischen Substanzen bei etwa 300 mg Jod/ml (nicht-ionische Kontrastmittel auch 370 mg Jod/ml) gemessen. Zum Vergleich wurde physiologische Kochsalzlösung und zwei hypertone Kontrollösungen injiziert. Metrizamid und alle ionischen Kontrastmittel verursachten das gleiche Maß an Proteinurie wie eine hypertone (1,8 osm/kg) Sorbitlösung. Das nicht ionische Kontrastmittel Iopromid bewirkte bei 300 mg Jod/ml keine, bei 370 mg Jod/ml eine gering erhöhte Albuminausscheidung. Es wird die Frage diskutiert, welche Kontrastmittel-Eigenschaften für die Nierentoxizität bei der Nierenangiographie verantwortlich sein könnten.

### Introduction

Renal tolerance of contrast material has become a major concern in the literature (8) although acute renal failure fortunately is only rarely observed and can mostly be avoided by the consideration of known risk factors (2). The mechanisms by which contrast media produce renal injury are unclear. Moreover, our knowledge of the properties of contrast agents responsible for kidney toxicity is poor. The situation is further confused by the fact that two different kidney toxicities exist with contrast material. One is observed after a high intravascular dosage. The kidney is probably damaged during the excretion of the contrast material in the tubules. Since low osmotic contrast agents reach higher concentrations in the tubules their "excretion tolerance" is not necessarily better than the tolerance of hypertonic contrast materials (7). The other type of kidney toxicity occurs during selective renal arteriography. In this case brief exposure of renal blood vessels to the undiluted contrast agent should be the reason for the toxicity and well tolerated low osmotic contrast media should cause less damage than strongly hypertonic angiographic agents.

The aim of the experiments reported in this paper was to compare various contrast media with regard to their tolerance during nephroangiography in the rat. Since this comparison includes sodium and meglumin salts, high osmotic and low osmotic, ionic and nonionic agents it should be possible to identify certain properties of the contrast molecules responsible for kidney toxicity in renal arteriography.

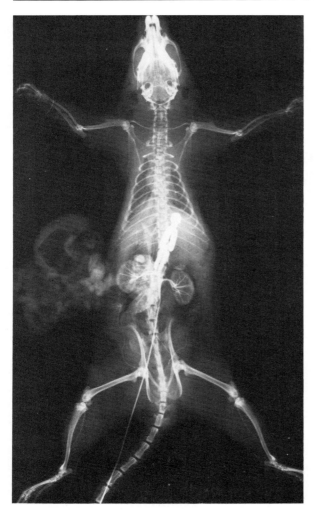

Fig 1 Renal arteriogram during the injection of contrast material at a dosage of 400 mg iodine/kg in the anaesthetized rat. The clamp prevents the escape of contrast material in the cranial direction. It is removed immediately after injection

## Material and Methods

### Test solutions

The following solutions were injected either to perform nephroangiography or to control the experimental conditions:

a) hypertonic contrast media (osmolality between 1.5 and 1.8 osm/kg water):
meglumine diatrizoate (Angiografin, Schering AG)
sodium diatrizoate (Urovison-Na, Schering AG)
meglumine iothalamate,
meglumine ioxithalamate (Telebrix 300, Guerbet)
meglumine ioglicate (Rayvist 300, Schering AG)

b) low osmotic ionic contrast medium:
sodium-meglumine ioxaglate (Hexabrix, Guerbet), 0.6 osm/kg water.

c) nonionic contrast media:
metrizamide (Amipaque, Nyegaard) 0.48 osm/kg water at 300 mg iodine/ml,
iopromide (Schering AG) 0.63 osm/kg water at 300 mg iodine/ml and
0.81 osm/kg water at 370 mg iodine/ml,
iohexol (Omnipaque, Nyegaard/Schering AG) 0.69 osm/kg water at 300 mg iodine/ml and 0.98 osm/kg water at 370 mg iodine/ml,
iopamidol (Bracco) 0.62 osm/kg water at 300 mg iodine/ml and
0.80 osm/kg water at 370 mg iodine/ml.

d) control solutions:
0.9% sodium chloride, 0.3 osm/kg water;
sorbitol 27.25 g/100 ml, 1.8 osm/kg water;
mannitol/electrolyte solution, 0.93 osm/kg water

### Animals

Each of the experiments was performed in 5 Wistar rats, 3 males and 2 females weighing 225–483 g.

### Experiments

The experiments were performed according to Holtas and coworkers (3) with some modifications. The rats were anaesthetized with pentobarbital sodium 50 mg/kg b.w. i.p. A catheter was introduced into the urinary bladder and the urine was sampled for one hour. Only rats in which a constant flow was observed were used for the experiments. Thereafter the A. mesenterica was blocked by ligature of the duodenum. A second catheter was introduced into the A. abdominalis, the tip being located just below the A. renales. During the injection of the contrast medium or control solutions the aorta was blocked in the cranial direction to prevent the escape of contrast material. The dosage was 400 mg iodine per kg body weight or an equal volume of saline, the injection rate 1 ml/min. The injection was performed under fluoroscopic control to guarantee complete filling of both kidneys (Fig 1).

Immediately after injection the blockade of the upper aorta was released. Urine samples were collected up to 30 min p. inj., 30 min to 60 min, 1 h to 2 hours p. inj. and in a part of the experiments 2–3 hours p. inj. The amount of albumin excreted during the respective periods of time was determined by immunoelectrophoresis according to

Laurell (6) using a rabbit anti-rat-albumin obtained from Miles-Yeda Ltd./Israel and the LKB 2117 Multiphor equipment from LKB-Bromma, Sweden.

## Results

### Comparison of Contrast Media and Hypertonic Solutions (Table 1)

In a first series of experiments various ionic hypertonic contrast media were compared in renal arteriography using proteinuria as a criterion for toxicity. The contrast media investigated differed with regard to the sodium or meglumine content, the iodinated acid and the osmotic pressure. As a control either the same volume of isotonic saline or a hypertonic solution of sorbitol (osmolality equal to conventional ionic contrast media) was injected. Compared to the preinjection values no increase in albumin excretion was observed following the injection of saline. The injection of hypertonic sorbitol and the injection of all contrast media produced marked albuminuria. No difference could be detected between the effects caused by the meglumine or sodium salt, the different iodinated compounds and even the low osmotic agent meglumine sodium ioxaglate.

The second set of experiments compared the new nonionic contrast agent iopromide with sodium

Table 1  Albuminuria up to 2 hours following selective renal arteriography in the rat using various contrast agents at a dosage of 400 mg iodine/kg bodyweight or equal volumes of control solutions and an injection rate of 1 ml/min

| Solution/contrast medium injected | iodine concentration (mg/ml) | excretion of albumin (mg, 0–2 hrs p. inj.) |
|---|---|---|
| 0.9 sodium chloride | – | 0.24±0.10 |
| sorbitol | – | 1.85±1.02 |
| meglumine diatrizoate | 306 | 2.06±1.44 |
| sodium diatrizoate | 300 | 2.52±3.16 |
| meglumine iothalamate | 300 | 2.25±2.06 |
| meglumine ioxithalamate | 300 | 3.27±1.86 |
| meglumine ioglicate | 300 | 2.15±1.23 |
| sodium megl. ioxaglate | 320 | 1.77±0.87 |
| | | |
| 0.9% sodium chloride | – | 0.14±0.08 |
| sodium-diatrizoate | 300 | 1.94±1.03 |
| metrizamide* | 300 | 2.99±1.94 |
| iopromide | 300 | 0.31±0.22 |
| | | |
| 0.9% sodium chloride | – | 0.44±0.19 |
| mannitol + electrolytes | – | 0.69±0.37 |
| iopromide | 370 | 1.03±0.44 |
| iohexol | 370 | 1.93±0.94 |
| iopamidol | 370 | 2.01±1.05 |

\* n = 4

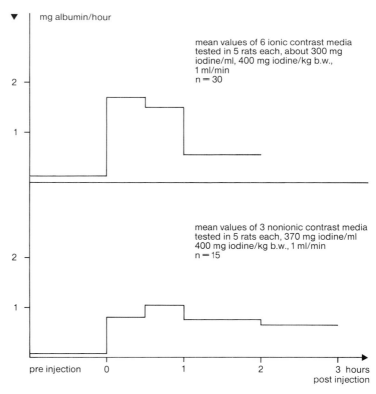

Fig 2  Time course of renal excretion of albumin following nephroangiography in the rat

diatrizoate and metrizamide. Iopromide caused distinctly less albuminuria than metrizamide and diatrizoate. At the concentration tested no difference between iopromide and the injection of 0.9% saline could be detected.

The next investigation comparing iopromide, iopamidol and iohexol was performed using solutions with 370 mg iodine/ml instead of 300 mg iodine/ml. It included a mannitol-electrolyte control with osmotic pressure similar to that of the contrast agents.

The results indicate that at least iopamidol and iohexol cause more albuminuria than saline (300 mosm/kg) and the mannitol solution having 930 mosm/kg (student's t-test). Iopromide caused more albumin excretion than 0.9% saline ($p < 0.05$). It was not significantly different from the hypertonic mannitol nor from the other contrast media.

### Time Course of Albumin Excretion

The increase in the excretion of albumin started immediately after the injection of the test solutions (Fig 2). A maximum was reached at about 1 hour p. inj. Thereafter the excretion of albumin slowly decreased. No distinct difference could be detected between ionic and nonionic contrast media in this respect.

## Discussion

The experimental method used to investigate tolerance of various contrast agents in nephroangiography in rats has been developed by Holtas and coworkers (3). The authors published results concerning metrizamide, meglumine diatrizoate, meglumine sodium diatrizoate (Urografin), iohexol and an experimental nonionic agent, C-29 (1, 4). The method has been shown to be able to detect significant albuminuria and to differentiate between contrast agents. The results up to now are in agreement with clinical experience in selective nephroangiography in as far as albuminuria is observed in clinical practice too and metrizamide seems to be no less injurious in this respect than diatrizoate in spite of its lower osmolality (5). Although the method was slightly changed, our results with diatrizoate, metrizamide and iohexol agree with the findings of Holtas (4).

Compared to the preinjection values the perfusion of the kidneys with a bolus of 0.9% sodium chloride solution produced at most a minor increase in albumin excretion if any. The injection of hypertonic sorbitol (1.8 osm/kg water) was followed by a substantial increase in albuminuria which was similar to that observed after the injection of hypertonic conventional contrast media. The toxic action of these contrast agents might therefore be explained by their hypertonicity. On the other hand the mannitol solution (0.9 osm/kg water) with an osmolality similar to low osmotic contrast media at about 370 mg/ml does not cause significant albuminuria. Since the low osmotic contrast agents sodium-meglumine ioxaglate (320 mg iodine/ml), metrizamide (300 mg iodine/ml), iohexol and iopamidol cause distinctly more albuminuria than the osmotic mannitol control these products would appear to act by a mechanism other than hypertonicity, e.g. chemotoxicity. Iopromide-370 is the only contrast medium tested, which did not produce significantly ($p > 0.05$) more albuminuria than the osmotic control although the difference compared to 0.9% saline was statistically significant and the difference between iopromide and iohexol or iopamidol was not. Absolutely no albuminuria could be detected with iopromide at an iodine concentration of 300 mg/ml.

The fact that sodium diatrizoate was not more deleterious than meglumine diatrizoate in nephroangiography in the rat is in agreement with other investigations in the dog (9) and with clinical experience (10). This result is very surprising. Sodium salts are less suitable in all other angiographic examinations. They produce pain, blood-brain-barrier breakdown and cardiovascular disturbance. Furthermore, the otherwise extremely well tolerated low osmotic nonionic agent metrizamide causes the same degree of albuminuria as the hypertonic sodium diatrizoate. This indicates that toxicity in renal arteriography occurs via mechanisms quite different from those influencing tolerance in other tissues.

# References

1 Golman, K., S. Holtas: Proteinuria produced by urographic contrast media. Invest. Radiol. 15: 61–66, 1980
2 Harkonen, S., C. Kjellstrand: Contrast nephropathy. Amer. J. Nephrol. 1: 69–77, 1981
3 Holtas, S., T. Almen, K. Goldman, L. Tejler: Proteinuria following nephroangiography. V. Influence of calcium and magnesium ions in non-ionic contrast media. Acta radiol. Diagn. 21: 397–400, 1980
4 Holtas, S., K. Golman, C. Törnquist: Proteinuria following nephroangiography. VIII. Comparison between diatrizoate and iohexol in the rat. Acta radiol. (Stockh.) Suppl. 362: 53–55, 1980
5 Krakenes, J., S. Elsayed, J. Göthlin, M. Farstad: Proteinuria after selective nephroangiography in man. Comparison of three media. Acta radiol. Diagn. 21: 401–406, 1980
6 Laurell, C. B.: Quantitative estimation of proteins by electrophoresis in agarose gel containing antibodies. Anal. Biochem. 15: 45–52, 1966
7 Moreau, J. F., D. Droz, L. H. Noel, J. Leibowitch, P. Jungers, J. R. Michel: Tubular nephrotoxicity of water soluble iodinated contrast media. Invest. Radiol. 15: 54–60, 1980
8 Mudge, G. H.: Nephrotoxicity of urographic radio contrast drugs. Kidney Int. 18: 540–552, 1980
9 Talner, L. B., H. N. Rushmer, M. N. Coel: The effect of renal artery injection of contrast material on urinary excretion. The effect of renal artery injection of contrast material on urinary excretion. Invest. Radiol. 7: 311–322, 1972
10 Talner, L. B., S. Saltzstein: Renal arteriography. The choice of contrast material. Invest. Radiol. 10: 91–99, 1975

# Enzymuria after Administration of Water-soluble X-ray Contrast Media

H. G. Hartmann

## Summary

X-ray contrast media which contain iodine and are eliminated via the kidneys, lead to a reversible tubular irritation if administered parenterally even in the absence of previously existing kidney parenchymal damage. The tubular alteration can be confirmed by an increase in urinary enzyme excretion.

In human beings the cytoplasmic LDH and the brush-border AP prove to be more sensitive indicators than the LAP and Gamma-GT values used so far. It was not possible to demonstrate a lesion of a specific tubular cell compartment.

The osmolarity of the x-ray contrast media and their administration route – intravenous or high-pressure intraarterial injection – do not have a decisive influence on the mechanism which damages the tubular epithelium. There is an almost proportional relationship between enzymuria and the given dose of the contrast substances.

Our studies show that we were able to detect that lysosomal enzymes like NAG, ASA, cannot be employed as specific indicators of renal tubular damage induced by the contrast medium.

## Zusammenfassung

Nierengängige, jodierte Röntgenkontrastmittel führen nach parenteraler Verabreichung auch bei nicht bestehender Nierenparenchymschädigung zu reversiblen tubulären Reizungen. Die tubulären Veränderungen konnten durch gesteigerte Enzymausscheidung im Urin nachgewiesen werden.

Soweit bisher bekannt, sind beim Menschen die LDH des Zytoplasmas und die AP des Bürstensaums empfindlichere Indikatoren als die Werte von LAP und Gamma-GT. Der Nachweis der Schädigung eines bestimmten tubulären Zellgebietes konnte nicht erbracht werden.

Die Osmolarität der Röntgenkontrastmittel und die Art ihrer Darreichung – intravenös oder als intraarterielle Hochdruckinjektion – sind nicht ausschlaggebend für den schädigenden Mechanismus auf das tubuläre Epithel. Es wurde eine fast proportionale Beziehung zwischen dem Grad der Enzymurie und der Kontrastmitteldosis beobachtet.

Gemäß unserer Studien konnten wir nachweisen, daß lysomale Enzyme, wie NAG, ASA, nicht als spezifische Indikatoren verwendet werden können, um kontrastmittelbedingte Nieren-Tubulusepithelschäden nachzuweisen.

## Introduction

Acute renal failure due to x-ray contrast media are well documented in the literature (3, 6, 10, 17, 19, 24). The intravascular route seems to be a greater hazard than oral administration. After intravenous urography and computed tomography, acute damage of the kidney is to be expected at an incidence rate of 0.15%. Angiography, with an incidence rate of 0.5% of acute renal failure, represents an even more dangerous diagnostic procedure. (14). Typically oliguria or anuria is observed about 24 hours after the roentgen contrast exposure and a subsequent rise in serum creatinine level is measured. Within the next few days the kidney function returns to normal. Repeated dialysis treatments are seldom necessary. With the available parameters the physicians have difficulties in recognising milder kidney damage, especially if there are no appreciable changes in the creatinine level. More sensitive laboratory tests are necessary for a better understanding of the nephrotoxic effects of the water-soluble radiographic media. During the last few years it has been demonstrated that the best indicator for the early detection of kidney damage is the increase in tubular enzyme excretion via the urine (1, 13).

By measuring tubular enzymes in urine after the intravascular administration of x-ray contrast media of triiodised benzoic acid derivative type which are eliminated via the kidneys, we tried to answer the following clinical questions:

1) Whether the products mentioned induce an augmented excretion of all types of enzymes or only of enzymes of the specific cell-compartments;
2) Whether the enzymuria depends on the dose of contrast media injected;
3) What influence do the different contrast media of varying osmolarity have on kidney damage;
4) Does the route of administration of x-ray contrast media, e.g. intravenous or intraarterial, have any bearing on the effects?

## Clinical and Biochemical Investigation Methods

All the patients had benign arterial hypertension without reduced kidney function. In this context of hypertension diagnosis, urography and angiography were indicated. We examined 70 patients of either sex, 36 men and 34 women at an average age of 45 years (24–70 years), with non-ionic roentgen contrast media like metrizamide (Amipaque), or with ionic products like meglumine diatrizoate (Urovist, Angiografin) and meglumine iothalamate (Conray).

Group A: Each of 10 patients received 40.5 g metrizamide as an i.v. 60 ml rapid infusion. The osmolarity of the solution was 480 mosm/kg water.

Group B: Each of 10 patients was given the pronounced hyperosmolar (osmolarity 1530 mosm/kg water) meglumine diatrizoate intravenously as a single dose of 39 g in 60 ml solution over a period of 5 minutes.

Group C: Each of 10 patients received a 200-ml i.v. infusion of 130 g meglumine diatrizoate with an osmolarity of 1530 mosm/kg water over a period of 10 minutes.

Group D: Each of 10 patients was given 250 ml meglumine iothalamate solution containing 60 g substance, with an osmolarity of 572 mosm/kg water, via a peripheral vein, over a period of 10 to 15 minutes.

Group E: 20 patients underwent aortography. At the same time most of them also underwent selective renovasography. On an average, 150 ml of 65% meglumine diatrizoate solution (Angiografin) with an osmolarity of 1530 mosm/kg water was used.

Group F: Each of 10 patients received an infusion of 200 ml hyperosmolar sorbit solution (osmolarity 1530 mosm/kg water) in about 10 minutes.

The followup in all patients was similar. After the exclusion of any previously existing kidney lesions by careful review of the case history, clinical findings as well as on the basis of conventional biochemical investigation findings (serum-creatinine, urine examination), each patient collected his 24-hour urine (6 to 6 o'clock) in plastic bags storing them in a refrigerator at 3–6°C. Provided the patients of our trial series had normal levels of endogeneous creatinine clearances (more than 80 ml/min./1.73 m$^2$ body surface) and 24 hours enzymuria (LDH: Lactatdehydrogenase, EC 1.1.1.27, ≤14.21 U/24 hrs, LAP: Leucinarylamidase, EC 3.4.11.2, ≤7.3 U/24 hrs, AP: Alkalische Phosphatase, EC 3.1.3.1, ≤2.41 U/24 hrs, gamma-GT: γ-Glutamyltransferase, EC 2.3.2.2, ≤42.3 U/24 hrs, NAG: N-Acetyl-β-Glucosaminidase, EC 3.2.1.30, ≤11.2 U/24 hrs, ASA: Arylsulfatase A, EC 3.1.6.1, ≤2.7 U/24 hrs), they were allotted to one of the above-mentioned groups. We evaluated the 24-hour enzymuria on the day before exposure to the contrast agent or sugar solution (basic enzymuria = zero value), on the day the substances were administered (exposure day = 1st evaluating day) and on following two days (2nd and 3rd evaluating day). On the clinical side we took precautions to avoid any adulteration of enzyme excretion due to diuretics, antibiotics and salicylates during the evaluation period. As far as possible the same type of diet and fluid intake were maintained.

We analysed serum and urine creatinine after Jaffé (20). The urine analysis was done with dipsticks (Combur 8-Test). After preparing the urine with gelfiltration (27), we measured in the eluate the activities of the cytoplasmic LDH after Güttler et al. (16), the brush-border enzymes LAP after Nagel et al. (18), AP after Amador et al. (2), Gamma-GT after Szasz (25) and the lysosomal enzymes NAG modified after Thomas (26), ASA after Baum et al. (5), in 24-hour urine standardized to that of a normal person with a body surface of 1,73 m$^2$.

To evaluate the question whether the roentgen contrast media as well as the high-percentage sugar solution could influence the enzyme activities in the urine at every individual evaluating step, we employed Friedman's Test. The differences in the individual days was confirmed by Wilcoxon-Wilcox-Test (21).

## Results

200 ml of hyperosmolar sorbit solution brings about an osmotic diuretic effect for several hours. No increase in the enzymes in 24-hour urine was found (Figs 1–3). All the investigated contrast solutions, independent of their physico-chemical properties and their administration methods increased the enzymuria to different extents. The least change was shown after giving 40.5 g of non-ionic, weakly hyperosmolar metrizamide.

Significant differences were seen in the urine enzymes of LDH, AP, and Gamma-GT (significance level alpha 5%) during the period of evaluation. The maximum variation in the enzyme excretion increase was found on the exposure day (↑ Gamma-GT around 32%) and on the following day (2nd evaluating day, ↑ LDH around 58% and that of AP around 76%). Very clearly pathological 24-hour enzymuria could be measured only for AP on exposure day and on the following day (Fig 2). On the second day after the administration of metrizamide all the elevated enzyme levels returned to normal. There was no evidence of a significant change in the lysosomal urine enzymes like NAG,

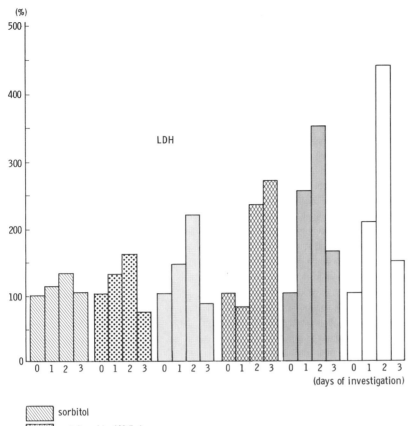

Fig 1  LDH excretion in 24-hour urine after administration of a hyperosmolar sugar solution (sorbitol) and different non-ionic (metrizamide) and ionic (meglumine diatrizoade, meglumine iothalamate) x-ray contrast media of variable amounts. Day 0 = basic enzymuria, Day 1 = day of exposure to sugar solution or contrast substances, 2 and 3 = first and second day after administration of the drugs. The differences between day 0 and day 2 are statistically significant for the ionic roentgen contrast media (alpha = 1%)

ASA and also that of brush-border LAP after giving Amipaque intravenously.

However, there was a stronger increase and as a result, more often pathological enzyme activities after administering ionic contrast media. Both test substances, independent of their concentration in the injection fluid – meglumine diatrizoate as a 65%, meglumine iothalamate as a 24% solution – resulted in a similar type of enzyme excretion. The strongest enzyme activity levels were measured on the day after administration of contrast agent (2nd evaluating day) in the case of meglumine diatrizoate and on the following day in case of meglumine iothalamate (Figs 1, 2, 3). The increase in the level of LDH reached after administering 39 g meglumine diatrizoate i.v. 117%, after 130 g intravenously 313% and after the intraarterial high-pressure injection of an average of over 100 g of the same material the elevation was about 245%. 60 g of meglumine iothalamate (Conray), brought about an increase in LDH (116%) (Fig 1) similar to that caused by the low dose of Urovist. The large amount of hyperosmolar roentgen media resulted in a more marked rise in the excretion of LDH. It was not possible to show any influence of the method of intravenous or intraarterial administration. On the 2nd day after administering ionic contrast media the LDH activities reverted to nearly normal values. Over the observation period of 4 days the changes in the 4 test series were of 1% level significance.

The reactions of the brush-border enzymes are different. The AP and the LAP seem to be more sensitive than Gamma-GT. On the day after the exposure (2nd evaluating day) to stronger hyperosmolaric substances the AP value lies in the 3 groups with the greater amount of roentgen contrast media in the same order with an percentage increase of about 250% (Fig 2), whereas Gamma-GT shows little change in its activity, especially in

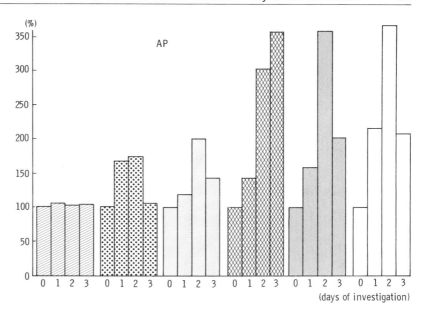

Fig 2 AP 24-hour enzymuria after sugar solution and contrast media. Same conditions as Fig 1. Level of sicnificance for all the x-ray substances alpha = 1%

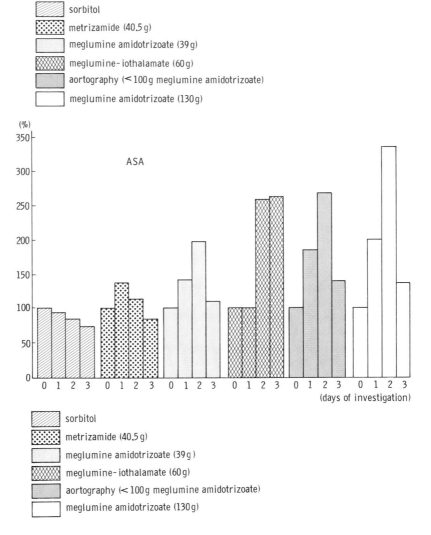

Fig 3 ASA activity in 24-hour urine. Same conditions as Fig 1 and 2. Significant increase in enzymuria on the day after the contrast medium exposure

the lower dose of 39 g Urovist. The measured values lie in the same range as the non-ionic Amipaque (increase of 36%). The LAP depends more clearly upon the dose of the hyperosmolar roentgen material. The lowest quantity results in a low (93%), the largest quantity of meglumine diatrizoate in the highest increase (300%) of enzyme activity.

Of the two lysosomal enzymes evaluated the changes observed after the administration of ionic contrast agents are more obvious in the case of ASA than in that of NAG. In all these 4 test groups the ASA just reached the pathological levels on the second evaluating day (Fig 3). After 39 g and 130 g Urovist the increase was about 100% and 236% respectively, after 60 g Conray the evaluation was 164% and after aortography with over 100 g Angiografin the change in ASA excretion was 169%.

All the measured enzymes showed as early as on the second day after the administration of meglumine diatrizoate a stronger tendency to return to normal, an expression of the reversibility of the tubular irritation. After Conray the reversibility seems to be slower because the measured enzymes are still high on the 3rd evaluating day (Figs 1–3). A real impairment of the kidney functions in terms of decreased capacity to excrete creatine could not be proved. Only in a few cases we were able to confirm a slight increase in the serum creatinine level to a maximum of 0.4 mg/dl. During the observation period the statistical evaluation of the endogenous creatinine clearance showed no significant deviation.

## Discussion

In previous years, different investigators have already undertaken urinary enzyme analysis after the administration of hyperosmolar x-ray contrast media. The primary interest was in the brush-border enzyme LAP (7, 8, 23, 28). Intravenous administration of ionic, hyperosmolar contrast media which are eliminated via the kidneys, to patients with previous kidney parenchymal damage, leads to increased LAP excretion as compared to healthy individuals (9).

Bartels et al. (4) compared the brush-border enzymes LAP and Gamma-GT as indicators for their sensitivity to tubular irritation after i.v. pyelography in children and came to the conclusion that the LAP clearly reacts more strongly than the Gamma-GT. Of the lysosomal urinary enzymes, after the administration of contrast media, alpha-glucosidase and lysozyme are the only ones which have been studies until now. The increased level of the previously mentioned enzymes could not be statistically established (15).

We analysed the usefulness of the cytoplasmic enzyme LDH, the brush-border enzymes LAP, Gamma-GT, AP and the lysosomal enzymes NAG, as well as the ASA in urine after the parenteral application of a non-ionic, weakly hyperosmolar contrast substance (metrizamide) as well as ionic more strongly hyperosmolaric contrast agents (diatrizoate and iothalamate) in patients with essential benign hypertension.

In the region of the nephrons, the ubiquitous LDH proved itself to be the most sensitive indicator among the analysed enzymes for irritations due to x-ray materials. The lowest elevation in the excretion of LDH was registered after giving non-ionic metrizamide. With the application of larger quantities, the hyperosmolar ionic substances induced an augmented enzymuria. There was an increase of 331% in LDH on the day after the administration of the largest amounts of these agents. On the other hand the infusion of 39 g of the same material leads to a rise of only 117% of the enzyme in urine.

Surprisingly the direct intraaortal as well as intrarenal artery injection of roentgen contrast medium under pressure do not cause any additional toxic effect to the kidney parenchyma, compared to the peripheral i.v. route. The i.a. method using an average of more than 100 g meglumine diatrizoate results in an increased LDH excretion of around 245%.

In particular, the changes in the enzyme activities of the lumenal plasma membranes originated from the proximal convoluted tubules, the so-called brush-border enzymes LAP, Gamma-GT and AP were retained in the same sense. The irritation of the proximal convoluted tubules as a result of contrast media was best recorded in the case of the AP. This enzyme increased significantly even at the lower doses of non-ionic Amipaque and ionic Urovist. With all the investigated diagnostic drugs there was a consistent increase in enzymuria of AP to the pathological level. The LAP shows a similar size of increase with ionic products. Even then the pathological enzymuria could be detected only after the administration of the higher quantity of material over 100 g meglumine diatrizoate.

The Gamma-GT is a less sensitive brush-border enzyme, according to our investigation. The changes in percentage vary with dose between 32% and 174% in the case of ionic agents. Very clearly the pathological enzyme activities could be barely noted by giving the high-test quantity of x-ray contrast media. There was no augmented excretion of the lysosomal enzymes ASA and NAG after the administration of non-ionic Amipaque. All the ionic contrast solutions, independent of the dose, cause a similarly strong output of ASA and NAG. The increase should be statistically secured, even though in none of the trial series any pathological enzymuria was definitely confirmed.

Our findings confirm the statements in the available literature (4, 8, 15, 23, 28), that in the absence of severe previous damage to the kidney parenchyma, the parenteral administration of conventional roentgen contrast media could result in a slight enzymuria only.

Furthermore, our findings show that the cytoplasmic LDH and the brush-border enzyme AP are more sensible parameters for the x-ray substance dependent irritations of the nephron, compared with the lysosomal tubulus enzymes ASA and NAG or the brush-border enzyme LAP and Gamma-GT.

The drugs which we tested for their tubular toxic properties, were eliminated with the urine to over 80% within 24 hours. On the other hand, the maximum enzymuria was found mostly in the 24-hr urine of the day after the administration of the drugs. For an explanation of this phenomenon we referred to the investigation results of Salvesen and Frey (22). They informed that iodine containing x-ray contrast media in vitro have an effect of weakening the activities of different enzymes like cholinesterase, glutamic-oxaloacetic transaminase and glucose-6-phosphate dehydrogenase. In our own studies we were able to demonstrate that metrizamide, meglumine-diatrizoate and meglumine iothalamate in concentrations up to 100 g/l urine, do not induce any suppression of the enzyme activities of LDH, LAP, Gamma-GT, AP, ASA and NAG. As an explanation for the belated maximum enzymuria we expect a slow release in the urine of the enzymes from the tubular cells damaged by contrast material.

Controversial statements about the aetiology of enzymuria after the administration of x-ray contrast media have been published. Due to the speedy reversibility of the augmented urinary excretions (mostly after 48 hours at the latest), Bignion (8) suspects either a direct effect on the tubules or an indirect effect on haemodynamic circulation through the hyperosmolality of the solutions. Burchardt (9) sees in the osmotic nephropathy of the proximal tubules the morphological correlations for the transitory increased LAP excretion. In his studies it is particularly marked in primarily or secondarily parenchymal damaged kidney disease. The enzyme output is stronger after giving a hyperosmolar solution.

These findings contrast with our own results, with clinical tests on healthy kidneys and with the findings of Bartels (4). These show that there is no proof that the enzymuria depends on the osmolality of x-ray contrast preparations. Hence, the augmented enzymuria should not be considered with reference to the different osmotic properties of the solutions; instead, it should be interpreted as an incidence of direct action on the tubular epithelium. This thesis is also supported by the findings of Danford et al. (11). According to them, the excretion of PAH in dogs was much more disturbed after giving the x-ray contrast media than after giving hypertonic saline solutions.

According to De Duve (12), the augmented enzymuria could be interpreted as a result of overfeeding of the reabsorption mechanism of the tubular apparatus. Finally there is an increased excretion of the so-called telelysosomes with effusion of the intracellular enzymes into the tubular lumen.

## References

1 Adelman, R. D., G. Conzelman, W. Spangler, G. Ishizaki: Comparative nephrotoxicity of gentamycin and netilmicin: Functional and morphological correlation with urinary enzyme activities. In Dubach, U. G., U. Schmidt: Diagnostic Significance of Enzymes and Proteins in Urine. Huber, Bern, 1979 (p. 166)

2 Amador, E., T. S. Zimmermann, E. C. Wacker: Urinary alcaline phosphatase activity. J. Amer. med. Ass. 185: 133, 1963

3 Ansari, Z., D. S. Baldwin: Acute renal failure due to radiocontrast agents. Nephron 17: 28, 1976

4 Bartels, H., E. W. Hempfing, P. Müller-Wiefel, H. D. Zwad: Der Einfluß der intravenösen Pyelographie auf die Ausscheidung von Leucin-Arylamidase und Gamma-Glutamyl-Transpeptidase im Urin bei Kindern. Mschr. Kinderheilk. 123: 424, 1975

5 Baum, H., K. S. Dodgon, B. Spencer: The assay of arylsulphatase A and B in human urine. Clin. chim. Acta 4: 453, 1959

6 Bennett, W. M., F. Luft, G. A. Porter: Pathogenesis of renal failure due to aminoglycosides and contrast media used in roentgenography. Amer. J. Med. 69: 767, 1980

7 Bergmann, H., F. Scheeler, S. Estrich, M. Schmidt: Der Nachweis tubulärer Funktionsstörungen der Niere durch Bestimmung der Aminopeptidase-Aktivität im Harn. Klin. Wschr. 42: 275, 1964

8 Bignion, H., G. Gluhovschi, N. Manescu, C. Zosin: Durch Kontrastmittel verursachte Veränderungen der Leucyn-Aminopeptidasen-Aktivität im Harn. Fortschr. Röntgenstr. 119: 343, 1973

9 Burchardt, U.: Alaninaminopeptidase-Ausscheidung mit dem Harn und osmotische Nephropathie. Z. Inn. Med. 30: 65, 1975

10 Byrd, L., R. L. Sherman: Radioconctrast-induced acute renal failure: a clinical and pathophysiologic review. Medicine (Baltimore) 58: 270, 1979
11 Danford, R. O., L.-B. Talner, A. J. Davidson: Effect of graded osmolalities of Saline solution and contrast media on renal extraction of PAH in the dog. Invest. Radiol. 5: 301, 1969
12 De Duve, C.: In A. Rueck, M. Cameron: Ciba Symposium on Lysosomes. Churchill, London 1963 (p. 126)
13 Dupond, J. L., R. L. Leconte des Floris, R. Gibey, J.-C. Henry: Intérêt du dosage de la N-Acetyl-Beta-D glucosaminidase dans la surveillance des traitements antibiotiques nephrotoxiques. Nouv. Presse méd. 6: 1881, 1977
14 Editorial: Radiocontrast-induced renal failure. Lancet II: 835, 1979
15 Guaneri, G. F., L. Faccini, M. Chersicla, E. Beltram, G. Battilana, S. Milani, M. Bazzocchi, M. P. Mucci, S. Lin, L. Campanacci: Urinary Enzymes (Alpha-Glucosidase and Lysosyme) Protein Pattern and Beta$_2$-Microglobulin as Indexes of Tubular Damage. Encymes in Health and Disease. Inaug. Scient. Med. Int. Soc. Clin. Encymol. Karger, Basel 1978 (p. 193)
16 Güttler, F., J. Clausen: Urinary lactate dehydrogenase activity. Determination of the urinary LDH isozyme pattern as a supplement to the measurement of total urinary LDH activity. Enzym. biol. clin. 5: 55, 1965
17 Krumlovsky, F. A., N. Simon, S. Santhanam, F. Del Greco, D. Roxe, M. M. Pomaranc: Acute renal failure: Association with administration of radiographic contrast material. J. Amer. med. Ass. 239: 125, 1978
18 Nagel, W., F. Willig, F. H. Schmidt: Über die Aminosäurearylamidase – (sog. Leucinaminopeptidase)-Aktivität im menschlichen Serum. Klin. Wschr. 42: 447, 1964
19 Olden, R. A., J. P. Miller, D. C. Jackson, T. S. Johnsrude, W. M. Thompson: Angiographically induced renal failure and its radiographic detection. Amer. J. Roentgenol. 126: 1039, 1976
20 Popper, H., E. Mandel, H. Mayer: Zur Kreatininbestimmung im Blute. Biochem. Z. 291: 354, 1937
21 Sachs, L.: Angewandte Statistik, 5th Ed. Springer, Berlin 1978 (p. 422 and 426)
22 Salvesen, S., K. Frey: Protein binding of metrizamide and the effect on various enzymes. Acta radiol. (Stockh.) Suppl. 335: 247, 1973
23 Scherberich, J. E., D. Knappik, J. Kollath, W. Mondorf, W. Schoeppe: Elimination von Nierenantigenen vor und nach parenteraler Gabe von Röntgenkontrastmitteln. Verh. dtsch. Ges. inn. Med. 85: 950, 1979
24 Swartz, R. D., J. E. Rubin, B. W. Leeming, P. Silva: Renal failure following major angiography. Amer. J. Med. 65: 31, 1978
25 Szasz, G.: Gamma-Glutamyltranspeptidase-Aktivität im Urin. Z. klin. Chem. 8: 1, 1970
26 Thomas, G. H.: Beta-D-Galactosidase in human urine: Deficiency in generalized gangliosidosis. J. Lab. clin. Med. 74: 725, 1969
27 Werner, M., D. Maruhn, M. Atoba: Use of gelfiltration in the assay of urinary enzymes. J. Chromat. 40: 254, 1969
28 Zurwehme, D.: Ausscheidung der Aminopeptidase im Harn nach intravenöser Gabe von Röntgenkontrastmitteln. Med. Klin. 61: 1458, 1966

# Monitoring of Contrast Media Nephrotoxicity by Specific Kidney Tissue Proteinuria of Membrane Antigens[*][**]

J. Scherberich, S. Tuengerthal and J. Kollath

## Summary

To clarify the nephrotoxic potential of x-ray contrast media (CM), the excretion of kidney-specific membrane proteins in the urine was studied in 28 patients before and after intravenous urography (n=10) and kidney angiography (n=18). The rise of tubular indicator enzymes in urine such as alkaline phosphatases (E.C. 3.1.3.1), alanine aminopeptidase (E.C. 3.4.11-) and gamma-glutamyl transpeptidase (E.C. 2.3.2.2) as well as that of the major brush-border surface glycoprotein (SGP) of a molecular weight of 240.000 dalton, were used as parameters describing the extent of tubulotoxic lesions. Urinary concentration of brush-border SGP was measured by counter-immunoelectrophoresis, one-dimensional electroimmunoassay and radial immunodiffusion, using specific antisera against brush-border membranes of the human kidney cortex. Labelled antisera gave a specific immunofluorescence of the luminal epithelial portion of the proximal tubule only. Analysis of tubular membrane-associated antigens was performed in 24 hours urine samples collected before application of the CM, and in four 2 hours, 48 hours and 72 hours samples after CM. Iothalamate (1400 mosmol/kg) was used for i.v. urography, megluminamidotrizoate (approx. 1500 mosmol/kg) was applied for renal vasography. In all cases, a significant increase of tubular brush-border membrane antigens in urine after CM application was observed (2p < 0.001, Wilcoxon test). Enzyme maxima were reached within 10–24 hours after injection of CM, where patients after renal angiography had a significantly higher increase of urinary kidney enzymes than patients after i.v. urography (2p < 0.001). The increase in membrane-bound tubular enzymes was paralleled by an increased excretion rate of brush border SGP. Tissue proteinuria was significantly lower in cases with unconspicuous findings compared to those where a pre-existing renal disease became apparent (2p < 0.05, Mann-Whitney test). After renal angiography, CM of low osmolality (Iopamidol, n=14) induced a significantly lower output of kidney proteins compared with high-osmol. CM (amidotrizoate: n=19). The results obtained suggest that the quantitative determination of kidney-specific membrane proteins is a useful tool in monitoring the potential nephrotoxic effect of CM in patients.

## Zusammenfassung

Zur Beurteilung des nephrotoxischen Potentials von Röntgenkontrastmitteln (KM), wurde die Ausscheidung nierenspezifischer Membranproteine im Harn bei 28 Patienten vor und nach i.v. Pyelographie (n=10) und Nierenangiographie (n=18) untersucht. Als Parameter zur Beschreibung des Ausmaßes einer möglichen tubulotoxischen Läsion dienten der Anstieg sog. tubulärer Indikatorenzyme im Harn wie der Alanin-aminopeptidase (E.C. 3.4.11-), einer Gammaglutamyltranspeptidase (E.C. 2.3.2.2), einer alkalischen Phosphatase, sowie der des wesentlichen Oberflächenglycoproteins der Bürstensaum-Membran proximaler Tubulusepithelien (Mol. Gew. 240 000). Die Harnkonzentration des Bürstensaum-Glycoproteins ("SGP") wurde in der Überwanderungselektrophorese, der eindimensionalen Elektroimmundiffusion und der Radialimmundiffusion mit Hilfe spezifischer Antiseren gegen Bürstensaum Membranfragmente der Humanniere bestimmt. Markierte Antiseren gaben eine spezifische Immunfluoreszenz, die sich auf die luminalen Abschnitte der proximalen Tubuli beschränkte, was die Spezifität der Antikörper belegte. Die Bestimmung der Membranproteine im Harn erfolgte im 24-Std.-Harn vor Gabe von KM, sowie danach in 4×2-Std.-Portionen, 24 Std., 48 Std. und 72 Std. später. Iothalamat (Conray®) (1400 mosmol/kg) wurde zur i.v. Urographie, Megluminamidotrizoat (Angiografin®) (ungef. 1500 mosmol/kg) für die Nierenangiographie verwendet. In allen Fällen wurde eine gegenüber der Kontrollphase signifikant vermehrte Ausscheidung tubulärer Membranproteine nach KM-Gabe beobachtet (2p < 0,001, Wilcoxon-Test). Die Enzymmaxima wurden innerhalb 10–24 Std. nach der KM-Injektion erreicht, wobei Patienten nach Nierenangiographie signifikant mehr Nierenproteine eliminierten als Patienten nach i.v. Urographie (2p < 0,001). Die Ausscheidung tubulärer Membranenzyme verlief parallel der an Bürstensaum SGP Antigen. Die Nierenproteinurie war bei klinisch-radiologisch unauffälligen Befunden signifikant geringer, als bei Patienten mit retrospektiv präexistenter Nierenerkrankung (2p < 0,05, Mann-Whitney-Test). Die Verwendung von KM niedriger Osmolalität (Jopamidol [Solutrast®], n=14) zur Nierenangiographie zeigte eine signifikant verminderte Ausscheidung im Vergleich zu hochosmolalen KM (Amidotrizoat; n=19). Die Ergebnisse zeigen, daß die quantitative Bestimmung spezifischer Nieren-Membranproteine im Harn einen brauchbaren Parameter darzustellen scheint, das mögliche nephrotoxische Potential von KM unter klinischen Bedingungen zu beschreiben.

---

[*] Supported by a grant of the Riese-foundation, Frankfurt am Main.

[**] Parts of this paper were presented at the Symposion on Pediatric Nephrology Frankfurt am Main 1981

*Acknowledgements:* We thank Prof. Dr. W. Schoeppe and Prof. Dr. W. Mondorf, Frankfurt am Main for continued support and valuable discussions.

## Introduction

In recent years increasing attention has been focussed on the fact that administration of radiopaque agents used for diagnostic purposes might be responsible for acute functional impairment of the kidney (1, 5, 9, 10, 16). Clinical data have revealed that this is especially true in patients with pre-existing renal insufficiency, dehydratation, diabetes mellitus, peripheral vascular disease, multiple myeloma, hyperuricaemia, and hepatic dysfunction associated with severe hypalbuminaemia (3, 6, 7). Compared to intravenous pyelography and cholangiography, usually higher doses of x-ray contrast media exeeding 200 ml are given during coronary angiography, infusion pyelography, computer tomography and in the event of percutaneous transluminal catheter dilatation of vascular stenosis where often larger and repeated doses of radiocontrast agents are needed to document pre- and post-dilatation conditions (4, 15, 17). In general, the incidence of radiocontrast media-induced renal functional deterioration is between 2–6% and might rise to 50–90% in high-risk patients (5, 6). Histological data presented evidence that renal impairment is initiated more or less by severe tubular damage (7, 9, 11), probably followed by a negative tubuloglomerular feedback (high distal tubule sodium concentration), thus inducing decline of glomerular filtration rate. After injection of potentially nephrotoxic drugs the first sign of tubular cytotoxicity is an increasing disintegration of the luminal plasma membrane of the proximal epithelia (especially of the straight "S-3"-segment), which consists of numerous microvilli ("brush-border"); ref. 8, 12. Initially, brush-border surface proteins are released at an increased rate, followed by exfoliation of vacuolar blebs, indicating more severe tubular membrane lesions due to the nephrotoxin (14).

Tubular membrane proteins shedded into the lumen and excreted in urine can be measured quantitatively applying specific anti-kidney brush-border antibodies (12, 13). However, no immunoreactive brush-border antigens are eliminated under normal conditions.

In the present study we report on the effect of contrast agents on the proximal epithelial cell of the human kidney cortex. The results indicate that the appearance of kidney tissue constituents in urine is a sensitive indicator of tubular damage preceding significant functional derangement ("early-phase parameter"). Thus, estimation of kidney specific membrane-antigens in urine turned out to be a useful tool in monitoring the potential nephrotoxicity of drugs (13). In addition, kidney tissue proteinuria might be of value predicting the outcome of high-risk patients following application of radiocontrast media, and, furthermore, allows comparative pharmacological-toxicological studies on the nephrotoxic potential of different radiopaque compounds.

## Material and Methods

The excretion of kidney-specific membrane antigens of the proximal tubule was measured in the urine of patients before and after intravenous urography and renal angiography. Tissue proteinuria was analyzed in 24 hours' urine samples before administration of contrast media (blank), during four 2-hours' collection periods, and during a 48 and 72 hours' collection period later.

Intravenous pyelography was performed in 10 patients (6 females, 4 males; 19–74 years) using iothalamate (approximately 1400 mosmol/kg) in a dose of 0.57 ml/kg body weight.

Kidney angiography was carried out by retrograde femoral approach in a total of 18 patients (7 females, 11 males; 21–66 years); after initial flush aortography, 50 ml meglumine amidotrizoate (approx. 1500 mosmol/kg) were injected above the origin of the renal artery with a flow rate of 5–7 ml/sec.

In a second study the possible effect of contrast medium with high osmolality (amidotrizoate) on proximal tubular cell membranes was compared in 19 patients with that of contrast medium with low osmolality (Jopamidol, 600 mosmol/kg) in 14 patients. Further details will be presented elsewhere.

Kidney indicator enzymes such as alanine-aminopeptidase (AAP, E.C. 3.4.11), alkaline phosphatase (AP; E.C. 3.1.3.1) and gamma-glutamyl-transpeptidase (GGT; E.C. 2.3.2.3) were assayed as described previously (12). The concentration of the major brush-border surface glycoprotein ("SGP"-antigen) was measured by quantitative radial immunoassay and one-dimensional electro-immunoassay or by applying specific anti-brush-border antisera from the rabbit (12). The antibody was immobilized in agarose special grade (Beckton-Dickinson, Orangeburg, N. J.) and antigen concentration was determined through a purified brush-border antigen preparation used as a standard. Isolation of this antigen ("SGP") was carried out performing lectin-affinity chromatography and gelfiltration of solubilized brush-border glycoproteins as described earlier (12–14). Counter immunoelectrophoresis was used for screening excretion of brush-border antigens in urine (Rapidophor-system, Immuno, Heidelberg). Details of the production of kidney antisera, processing of urine samples, urinalysis by immunochemical techniques, staining of immunoprecipitates have been reported previously (12). The specificity of the antisera used in this study was documented by immunofluorescence microscopy, where 7μ cryosections of human kidney were incubated with brush-border antiserum (antibody against "SGP-antigen") for 60 min, washed in phosphate-buffered saline and incubated with fluoresceine isothiocyanate-labelled anti-rabbit gammaglobulin. Tissue sections were then viewed in a Zeiss microscope using epi-illumination (KBR 500 filter, HBO burner); Kodak Ektachrome 400 ASA films were used for documentation.

Statistic calculations were performed with a Hewlett-Packard microcomputer (Wilcoxon test, Mann-Whitney test).

## Results

### Kidney-Tissue Proteinuria after Intravenous Urography

In all 10 patients studied, compared to the control period, a significant increase of alanine amino-peptidase, alkaline phosphatase, and gamma-glutamyl transpeptidase activity was found within the first 24 hours in urine samples after i.v. urography ($2p < 0.005$, Wilcoxon test). The maxima of urinary enzyme activities were attained between the 4th and 8th hour after administration of contrast medium (iothalamate); see Table 1; Fig 1. The elimination of major immunoreactive brush-border surface antigen ("SGP") was similar to that of tubular marker enzymes AAP, AP and GGT.

Table 1 Excretion of tubular indicator enzymes alkaline phosphatase, alanine-aminopeptidase and gamma-glu-transpeptidase in urine before (= A) and after (=B, 2nd – 24th hour) administration of contrast medium

*IV Urography* (n = 10), Iothalamat, 1400 mosmol/kg

|  | A | B |
|---|---|---|
| Alkaline Phosphatase | 5,9±5.0 | 15.5± 8.7 |
| Alanine-Aminopeptidase | 3.0±0.25 | 9.4± 6.6 |
| Gamma-glutamyltranspeptidase | 14.2±9.8 | 41.3±33.7 |

*Kidney Angiography* (n = 13); meglumine-amidotrizoate (1500 mosmol/kg)

| Alkaline Phosphatase | 6.0±3.6 | 26.2± 8.2 |
| Alanine-Aminopeptidase | 3.2±2.5 | 16.3± 9.8 |
| Gamma-glutamyltranspeptidase | 12.0±6.8 | 69.0±40.2 |

(mU/min)

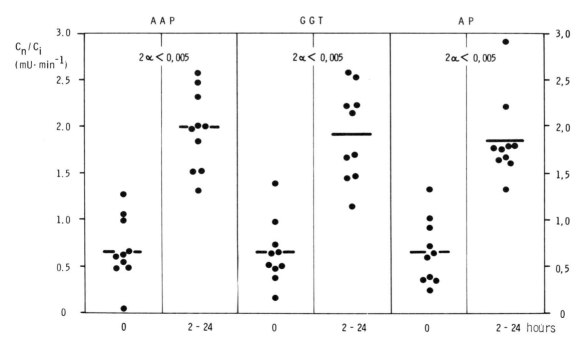

Fig 1 Excretion profile of kidney brush-border associated enzymes alanine-aminopeptidase (AAP), gamma-Glu-transpeptidase (GGT) and alkaline phosphatase (AP) in the urine of patients following intravenous pyelography (iothalamate); significant rise in enzyme activity within the first 24 hours after administration of contrast media (Wilcoxon test). $C_n$ = mU/min; $C_i$ = mean value of $\Sigma C_n$ (n = 10)

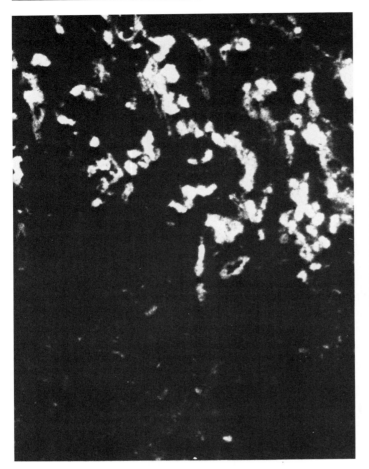

cortex

medulla

Fig 2 Specificity of the antibody used for monitoring of kidney cell-membrane antigens in urine before and after administration of x-ray contrast media. Incubation of cryosections from human kidney with the antibody revealed a specific immunofluorescence (sandwich technique) of the luminal plasma membrane of the proximal tubule only. Glomeruli, distal tubule and interstitium were negative. Membrane antigens from this histologically defined nephron segment in urine indicate tubular injury due to nephrotoxic events. Magnification × 60. FITC labelled anti-rabbit gammaglobulin

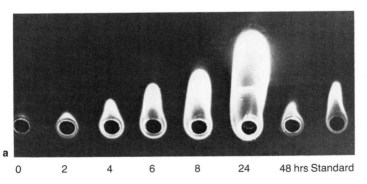

a  0   2   4   6   8   24   48 hrs Standard

Fig 3 Excretion of brush border membrane antigens before and after kidney angiography as monitored by sensitive immunological techniques. Fig. 3 A shows a one-dimensional electroimmunoassay of urine samples before (o) and after administration of the contrastmedia (patient with renal adenocarcinoma). Fig. 3 B gives an example of the excretion of kidney membrane antigens applying counter immunoelectrophoreses. Note increase of kidney tubule associated antigens after injection of contrast media within the first 24 hours. Staining for alanine aminopeptidase and protein; anti-brush-border antibody totally absorbed against normal serum proteins from the rabbit

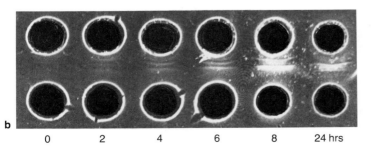

antibody against
kidney brush border

urine samples

b  0   2   4   6   8   24 hrs

Urinary concentration of "SGP-antigen" rose significantly after urography (2p < 0.005, Wilcoxon test). In 3/10 patients a rise of serum creatinine concentration was observed (mean increment 0.9 mg/dl ± 0,41 mg/dl). Retrospectively the excretion of kidney components following i.v. pyelography was significantly lower in cases with unconspicuous findings compared to those patients where a pre-existing renal disease became apparent (2p < 0.05, Mann-Whitney test).

The specificity of the antisera used for monitoring kidney membrane antigens in urine is shown in Fig 2; immunofluorescence is restricted to the luminal portion of the epithelia from the proximal tubule.

## Kidney-Tissue Proteinuria after Renal Angiography

In connection with the criteria of two-hours' collection periods after administration of contrast medium (amidotrizoate), 13/18 patients (6 females, 7 males) could be evaluated for kidney-specific proteins in the urine. In all cases a significant rise in AAP, AP and GGT activity was observed (2p < 0.0001). Compared to cases with intravenous pyelography, the absolute concentrations of tubular-indicator enzymes in urine were higher in patients after renal angiography (Table 1).

In similar manner, excretion of brush-border "SGP"-antigen was elevated compared to the control period (2p < 0.001), see Figs 3 and 4. In 3 of 16/18 patients, creatinine concentration in serum increased after angiography (mean rise 0.96 mg/dl ± 0.38 mg/dl).

In addition, after renal vasography, contrast media of low osmolality induced a lower output of brush-border proteins compared with contrast medium of high osmolality (see material and methods): urinary enzyme activities of both groups were significantly different: AP (mU/24 hours) 2p < 0.0098, AAP: 2p = 0.0016; GGT: 2p = 0.00015 (Mann-

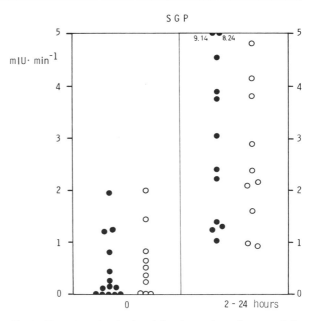

Fig 4 Excretion of major brush-border surface glycoprotein in patients after intravenous pyelography and kidney angiography, respectively, measured by radial-immunoassay. "SGP"= surface glycoprotein; compared to the control period (0) injection of contrast media (iothalamate, meglumine amidotrizoate) caused significant rise of the tubular membrane antigen in the urine. ● = samples obtained from 14 patients before and after kidney angiography (2p<0.001); ○ = samples of 10 patients before and after intravenous urography (2p<0.005). Wilcoxon test

Table 2 Excretion of kidney tubule ala-aminopeptidase, gamma-Glu-transpeptidase and alkaline phosphatase in patients 24 and 48 hours after administration of low osmol CM (Solutrast) and high osmol CM (Amidotrizoate) (renal angiography). Two days after angiography (24th – 48th hour) enzymuria of brush border proteins following amidotrizoate is significantly higher compared to that after injection of Jopamidol (n = 14; Angiografin group: 19 patients). In the case of low osmol CM excretion of tubular proteins returns to normal one day earlier; observation period 0–96 hours. Test according to Mann-Whitney; ns = not significant

| Enzyme excretion (ratio) | Jopamidol: Amidotrizoate 24 hours after angiography | Jopamidol: Amidotrizoate 48 hours after angiography |
|---|---|---|
| *Ala-aminopeptidase* | | |
| mU · ml⁻¹ | n.s. | 2p = 0.0016 |
| mUmin⁻¹ | n.s. | 2p = 0.027 |
| *Gamma-Glu-transpeptidase* | | |
| mU · ml⁻¹ | n.s. | 2p = 0.00015 |
| mU · min⁻¹ | n.s. | 2p = 0.0024 |
| *Alkaline Phosphatase* | | |
| mU · ml⁻¹ | n.s. | 2p = 0.0098 |
| mU · min⁻¹ | n.s. | 2p = 0.037 |

Whitney test, see Table 2). After injection of low osmol. contrast medium (600 mosmol/kg), enzymuria returned 24 hours earlier to normal. Details of this study will be presented elsewhere in connection with changes of the complement system.

## Discussion

The aim of the present study was to gain a better insight into the nephrotoxicity of x-ray contrast media (=CM) used in diagnostic pyelography and renal angiography. The results obtained showed that the administration of CM induced an increased structural imbalance of the proximal tubular cell: tubular marker enzymes AAP, AP and GGT, closely bound to the brush-border membrane, were excreted at an increased rate in urine after injection of the drug. Previous studies presented evidence that AAP as well as part of GGT is localized on the brush-border membrane surface while AP is more tightly bound to the membrane core (12). The elimination of the major brush-border glycoprotein (molecular weight 240 000) was closely related to that of AAP, AP and GGT, indicating a similar cytotoxic mechanism. Further studies revealed that intravascular injection of CM can also lead to shedding of macromolecular membrane vesicles which are fragmented from the apical plasma membrane of the proximal tubule (14). Exfoliation of the brush-border into the tubular lumen ("obstructing blebs") especially of the S-3 segment, might cause complete cell necrosis, while cells from the proximal S1 and S 2 segment seem to be more resistant to nephrotoxic influence. Apparently, the increased elimination of membrane proteins in urine is a direct correlate of structural tubular lesions due to the effect of the CM. In patients with pre-existing renal disease the output of kidney proteins was more pronounced than in uncomplicated cases ($2p < 0.05$). This observation parallels clinical data that patients with impaired renal function might more easily develop acute renal failure due to the administration of contrast media (3, 6, 15, 16). Under such circumstances hydratation of the patient and infusion of 20% mannitol seem to protect the kidney to a certain extent (2). Several data indicate that osmolality of CM plays a dominant role for tubulotoxic side effects (11). The studies of Rohrbach on epithelial morphology after administration of CM of different osmolality are supported by our observations, where kidney-membrane proteinuria was significantly lower in patients after administration of non-ionic low-osmol. CM (renal angiography). Further detailed studies will be required. Nevertheless, the present data allow to assume that the determination of specific kidney antigens in urine provides a sensitive tool describing the nephrotoxic potential of CM and helps to predict the outcome of high-risk patients.

## References

1 Ansari, Z., D. S. Baldwin: Acute renal failure due to radiocontrast agents: Nephron 17: 28, 1978
2 Anto, H. R., S.-Y. Chou, J. G. Porush, W. B. Shapiro: Infusion intravenous pyelography and renal function: effect of hypertonic mannitol in patients with chronic renal insufficiency: Arch. intern. Med. 141: 1652, 1981
3 Berezin, A. F.: Acute renal failure, diabetes mellitus, and scanning: Ann. intern. Med. 86: 829, 1977
4 Feldman, J. A., S. Goldfarb, D. K. McKurdy: Recurrent radiographic dye-induced acute renal failure. J. Amer. med. Ass. 229: 72, 1974
5 Harkonen, S., C. Kjellstrand: Contrast nephropathy: Amer. J. Nephrol. 1: 69, 1981
6 Krumlowsky, F. A., N. Simon, S. Santhanam, F. de Greco, D. Roxe, M. M. Pomeranc: Acute renal failure-association with administration of radiographic contrast media. J. Amer. med. Ass. 239: 125, 1978
7 McEvoy, J., M. G. McGoven, R. Kumar: Renal failure after radiological contrast media: Brit. med. J. IV: 717, 1970
8 Mondorf, W., J. E. Scherberich, T. Stefanescu, P. Mitrou, W. Schoeppe: The elimination of brush-border membrane proteins in urine caused by toxic alterations of the tubular cell. Contr. Nephrol. 24: 99, 1981
9 Mudge, G.: Nephrotoxicity of urographic radiocontrast drugs: Kidney Int. 18: 540, 1980
10 Radiocontrast-induced renal failure (editorial). Lancet II: 835, 1979
11 Rohrbach, R., D. Weingard: Zur Nephrotoxizität wasserlöslicher Kontrastmittel bei der Nierenangiographie (Abstr.). Nieren- u. Hochdruckkrankh. 5: 219, 1980
12 Scherberich, J. E., W. Mondorf: Excretion of brush-border antigens as a quantative indicator of tubular damage: Curr. Probl. clin. Biochem. (Bern) 9: 281, 1979
13 Scherberich, J. E., W. Mondorf, W. Schoeppe: Side effects of antimicrobial therapy: nephrotoxic potential of antibiotics (aminoglycosides, cephalosporins) as monitored by brush-border tissue-proteinuria. In Losse. H., A. W. Asscher, A. E. Lison: Pyelonephritis, Vol. IV. Thieme, Stuttgart 1980 (pp. 176)
14 Scherberich, J. E., C. Gauhl, W. Mondorf, G. Heinert, J. Schneider, W. Schoeppe: Pathobiochemische Hintergründe der Ausscheidung von Tubulusmembranenzymen und anderen Nierenantigenen im Harn: I. Int. Symposium. Harnenzyme. Universität Halle-Wittenberg 1982
15 Swartz, R. D., J. E. Rubin, B. W. Leeming, P. Silva: Renal failure following major angiography. Amer. J. Med. 65: 31, 1978
16 Teruel, J. L., R. Marcen, J. M. Onaindia, A. Serrano, C. Quereda, J. Ortuno: Renal function impairment caused by intravenous urography. Arch. intern. Med. 141: 1271, 1981
17 Weinrauch, S. D., R. W. Healy, O. S. Leland, H. H. Goldstein, S. D. Kassiesieh, J. A. Libertino, F. J. Takacs, J. A. Delia: Coronary angiography and acute renal failure in diabetic azotaemic nephropathy: Ann. intern. Med. 86: 56, 1977

# Urinary β-2-Microglobulin Determinations in Assessment of Tubular Dysfunction after X-ray Contrast Media Application

U. Uthmann, H. P. Geisen and E. Glück

## Summary

Clinical studies and experiments have demonstrated that x-ray (roentgen) contrast media (RCM) may cause renal failure. Histologic findings after renal angiography showed a vacuolisation of the proximal tubular region as a first sign of renal reaction.
Creatinine levels, which are the common parameter for renal dysfunction, are primarily not influenced by lesions in the proximal tubular region. Therefore, they seem to be of little help in the early detection of renal dysfunction after RCM. We studied the urinary excretion of β-2-microglobulin, an endogenously produced polypeptide, which is nearly completely catabolized in the proximal tubular region. In a randomised series we determined serum and urinary levels after application of physiological saline as control and two different RCM.
After physiological saline the β-2-microglobulin excretion did not exceed the normal range, while after RCM a significant rise of β-2-microglobulin excretion was seen in 14 out of 20 cases. After the high-osmolality RCM, the rises in β-2-microglobulin excretion were higher and more frequent than in the low-osmolality RCM. The determination of urinary β-2-microglobulin excretion seems to be the adequate method to detect early renal dysfunction after RCM application. It may contribute to further knowledge of the mechanisms leading to RCM-induced renal failure.

## Zusammenfassung

Experimentelle und klinische Studien haben gezeigt, daß Röntgenkontrastmittel (RKM) zum Nierenversagen führen können. Histologisch findet sich als erstes Zeichen der Nierentoxizität eine Vakuolisierung der proximalen Tubuluszellen. Primär werden diese Veränderungen nicht durch einen Anstieg des Serumkreatinins wiedergegeben, so daß dieser Parameter für die Früherkennung einer Nierendysfunktion von geringem Wert ist. Wir untersuchten die Ausscheidung des endogen produzierten Polypeptids β-2-Mikroglobulin, das nahezu vollständig in der proximalen Tubulusregion abgebaut wird. In randomisierten Serien bestimmen wir den Gehalt im Serum und Urin nach Gabe von 2 unterschiedlichen RKM und physiologischer Kochsalzlösung als Kontrolle.
Nach physiologischer Kochsalzlösung überschritt β-2-Mikroglobulin nicht den normalen Ausscheidungsbereich, während die RKM in 14 von 20 Untersuchungen einen signifikanten Anstieg verursachten. Nach dem hochosmotischen wurden im Vergleich zu dem niedrigosmotischen RKM höhere und häufigere Anstiege der β-2-Mikroglobulinausscheidung beobachtet. Die Bestimmung der Ausscheidung von β-2-Mikroglobulin im Urin scheint eine brauchbare Methode zur frühen Entdeckung einer renalen Dysfunktion nach RKM-Applikation zu sein und kann zur Klärung des Mechanismus eines RKM-induzierten Nierenversagens beitragen.

## Introduction

Renal failure following x-ray (roentgen) contrast media (RCM) injection has been described, beginning with the intravascular application of radiographic contrast media. Case reports (1, 2), retrospective evaluations (3, 8, 20) and experimental studies have appeared (9, 10, 14, 26). In recent years the increased use of RCM in computed tomography, angiography and intravenous pyelography together with an increased awareness of drug toxicity have resulted in prospective studies on changed renal function following the application of contrast media (4, 13, 22). Case reports and retrospective studies showed that diabetic nephropathy, multiple myeloma and renal insufficiency of other origin increased the risk of RCM-induced renal failure (1, 2, 16, 19).
Partly irreversible renal failure has been described not only after i.v.p.s. and angiography, but even after cholangiography (27).

In most instances the criterion used to identify renal failure was a rise in serum creatinine levels. Massive proteinuria has also been described following angiography. Both high and low molecular proteins were identified in these cases (3, 10, 11, 21).
The histological finding of biopsy material obtained after intravascular application of RCM was a massive vacuolisation in the proximal tubular region (14, 17, 26). Contrary to typical osmotic nephrosis, these changes were found in the basal region of tubular cells close to peritubular capillaries. Vacuolisation of mitochondria and lysosoma was however also found (26). Glomerular and distal tubular changes were few in these specimens.
Renal plasma flow and glomerular filtration rate can be estimated with serum creatinine and creatinine clearance, but this function is not immediately

influenced by the morphological changes, which were found after RCM application. The adequate diagnostic procedure to assess these early changes in the tubular region should be the determination of an endogenic substance with free glomerular passage and complete tubular reabsorption. The determination of β-2-microglobulin in serum and urine could meet these demands.

β-2-microglobulin (β-2-m) is a polypeptide of 100 amino acids with a molecular weight of 11800 Dalton, a molecular radius of 16 Å and a disulfide binding between the 25$^{th}$ and 81$^{st}$ amino acid. β-2-microglobulin is known since 1968 and found on the surface of all nucleated cells as the constant light chain of HLA-antigenes. It is set free in normal cell turnover. The catabolism is via the kidney by complete glomerular filtration, reabsorption in the proximal tubular region and hydrolisation to amino acids, which are then returned to circulation (15, 28). The normal plasma and urine levels in healthy subjects are constant between 1.4 to 3.0 mg/l for serum levels and under 250 µg/l urine or 400 µg/24 h urine excretion.

Extensive knowledge about the diagnostic value of β-2-microglobulin determinations in serum and urine have been acquired following renal transplantation and renal surgery. Furthermore β-2-m levels have been assessed following cadmium, lead and aminoglycoside nephrotoxic damage and in kidney injury due to cytostatics. It has been reported that lesions of the proximal tubular region were detected earlier by determining the β-2-microglobulin excretion in urine than by any other clinical laboratory test (5, 12, 23, 25). The aim of this study was to determine the β-2-microglobulin excretion in urine following the application of different tri-iodine RCM. The study used a randomized, selected population, and compared this with a control group receiving physiological saline only.

## Methods

The study includes 3 groups of 10 patients each. Two groups received an intravenous injection of one of two different radio contrast media and the controls were given the same volume of physiological saline. The sequence was randomised and neither the examiner nor the person doing the laboratory determinations knew which patient had been placed into which group. Patients serving as controls had no radiological examinations during the time of urine collection and β-2-microglobulin determination. The radio contrast media used were: Urovist 65% (ionic monomer) and Hexabrix 59% (ionic dimer). The iodine content of the

Table 1  Characteristics of injected x-ray contrast media and physiological saline as control

| Substance | Volume/Injection | Ratio iodine atomes -osmot. active molecules | Iodine content mg/ml | Osmality |
|---|---|---|---|---|
| Na Cl 0.9% (Physiol. saline) | 50 ml | – | – | 300 mosmol/kg H$_2$O at 37°C |
| Ioxaglate (Hexabrix 59%) | 50 ml | 6–2 | 320 | 580 mosmol/kg H$_2$O at 37° C |
| Diatrizoate (Urovist 65%) | 50 ml | 3–2 | 306 | 1580 mosmol/kg H$_2$O at 37° C |

Table 2  Reasons for i.v.p. in 30 examined persons

| Reason for radiological examination | Control (Physiol. saline) | Ioxaglate (Hexabrix 59%) | Diatrizoate (Urovist 65%) |
|---|---|---|---|
| Urolithiasis | 2 | 2 | 3 |
| Benign prostatic hypertrophy | 1 | 3 | 1 |
| Microhematuria | 1 | 2 | 1 |
| Epididymitis | 2 | 1 | 1 |
| Hypertension | 2 | 1 | 1 |
| Varicocele | 1 | 1 | 1 |
| Renal trauma | – | – | 2 |
| Urethral stricture | 1 | – | – |

injected contrast media was 15 g per injection. This is equivalent to 50 ml Hexabrix or Urovist 65%. The osmolality of the contrast media was 580 mosm/kg $H_2O$ at 37°C for Hexabrix, and 1580 mosm/kg $H_2O$ at 37°C for Urovist 65%. The osmolality of physiological saline is 300 mosm/kg $H_2O$ at 37°C, which is iso-osmolar to human plasma (Table 1).

Thirty men between 26 and 70 years of age were examined. The medium age was 44 years at the time of examination. Patients were referred for the radiological evaluation due to urolithiasis (7 each), micturition problems (5 each), microhaematuria (4 each), epididymitis (4 each), hypertension (4 each), varicocele (3 each), suspected renal trauma (2 each) and urethral stricture (1 each) (Table 2). Patients were excluded from the study when one of the following criteria applied: below 20 or above 70 years of age, insulin-treated diabetes mellitus, renal insufficiency with creatinine levels above 1.8 mg/dl. Furthermore, patients were excluded when contra-indication existed against the use of x-ray contrast media.

At injection of x-ray contrast media and at 3 and 24 hours after injection, blood samples were taken. β-2-microglobulin, creatinine and BUN were determined from these samples. Urine was collected at intervals of 0 to 3, 3 to 6, 6 to 12 and 12 to 24 hours after injection of radiographic contrast media. For determination of the initial levels we either collected urine for 24 hours prior to contrast media application, or obtained spontaneously voided urine. In the second case we determined the specific weight to estimate the approximate 24 hours' urine excretion. A specific weight over 1020 suggested a urine volume of 1000 ml per 24 hours, a specific weight between 1015 and 1020 indicated a urine volume of 1200 ml/24 hours, a specific weight between 1012 and 1015 resulted in a urine volume estimation of 1500 ml/24 hours, and a specific weight below 1012 indicated that the urine volume was close to 1800 ml/24 hours.

β-2-microglobulin, creatinine and BUN were determined from the urine as well as from the blood samples. When collecting the urine we brought the pH above 6, which was achieved by putting some drops of a 2 n sodium hydroxide into the collecting vessels. At a pH below 6 a time, temperature and pH dependent lysis of β-2-microglobulin takes place.

β-2-microglobulin was determined with a commercial radio-immuno-assay (Deutsche Pharmacia, Freiburg, F.R.G.). Each series of determinations used four standards. When standards differed, or when improbable results were obtained the determinations were repeated.

Results were tested two tailed by means of a Kruskal-Wallis test with alpha = 0.005 and a critical point of $psi^2$ distribution of 5.991. This means that only a result over 5.991 reveals a significant difference. T was found to be 13.26, which is far above the critical point.

## Results

We identified a slight renal function reduction in 2 of the 30 patients. At time of radio contrast media application the mean serum creatinine level was 1.1 mg/dl and varied from 0.7 to 1.8 mg/dl. One of these patients had a slight elevation of the serum creatinine of 1.7 mg/dl at the time of RCM injection caused by an unknown pre-existing impairment of renal function. The other patient showed a rise in the serum creatinine level from 0.9 to 1.6 mg/dl, following application of the contrast media. This was accompanied by a rise in urinary β-2-microglobulin excretion, as well as a decline in the urinary creatinine excretion per unit time.

The creatinine excretion per collecting interval, normalized to a 24-hours' interval for easier comparison decreased for 11 patients and rose in 19 patients. The maximum decline was −2.3 g/24 h and the maximum increase was +4.36 g/24 h.

## Controls

The 10 control patients had a serum creatinine range from 0.7 to 1.3 mg/dl. Injection of 50 ml

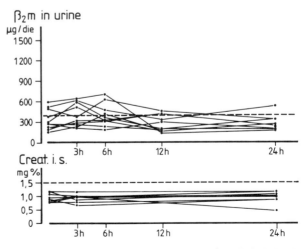

Fig 1  β-2-microglobulin excretion at intervals 0–3, 3–6, 6–12 and 12–24 h after injection of physiological saline in the control group corrected to excretion/24 h.
Creatinine serum levels in the same patients during the same period

physiological saline failed to influence the serum creatinine level. In 2 cases we found a slight decline in urinary creatinine excretion, which was less than 500 mg per 24 hours. Controls had normal β-2-microglobulin levels at the time of physiological saline injection. Three patients had values at the upper limit of normal. The maximal rise of β-2-microglobulin serum levels was 1.2 mg/l. The upper limit of 3.0 mg/l was not attained in these cases.

Three patients showed a β-2-microglobulin urinary excretion, which was above the upper limit of 400 µg/24 h following injection of 50 ml physiological saline. These patients had values of 497, 549 and 607 µg/24 h. Return to normal levels occured within the observation period in 2 patients, while the elevated excretion persisted in one. Seven patients had normal β-2-microglobulin excretion at time of injection. In 4 determinations a slight increase was seen which exceeded the methodical variation only once (Fig 1).

## Diatrizoate (Urovist 65%)

The serum creatinine levels of 10 patients examined after injection of 50 ml Urovist 65% varied from 1.0 to 1.7 mg/dl. In one patient a value of 1.7 mg/dl at the time of injection of contrast media later rose to 2.2 mg/dl at 3 hours and remained elevated at 24 hours. The creatinine level at 72 hours declined to 1.8 mg/dl.

The serum creatinine level was unaffected in 9 patients. The creatinine excretion declined more than 500 mg/24 h in 2 patients. The absolute creatinine excretion was however within normal limits. No other signs of impaired renal function were seen.

Two patients had β-2-m serum levels of 4.4 and 5.6 mg/l at the time of Urovist injection. These values exceeded the normal upper limits. The β-2-microglobulin serum level of 5.6 mg/l was found in the patient with a serum creatinine of 1.7 mg/dl and impaired renal function. This patient also had a high β-2-microglobulin urinary excretion of 6410 µg/24 h prior to application of RCM. Following radiographic media injection the excretion rose to 44400 µg/24 h. At the time of the last collecting period the β-2-m excretion declined to 9500 µg/24 h, still far above the upper limit of 400 µg/24 h.

Five of the 10 examined patients had a slight elevation of β-2-microglobulin excretion prior to radiographic contrast media injection (540–6410 µg/24 h). In 4 of these patients we noted an increase in β-2-microglobulin excretion in excess of 200% following application of the contrast media. Another 4 patients with a normal excretion rate prior to contrast media application also had increased β-2-microglobulin urinary excretion in excess of 400 µg/24 h or 200%. At the end of the collecting intervals 7 patients had a normal β-2-microglobulin urinary level while 4 continued to have a β-2-microglobulin excretion far above the upper limit (886, 9500, 840, 855 µg/24 h) (Fig 2).

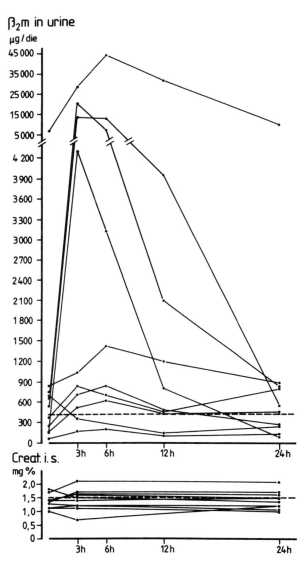

Fig 2  β-2-microglobulin excretion in the intervals 0–3, 3–6, 6–12 and 12–24 h after injection of Diatrizoate (Urovist 65%) corrected to excretion/24 h.
Creatinine serum levels determined in the same patients at injection and 3 and 24 h after injection

## Ioxaglate (Hexabrix 59%)

The initial serum creatinine levels of 10 patients who received Ioxaglate 59% (Hexabrix) varied from 0.8 to 1.7 mg/dl. 24 hours after radiographic contrast media injection one patient had a significant rise in serum creatinine from 0.7 mg/dl to 1.6 mg/dl. The impaired renal function also caused the creatinine excretion to decline from 3.3 to 1.88 g/24 h, and the β-2-microglobulin urinary excretion to rise from 150 µg/24 h to 670 µg/24 h.

A decreased creatinine excretion in excess of 500 mg per 24 hours was seen in 3 patients only, whose absolute values were still in the normal range. These 3 patients had a very low urinary volume during the collecting periods, so that urine collection may have been inadequate. Three patients had elevated β-2-m serum levels at the time of contrast media application with values between 4.1 and 4.8 mg/l. One of these patients had an elevated serum creatinine (1.5 mg/dl) and thus had a previously unknown decrease of renal function, which also caused the urinary β-2-microglobulin to be highly elevated at 12100 µg/24 h.

Three out of 10 patients had an elevated β-2-microglobulin excretion per unit time at the time of injection. Two of these demonstrated a significant rise in urinary β-2-m excretion. Within 12 to 24 hours after Ioxaglate injection the β-2-m excretion returned to normal again in these patients. Four patients with normal β-2-m excretion at injection also had a β-2-microglobulin excretion in excess of 200% of the initial values or 400 µg/24 h. The β-2-microglobulin excretion remained elevated in one patient throughout the period of observation (Fig 3).

We evaluated statistically the integrals of β-2-microglobulin excretion in 24 hours. The Kruskal-Wallis test shows a significant difference between the three groups. ($x^2=13,36$). The average values of ranks were 9.19 in the control, 14.79 in the Hexabrix group and 23.31 in the Urovist group. If we refer these values to measured β-2-microglobulin excretion we see that after Urovist the β-2-microglobulin excretion was between 445 and 21484 µg/24 h with a median value of 3600 µg/24 h. These values were much higher than after injection of Hexabrix (182 to 8893 µg/24 h with a median value of 450 µg/24 h), which still were far above the β-2-m excretion after physiological saline, which varied from 220 to 680 µg/24 h with a median value of 280 µg/24 h (Fig 4).

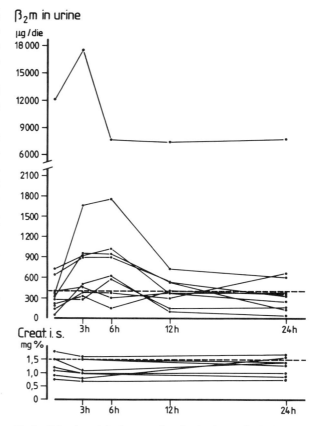

Fig 3  β-2-microglobulin excretion in the intervals 0–3, 3–6, 6–12 and 12–24 h after injection of Ioxaglate (Hexabrix 59%) corrected to excretion/24 h
Creatinine serum levels determined in the same patients at injection and 3 and 24 h after injection

## Discussion

The present study showed that significant differences exist in the urinary β-2-microglobulin excretion following injection of physiological saline and two radiographic contrast media. Each radiographic contrast medium contained a similar amount of iodine, but both had different chemical structure and highly different osmolality (Diatrizoate 65% and Ioxaglate 59%). The microglobulin excretion differences were equally evident when saline and the contrast media were compared as between the two iodinated media.

In spite of the low dose of radiographic contrast media injection (15 g iodine/application) an increase in β-2-microglobulin excretion was seen before, and even without change in serum and urinary creatinine levels. Since the serum β-2-microglobulin levels were sufficiently stable and below the tubular reabsorptive capacity, the rise in urinary microglobulin excretion must be explained as resulting from diminished tubular reabsorption. Our results are in agreement with the data reported by Tejler, Holtas and others, who found temporary proteinuria after angiography. They also agree with the biopsy findings of Moreau and Weingard, who described a tubular vacuolisation as a first reaction following injection of tri-iodinated x-ray contrast media (6, 10, 11, 17, 21, 26). β-2-micro-

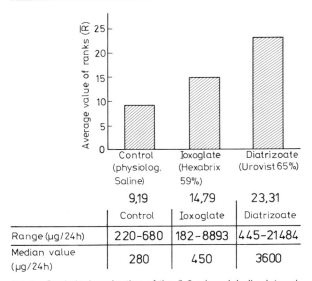

Fig 4 Statistical evaluation of the β-2-microglobulin determinations following application of the x-ray contrast media and range of β-2-microglobulin excretion in the three different groups

globulin determinations in the serum and urine appear to be more sensitive than creatinine determinations for early detection of x-ray contrast media-induced renal dysfunction. Similar results had been reported in the identification of renal damage due to ischemia, graft rejection and toxic substances, where β-2-microglobulin reveals dysfunction earlier than other routine laboratory tests (18, 23, 25).

Furthermore, our results show that different RCM having the same iodine content but differing in respect of their osmolality and chemical structure, cause different urinary β-2-m excretion. The osmolality of the two substances differs considerably (Diatrizoate 65%: 1600 mosm, Ioxaglate 59%: 580 mosm). This is a major factor in nephrotoxicity, and may be the most important one. In agreement with Moreaus and Weingards histological findings, we think that a different degree of tubular vacuolisation is effected by different osmolalities. The influence of different chemical structures of RCM was not subject of this investigation.

The β-2-microglobulin determination in serum and urine appears to be a more adequate and sensitive method to measure the nephrotoxicity of x-ray contrast media than the usual measurement of serum and urine creatinine levels. The lower nephrotoxicity in newly developed x-ray contrast media may also be compared by β-2-microglobulin excretion in urine. As x-ray contrast media have a diurectic effect one should always give the β-2-microglobulin excretion by amount of time, not by concentration alone, as a sudden rise in urine volume could mask an initial renal dysfunction.

Further investigations have to be initiated regarding the influence which chemical structure has on urinary β-2-microglobulin excretion as well as a study of urinary β-2-microglobulin excretion in patients who underwent a high-dosage x-ray contrast media application for instance in angiography. A study in a group of patients with diabetes and renal insufficiency who were both excluded from our first study has begun. It will be examined whether the decrease of tubular function is higher in these patients, compared to those with normal renal function.

## References

1 Barshay, M. E., J. H. Kaye, R. Goldmann, J. W. Coburn: Acute renal failure in diabetic patients after intravenous infusion pyelography. Clin. Nephrol. 1: 35, 1973
2 Bartels, E. D., G. C. Brun, A. Gammeltoft, A. Gjorup: Acute anuria following intravenous pyelography in a patient with myelomatosis. Acta med. scand. 60: 297, 1954
3 Byrd, L., R. L. Sherman: Radiocontrast-induced acute renal failure: a clinical and pathophysiologic review. Medicine 58: 270, 1979
4 Eisenberg, R. L., W. O. Bank, M. W. Hedgcock: Renal failure after major angiography. Amer. J. Med. 68: 43, 1980
5 Fleming, J. J., L. Parapia, D. B. Morgan, J. A. Child: Increased urinary β$_2$-microglobulin after cancer chemotherapy. Cancer Treat. Rep. 64: 581, 1980
6 Goldstein, E. J., D. A. Feinfeld, G. M. Fleischner, M. Elkin: Enzymatic evidence of renal tubular damage following renal angiography. Radiology 121: 617, 1976
7 Harkonen, S., C. M. Kjellstrand: Exacerbation of diabetic renal failure following intravenous pyelography. Amer. J. Med. 63: 939, 1977
8 Heideman, M., G. Claes, A. E. Nilson: Risk of renal allograft rejection following angiography. Transplantation 21: 289, 1976
9 Holtås, S., T. Almén, L. Tejler: Proteinuria following nephroangiography. Acta radiol. (Stockh.) 19: 33, 1978
10 Holtås, S., T. Almén, L. Tejler: Proteinuria following nephroangiography. Acta radiol. (Stockh.) 19: 401, 1978
11 Kirkland, J. A., M. R. Haslock: Transient proteinuria following intravascular injection of contrast media. Lancet 695, 1961/I
12 Kjellström, T., P.-E. Evrin, B. Rahnster: Dose-response analysis of cadmium-induced tubular proteinuria. Envir. Res. 13: 303, 1977
13 Kumar, S., J. D. Hull, A. J. Cohen, P. G. Pletka: Low incidence of renal failure after angiography. Arch. intern. Med. 141: 1268, 1981

14 Lélek, I.: Beitrag zur nierenschädigenden Wirkung der Kontrastmittel. Fortschr. Röntgenstr. 125: 259, 1976
15 Maack, T., V. Johnson, S. T. Kau, J. Figueiredo, D. Sigulem: Renal filtration, transport, and metabolism of low-molecular-weight proteins: A review. Kidney Int. 16: 251, 1979
16 Milman, N., P. Gottlieb: Renal function after high-dose urography in patients with cronic renal insufficiency. Clin. Nephrol. 7: 250, 1977
17 Moreau, J. F., D. Droz, J. Sabto, P. Jungers, D. Kleinknecht, N. Hinglais, J.-R. Michel: Osmotic nephrosis induced by water-soluble triiodinated contrast media in man. Radiology 115: 329, 1975
18 Schentag, J. J., M. E. Plaut, F. B. Cerra, P. B. Wels, P. Walczak, R. J. Buckley: Aminoglykoside nephrotoxicity in critically ill surgical patients. J. Surg. Res. 26: 270, 1979
19 Shafi, T., S.-Y. Chou, J. G. Porush, W. B. Shapiro: Infusion intravenous pyelography and renal function. Arch. intern. Med. 138: 1218, 1978
20 Swartz, R., J. E. Rubin, B. W. Leeming, P. Silva: Renal failure following major angiography. Medicine (Baltimore) 65: 31, 1978
21 Tejler, L., T. Almén, S. Holtås: Proteinuria following nephroangiography. Acta radiol. (Stockh.) 18: 634, 1977
22 Teruel, J., R. Marcén, J. M. Onaindia, A. Serrano, C. Quereda, J. Ortuna: Renal function impairment caused by intravenous urography. Arch. intern. Med. 141: 1271, 1981
23 Uthmann, U., H. P. Geisen, L. Röhl: Beta-2-Mikroglobulin im Urin, eine labordiagnostische Funktionskontrolle nach ischämischen Nierenschädigungen und Nierenparenchymeingriffen. Helv. chir. Acta 48: 513, 1981
24 Uthmann, U., K. Dreikorn, H. P. Geisen: Stellenwert der $\beta_2$-Mikroglobulin-Bestimmungen in Serum und Urin bei der Diagnostik von Funktionsstörungen nach Nierentransplantation. Nieren u. Hochdruckkrankh. 11: 84, 1982
25 Vincent, C., J. P. Revillard, H. Pellet, J. Traeger: Serum $\beta_2$ microglobulin in monitoring renal transplant. Transplant. Proceed. 9: 438, 1979
26 Weingard, D., R. Rohrbach: Zur Nephrotoxizität wasserlöslicher Kontrastmittel bei der Nierenangiographie. (Vorläufige Mitteilungen). Deutscher Stifterverband für Nierenforschung e.V., Informationsdienst 2: 1979
27 Whitcombe, J. B.: Renal tubular sludging of meglumine iodipamide (Biligrafin). Brit. J. Radiol. 51: 579, 1978
28 Wibell, L., F. A. Karlsson: The serum level of $\beta_2$ microglobulin ($\beta_2$m) a low molecular weight protein. Prot. Biol. Fluids 23: 343, 1975

# Vascular Tolerance

## Contrast Media and Pain: Hypotheses on the Genesis of Pain Occurring on Intra-arterial Administration of Contrast Media

B. Hagen and G. Klink

### Summary

It has been found that certain physiochemical properties of the contrast media in common use are responsible for the sensations of pain and heat which occur on intravascular administration. Not only the chemotoxicity, but also and in particular the high osmolality of ionic, monomeric contrast media plays an important role in the genesis of such local side effects, as has been convincingly demonstrated in numerous clinical and animal studies. Of the various theories on the origin of pain, vascular spasm and vasodilation are of more historical importance as causative factors. Recently gained histomorphological and neurophysiologic knowledge suggests that biochemical mechanisms play a primary role. A synoptic model is described which – in analogy to the processes in inflammatory and anaphylactic phenomena – conceives contrast medium induced pain as a cascade of biochemical processes taking place in the terminal vascular system and leading to depolarization of paravascular neuroreceptive terminals (chemosensitive receptor field).

### Zusammenfassung

Es hat sich gezeigt, daß bestimmte physiko-chemische Eigenschaften der gebräuchlichen Röntgenkontrastmittel für die bei intravasaler Applikation auftretenden Schmerz- und Hitzesensationen verantwortlich zu machen sind. Neben der Chemotoxizität spielt insbesondere die hohe Osmolalität ionischer, monomerer KM bei der Genese solcher lokaler Begleiteffekte eine wichtige Rolle. Dies wird klinisch wie tierexperimentell durch zahlreiche Studien überzeugend belegt. Unter den verschiedenen Theorien der Schmerzentstehung kommen dem Gefäßspasmus und der Gefäßdilatation als auslösenden Faktoren eine mehr historische Bedeutung zu. Nach neueren histomorphologischen und neurophysiologischen Erkenntnissen müssen primär Mechanismen biochemischer Natur diskutiert werden. Es wird ein synoptisches Modell vorgestellt, das vergleichbar den Vorgängen bei entzündlichen und anaphylaktischen Phänomenen den durch KM ausgelösten Schmerz als Kaskade von in der terminalen Strombahn ablaufenden biochemischen Prozessen begreift, die zur Depolarisation paravaskulärer neurorezeptiver Terminals (chemosensitives Rezeptorfeld) führen.

### Introduction

The systemic and local toxicity of iodinated radiographic contrast media (RCM) can be divided into its causes and effects (Table 1).
The effects can be described as phenomena of a haemodynamic, morphological and biochemical nature (Table 2). They may be clinically latent or manifest. If they are of nosological relevance, i.e. of an injurious nature, then they are classified as contrast medium adverse reactions.
The causes of the phenomena observed are of a physicochemical nature. The chemotoxicity of ionic RCM depends on the chemical properties of the basic iodinated substance (anion fraction) and on the nature and mixture of the cation fraction. In the case of non-ionic substances it is determined by the overall structure of the RCM molecule.

It has long been recognized that, of the specific physical properties of RCM such as their viscosity, interfacial tension and electrical charge, their

Table 1  Systemic and local RCM-toxicity

| Causes | Effects |
|---|---|
| • Osmolality | • Haemodynamics |
| • RCM - molecule (cationic - and anionic part) | • Blood cells |
| | • Protein - binding |
| • Lipophilia | • Metabolism |
| • Interfacial tension | • Endothelium damage |
| • Viscosity | • Pain and heat |
| • Electro - affinity | |

Table 2  Systemic and local RCM - toxicity

Chemotoxic effects

- Blood cells
  - → erythrocyte    (echinocytosis)
  - → thrombocyte    (thromboplastin, serotonine)
  - → leucocyte      (histamine)
  - → mast cell      (histamine)
- Vascular muscle cell (dilation)
- Endothelial cell
  - → contraction
  - → micro - vesicles, pinocytosis
  - → intercellular junctions
     (tight −, gap - junctions, desmosomes)
- Subendothelial collagen
  (activation of factor XII)
- Tubulus epithelium (micro - vesicles)
- Pain

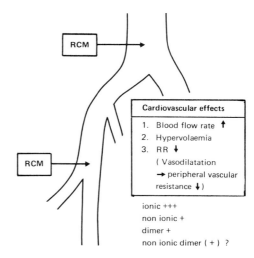

Fig 1  Cardiovascular effects following intravascular injection of RCM.
+++ strong effects, + slight effects

Table 3  Systemic and local RCM - toxicity

Osmotic effects

- Plasma volume (expansion)
- Erythrocyte (desiccocytosis)
- Endothelial cell (shrinkage)
- Intercellular space (opening)
- Pain

osmolality in particular is responsible for a number of side effects (Table 3):

1. It has, for example, been demonstrated that expansion of the plasma volume (hypervolaemia) and vasodilation with reduction of the peripheral vascular resistance and consecutive hypotension (Fig 1) was attributable to the hypertonicity of the RCM commonly used in the 50's and 60's (1, 21, 32).
2. The increase of pulmonary arterial pressure due to erythrocyte aggregation (2) was likewise ascribed to an osmotic effect, since dehydration (desiccocytosis) and loss of erythrocyte fluidity occur under the influence of intravascular injected RCM. Although erythrocytes are primarily desaggregated by RCM, microembolism-like aggregations and, hence, increased pulmonary resistance can occur in the processes just described because of the increase of viscosity in the terminal vascular system (4, 47).
3. Endothelial damage can be explained both by the chemotoxic properties of a contrast medium substance and by their osmotic pressure (14). Rapoport (41) described the osmotic opening of the blood-brain barrier following perfusion of the internal carotid artery with hypertonic solutions and ascribed this effect to shrinkage of the endothelial cells with simultaneous reversible opening of the intercellular clefts. Hyperosmolar contrast medium solutions are also said to cause such effects in the endothelia of the cerebrovascular system (42). These hypotheses appeared to be confirmed by electron-optical studies which revealed enlargement of the intercellular clefts and opening of "tight junctions" between the endothelium cells following perfusion with hyperosmolar RCM (6, 53, 60).
4. According to most workers, the sensations of pain and heat which occur on intravascular RCM perfusion of body regions with mainly striated muscles are also primarily a consequence of the high osmolality (14, 18, 19, 22, 34, 48, 52, 57, 58, 64).

The algogenic effect of osmotic substances has been known for a long time. Pain has been evoked, for example, by Armstrong et al. (3) using their cantharidin blister technique and by Wolff et al. (61) following intramuscular injection of hypertonic saline solutions (5% Nacl), whereby the hyperosmolarity of the substance was said to cause adequate stimulation of the nociceptive structures. However, the chemotoxicity of RCM is also reckoned to have a pain-inducing potential. It is, for example, known that sodium ions in the cation fraction of the RCM molecule can cause greater pain reactions than meglumine ions (52). Dahl et al. (10) recorded greater sensations of heat in patients given an injection of metrizoate with a sodium, calcium or magnesium-containing cation fraction than in those injected with meglumine-containing metrizoate.

Of all the suggestions made in the past for reducing the pain on intra-arterial injection of RCM, e.g. examination under general anaesthesia, premedication, dilution of the RCM solutions, slow injection and addition of local anaesthetics, only reduction of the osmolality appears to act causally on the conditions which play a role in the genesis of pain. We ourselves have demonstrated that both the dimeric, ionic substance ioxaglate (Hexabrix, Laboratoire Guerbet, in Germany: Byk Gulden) (19), and the non-ionic, monomeric substance iopamidol (Iopamiro, Bracco Research, in Germany: Solutrast, Byk Gulden) (18) cause significantly weaker sensations of pain and heat in arteriography of the extremities than the ionic, monomeric substance ioglicate (Rayvist, Schering AG) and ioxithalamate (Telebrix, Byk Gulden). At 1800 and 2100 mosm/kg $H_2O$, respectively, the osmolality of ioglicate and ioxithalamate is 3 times that of iopamidol and ioxaglate (600 mosm/kg $H_2O$) and 6 times that of blood (300 mosm/kg $H_2O$). The differences recorded between ioxaglate and iopamidol were not significant as regards the sensations of pain and heat whereas they were between the somewhat higher concentration (370 mg iodine per ml) and the lower concentration (300 mg iodine per ml) of iopamidol. The difference in osmolality between these two solutions is only 180 mosm/kg $H_2O$.

Table 4 Possible factors in the generation of pain after intravascular application of RCM

- Osmotic
- Chemotoxic
- Release of "neurovasoactive substances"
- Changes of ph and electrolytes
- Stretch of vessels (vasodilatation and hypervolaemia)
- Hypoxia and ischaemia
⟶ a. "osmotic plug" by the RCM
⟶ b. hyperviscosity (red cell deformation, a.-v. shunting)

Moreover, in a double-blind study we demonstrated that the addition of local anaesthetics (lidocaine/HCL) to conventional RCM likewise leads to a significant reduction of pain in comparison to the same substance without the addition of lidocaine, although the reduction is not as great as that achieved with the use of substances of low osmolality (19).

The following is a synopsis of the factors which possibly play a role in the genesis of pain after intravascular administration of RCM (Table 4 and Fig 2).

Fig 2 Synopsis of the multifactorial effect of RCM on blood cells, the vascular wall and pain receptors

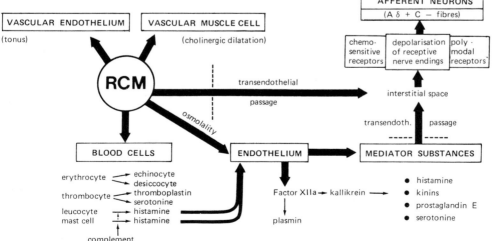
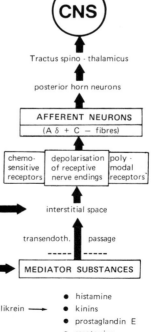

## Historical Review, the Role of Local Anaesthetics

Reports on the severe pain reactions recorded on intra-arterial injections of contemporary mono-iodinated and di-iodinated RCM appeared as early as the 1930's (33, 36, 45). The pain phenomena observed were so pronounced – particularly in angiography of the extremities – that general anaesthesia was frequently required. One of the assumptions of the time was that the pain was caused by arterial spasm on injection of RCM (24, 50, 59). In 1942, Leriche (29) established a direct analgesic effect of procaine on arterioles and capillaries, which led him to the assertion that vessels are "sensitive to pain". The idea of an influence of the autonomic nervous system on vascular tonus formulated so precisely by Leriche led to the development of "analgesic surgery" of vessels.

In 1939, Dimtza and Jaeger attempted to prevent or reduce vascular pain by bolus-like premedication with procaine or by the addition of procaine to the intraarterially injected RCM.

The relatively marked sensations of heat with simultaneous reduction of pain observed by some workers (16, 19, 48) are attributed to the vasodilatory effect of the added local anaesthetics (e.g. lidocaine/HCL). The analgesic effect observed by many workers led to hypotheses about the existence of a receptor in the vascular wall. The hypothetical assumption of an interaction between local anaesthetics and the osmotic RCM in the sense of competition at the receptor membrane of the sensitive nerve ending or, alternatively, in the form of a blockade of the centripetal pain impulse in the neuroaxon is based on the following conception: since substance such as lidocaine block the depolarising slow increase of permeability of the receptor membrane for sodium ions (13, 56), they are able to prevent the genesis and conduction of noxious impulses such as those provoked by osmotic RCM.

## Vascular Tone

For many workers, the marked vasodilation and – particularly in angiography of the extremities – the severe pain observed with classical tri-iodinated RCM up to the introduction of non-ionic material constituted evidence for a causal association between these two phenomena (25). The simultaneous induction of pain and dilation of the vessels known to be caused by "neurovasoactive" substances such as kinins (including the particularly potent bradykinin) and histamine (20) and the discovery of the vascular genesis of migrainous pain (62) appeared to confirm this hypothesis.

Reports on the absence of pain reactions on accidental intraarterial injection of iodipamide (8, 52) must therefore seem contradictory. Iodipamide, a substance with relatively high systemic toxicity ($LD_{50}$ = 3 g I/kg bodyweight in rats), is known to be a potent vasodilator. Because of its dimeric structure, however, the osmolality of this substance at an iodine content of 300 mg/ml is only 710 mosm/kg $H_2O$ (52).

Osmotic and chemotoxic vasodilation must be distinguished from passive stretching of the vascular wall as observed on mechanical action.

The irritation of mechanoreceptors due to mechanical stretch obviously causes real dilation pain. The stretch pain of the highly muscular arteries is demonstrated particularly impressively by the sometimes painful experience of the patient during maximum balloon dilation in angioplastic procedures. In this case, maximum, unphysiological mechanical irritation of the dilation receptors (mechanoreceptors) is caused "experimentally" in the adventitia of the distributing arteries. There is no reason to believe that the mechanism of passive dilation of all layers of the arterial wall and the active loss of tone of the muscle cell induced chemotoxically by cholinergic stimulation lead to identical effects at the receptor membrane. Cholinergic vasodilation (9) concerns primarily the highly muscular media – if at all, the adventitia with its network of receptive end organs is only slightly affected.

Moreover, consideration of the possible mechanism of the genesis of pain by the RCM perfusate suggests that pain is generated in the terminal vascular system and not at the level of the pre-arterioles.

In analogy to the processes observed in inflammatory and anaphylactic phenomena, mechanisms of a biochemical nature whose interaction with the neuroterminals of receptive organs in the interstitium of the terminal vascular system has long been known therefore may play a major role.

## Biochemical and Neurophysiological Aspects

Sako's assumption (46) that chemical irritation of the nerve endings in the adventitia of the vessels is responsible for the pain occurring after injection of RCM offers a useful conception to an understanding of the genesis of pain on intravascular administration of RCM.

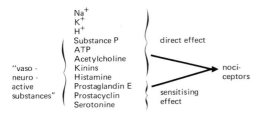

Fig 3   Pain producing substances

The existence of neural structures in the adventitia and muscles was first established anatomically by Dogiel in 1898 (12). This was later confirmed by Lazorthes (28) and Stöhr jun. (55) with the aid of modern microscopic methods and then formulated in particular by Sicuteri (51) for the terminal vascular system in connection with a study of the effect of polypeptide substances on pain receptors. According to Lim's studies (30, 31), there is good reason to believe that amyelinic, free-ending paravascular receptors accompanying the blood vessels up to their capillary network are ubiquitous. The afferent fibre systems proceeding from the vascular wall display a repertoire which is remarkably similar to the cutaneous innervation. Whether nociceptors (with thermo-, mechano- and chemosensitive differentiation) are involved or pure chemoreceptors whose excitation proceeds beneath the threshold value of normal nociceptive stimuli is unclear.

The relatively quick pain reaction following intra-arterial injection of bradykinin (17) and phenyldiguanide (5) suggests that the chemosensitive receptor field must be localized immediately around the capillaries, since otherwise the rapid onset of kininase activity would quickly break the bradykinin down.

The afferent pain conductors have been identified by means of precise measurements of individual fibres and microelectrode measurement of posterior horn neurons: they are exclusively quick-conducting, myelinated A-delta and amyelinic, slower-conducting C fibres (23).

In the evidence of histomorphological, neurofunctional and biochemical modalities, the following hypotheses appear to be important to understand the pathogenesis of pain following intra-arterial injection of RCM (Fig 2):

1. As a result of the action of contrast material on corpuscular blood components and on the endothelium of the vascular wall, phenomena comparable to the model of an inflammatory tissue reaction are set in motion like a cascade and lead to excitation of nociceptors (chemoreceptors).
   Similar to inflammatory tissue reactions, "biogenic amines" are first of all released from blood cells (basophilic leucocytes, mast cells and thrombocytes) and also directly by endothelial damage (27, 43, 44). The amines concerned are plasma kinins (including bradykinin, which is particular potent), histamine, serotonin and the prostaglandins (particularly $PGE_2$ and $PGI_2$). As "vasoneuroactive substances" (Fig 3), these agents have several properties in common: they act on smooth muscles, they greatly increase the permeability of cell membranes (and therefore also that of the vascular endothelium) and they cause pain in man (20).

2. A direct effect of RCM on neuroreceptive fibres of the vascular wall or of the interstitial space following transendothelial passage is purely speculative. It is, however, known that, due to transcapillary flux, RCM with their cationic and anionic moieties, are distributed up to a certain equilibrium in the interstices (extravascular and extracellular space) (11, 63). This phenomenon applies to a greater extent to ionic than to non-ionic RCM. It has further been shown that cations such as sodium penetrate into cells to a larger extent than cations such as meglumine (37). The size of the cation molecule appears to play an important role here. It is interesting in this connection that the character of the cation of a contrast medium can apparently influence the sensation of pain. For example, greater pain is registered on injection of pure sodium-containing salts than on injection of meglumine-containing RCM of the same osmolality (52).

3. Endothelial damage following intravasal perfusion with hyperosmolar iodinated solutions has been known since the studies of Zinner and Gottlob (65) and are largely confirmed by more recent studies (15, 38, 39). We know from studies of the ultrastructure of the vascular endothelium that it can synthesize neurovasoactive substances (7). The extent to which contrast medium-induced release of such substances takes place from the endothelium and subendothelial collagen remains to be seen.
   It can, however, be assumed that anything that will increase the contact time of RCM and the vascular endothelium (e.g. vascular diseases with the ischaemia syndrome) also leads to intensification of the induction of activator mechanisms (Factor 12 and plasmin) and to the release of histamine (27). The changes in the microcirculation described by Schmid-Schönbein (47) and Aspelin (4) and which can be registered on intra-arterial administration of RCM provide a good indication of the pro-

longed dwelling time of RCM in the terminal vascular system: membrane changes of the red cell, which are documented morphologically as an alteration of its shape (echinocytosis), occur as a result of contact with RCM.
At the same time, the fluidity of its contents can also be decreased, which implies a loss of deformability or an increase of rigidity. To a certain extent, the resultant increase of viscosity can be balanced out in the region of a healthy microcirculation with high shear rates.

If, however, the flow conditions are poor – as observed in obliterating changes with a post-stenotic fall of pressure –, then a vicious circle develops which can lead to complete stagnation of the blood-contrast medium mixture in the terminal vascular system. The resulting change of milieu with lowering of the pH due to reduced oxygen extraction, the longer-lasting and, hence, injurious action of the contrast medium on the endothelia with the release of biologically active substances such as the kallikrein-kinin-PG-system as well as the plasmin and complement system and the increase of capillary permeability caused by the release of histamine create the essential conditions for a multifactorial effect on the receptor. Local stasis and acidosis in the ischaemia syndrome lead in particular to the release of metabolites of arachidonic acid, whereby prostaglandins cause immediate but short-lasting hyperalgesia. It is a known fact that prostaglandins ($PGE_2$ and $PGI_2$) sensitize pain receptors to chemical, thermal and mechanical stimuli (35, 49).

What changes of a microcirculatory and biochemical nature ultimately bring about the considerable pain experienced on intra-arterial injection of hyperosmolar contrast media, has not yet been clarified.

Obviously we are faced with a complex interaction of the contrast medium itself or its moieties and biochemical modulation by neurovasoactive substances which, from an electrophysiological point of view, build up a receptor potential and, finally, lead to partial or total depolarisation of free-ending terminals of nociceptive structures.

## References

1 Almén, T.: Contrast agent design. J. theoret. Biol. 24: 216, 1969
2 Almén, T., P. Aspelin, B. Levin: Effect of ionic and non ionic contrast medium on aortic pulmonary arterial pressure. An angiocardiographic study in rabbit. Invest. Radiol. 10: 519–525, 1975
3 Armstrong, D., J. B. Jepson, C. A. Keele, J. W. Stewart: Observations on chemical excitants of cutaneous pain in man. J. Physiol. (Lond.) 120: 326–351, 1953
4 Aspelin, P.: Effect of ionic and non-ionic contrast media on red cell deformability in vitro. Acta radiol. Diagn. 20: 1–12, 1979
5 Bradley, B. E.: Activity from nervs innervating cat hindlimb vasculature. In: Art. Baroreceptors and Hypertension. Sleight, Oxford 1980 (pp. 80–87)
6 Brightman, M. W., M. Hori, S. I. Rapoport, T. S. Reese, E. Westergaard: Osmotic opening of tight-junctions in cerebral endothelium. J. comp. Neurol. 152: 317–325, 1973
7 Buonassisi, V., P. Colburn: Hormone and surface receptors in vascular endothelium. In: Advances in Microcirculation, Vol. IX. Karger, Basel 1980 (pp. 76–94)
8 Clauss, W.: Mündl. Mitteilung 1982
9 Coel, M. N., E. C. Lasser: A pharmacological basis for peripheral vascular resistance changes with contrast media injections. Amer. J. Roentgenol. 111: 802, 1971
10 Dahl, S. G., O. Linaker, A. Mellbye, K. Sveen: Influence of the cation on the side-effects of urographic contrast media. Acta radiol. Diagn. 17: 461–471, 1976
11 Dean, P. B.: Contrast media in body computed tomography. Invest. Radiol. 15: 164–170, 1980
12 Dogiel, S. A.: Arch. mikr. Anat. 52: 44, 1898
13 Fleckenstein, A.: Die periphere Schmerzauslösung und Schmerzausschaltung. Steinkopff, Frankfurt/M. 1950
14 Gonsette, R. E.: Animal experiments and clinical experiences with a new contrast agent (ioxaglic acid) with a low hyperosmolality. Ann. Radiol. 21: 271–273, 1978
15 Gottlob, R.: Die Auswertung endothelschädigender Wirkungen verschiedener angiographischer Kontrastmittel an einem Tiermodell. Fortschr. Röntgenstr. 135: 560–565, 1981
16 Guthaner, D. F., J. E. Silverman, W. C. Hayden, L. Wexler: Intra-arterial analgesia in peripheral arteriography. Amer. J. Roentgenol. 128: 737–739, 1977
17 Guzman, F., C. Braun, R. K. Slim, G. D. Potter, D. W. Rodgers: Narcotic and non-narcotics analgesics which block visceral pain evoked by intra-arterial injection of bradykinin and other algesic agents. Arch. int. Pharmacodyn., 149: 571–588, 1964
18 Hagen, B.: Iopamidol, ein neues nicht-ionisches Röntgenkontrastmittel. Radiologe 22: 581–585, 1982
19 Hagen, B., W. Clauss: Kontrastmittel und Schmerz bei der peripheren Arteriographie. Randomisierter, intraindividueller Doppelblindversuch: Ioglicinat, Ioglicinat-Lidocain, Ioxaglat Radiologe 22: 470–475, 1982
20 Handwerker, H. O.: Modulation der Erregung nociceptiver Afferenzen durch körpereigene Substanzen. In Kocher, R., D. Gross, H. E. Kaeser: Schmerzstudien Bd. III. Fischer, Stuttgart 1980 (S. 298–309)
21 Hilal, S. K.: Hemodynamic changes associated with the intra-arterial injection of contrast media. Radiology 86: 615–633, 1966
22 Holm, M., J. Praestholm: Ioxaglate, a new low osmolar contrast medium used in femoral angiography. Brit. J. Radiol. 52: 169–172, 1979
23 Iggo, A.: Activation of cutaneous nociceptors and their actions on dorsal horn neurons. In Bonica, J. J.: Pain –

Advances in Neurology. Raven Press, New York 1974 (pp. 1–9)
24 Jepson, R. P., F. A. Simeone: The actions of intra-arterial Diodrast, Thorotrast and sodium iodide on the peripheral pulse volume of the lower extremity. Surgery 33: 276, 1953
25 Kågström, E., P. Lindgren, G. Törnell: Circulatory disturbances during cerebral angiography. Acta radiologica 54: 3–16, 1960
26 Keele, C. A., D. Armstrong: Substances Producing Pain and Itch. Arnold, London 1964
27 Lasser, E. C.: New aspects of contrast media reactions: considerations, ideology, and prophylaxis. In Felix, R., E. Kazner, O. H. Wegener: Contrast Media in Computed Tomography. Excerpta Medica, Amsterdam 1981 (pp. 33–37)
28 Lazorthes, G.: Le système neurovasculaire. Masson, Paris 1949
29 Leriche, R.: Intra-arterial and intravenous injection of novocaine as general method of vasodilatation caused by action on endothelium. Progr. méd. (Paris) 70: 443, 1942
30 Lim, R. K. S.: Pain. Ann. Rev. Physiol. 32: 269, 1970
31 Lim, R. K. S., F. Guzman, D. W. Rodgers, K. Goto, C. Braun, G. D. Dickerson, R. J. Engle: Site of action of narcotic and non narcotic analgesics determined by blocking Bradykinin-evoked visceral pain. Arch. int. Pharmacodyn. 152: 25–58, 1964
32 Lindgren, P.: Hemodynamic responses to contrast media. Invest. Radiol. 5: 424–435, 1970
33 Löhr, W., W. Jacobi: Die Arteriographie und die kombinierte Encephaloarteriographie. Fortschr. Röntgenstr. 48: 385, 1933
34 Meves, M., H. Kiefer: Klinische Erfahrungen mit Ioxaglat, einem neuen Kontrastmittel für die Angiographie. Fortschr. Röntgenstr. 133: 657–659, 1980
35 Moncada, S., S. H. Ferreira, J. R. Vane: Pain and Inflammatory Mediators. Springer, Berlin 1978
36 Moniz, E.: Die zerebrale Arteriographie und Phlebographie. Springer, Berlin 1940
37 Mützel, W.: Properties of conventional contrast media. In Felix, R., E. Kazner, O. H. Wegener: Contrast Media in Computed Tomography. Excerpta Medica, Amsterdam 1981 (pp. 19–26)
38 Nyman, U., T. Almén: Effects of contrast media on aortic endothelium. Experiments in the rat with non ionic and ionic monomeric and monoacidic dimeric contrast media. Acta radiol. Suppl. 362: 65–71, 1980
39 Raininko, R.: Endothelial permeability increase produced by angiographic media. Fortschr. Röntgenstr. 131: 433–438, 1979
40 Raininko, R.: Histamine release and endothelial leakage from an intravascular contrast medium. Fortschr. Röntgenstr. 134: 445–449, 1981
41 Rapoport, S. I.: Effect of concentrated solutions on blood brain barrier. Amer. J. Physiol. 219: 270–274, 1970
42 Rapoport, S. I., H. K. Thompson: Osmotic opening of the bloodbrain barrier in monkey without associated neurological deficits. Science 180: 971, 1973
43 Ring, J., C. M. Arroyave: Alteration of human blood cells and changes in plasma mediators produced by radiographic contrast media. Z. Immun.-Forsch. 155: 200–211, 1979
44 Rockoff, S. D., C. Kuhn, M. Chraplyvy: Contrast media as histamine liberators. V. Comparison of in vitro mast cell histamine release by sodium and methylglucamine salts. Invest. Radiol. 7: 177, 1972
45 Saito, M., K. Kamikawa, K. Yanagizawa: A new method of blood vessel visualization (arteriography, venography, angiography) in vivo. Amer. J. Surg. 10: 225, 1930

46 Sako, Y.: Hemodynamic changes during arteriography. J. Amer. med. Ass. 183: 121–124, 1963
47 Schmid-Schönbein, H., P. Aspelin: Der Einfluß hypertoner Röntgenkontrastmittel auf die Mikrorheologie menschlicher Erythrozyten. In Zeitler, E.: Neue Aspekte des Kontrastmittel-Zwischenfalls. Symposium Berlin 1977
48 Schmidt, K. R., K. J. Pfeifer, H. Welter, H. Ingrisch, G. Heyde: Untersuchungen zur Schmerzverminderung bei der Extremitätenangiographie. Fortschr. Röntgenstr. 130: 200–204, 1979
49 Schrör, K.: Periphere biochemische Mechanismen der Schmerzentstehung – die Bedeutung von Prostaglandinen für den myocardialen Ischämieschmerz. In Kocher, R., D. Gross, M. E. Kaeser: Schmerzstudien, Bd. III. Fischer, Stuttgart 1980 (S. 310–322)
50 Shaw, R. S.: Vascular response to intra-arterial Diodrast und Urokon during arteriography. Surgery 39: 385–388, 1956
51 Sicuteri, F., M. Fanciulacci, G. Franchi, B. L. Del Bianco: Serotonin-Bradykinin potentiation in the pain receptors in man. Life Sci. 4: 309–316, 1965
52 Speck, U., H. M. Siefert, G. Klink: Contrast media and pain in peripheral arteriography. Invest. Radiol. 15: 335–339, 1980
53 Sterrett, P. R., J. M. Bradley, G. T. Kitten, H. F. Janssen, L. S. Holloway: Cerebrovasculature permeability changes following experimental cerebral angiography. A light and electron microscopic study. J. neurol. Sci. 30: 385, 1976
54 Stöhr jr., P.: Acta neuroveg. (Wien) 1: 74, 1950
55 Stöhr jr., P.: Lehrbuch der Histologie und der mikroskopischen Anatomie. Springer, Berlin 1951
56 Taylor, R. E.: Effect of procaine on electrical properties of squid axon membrane. Amer. J. Physiol. 196: 1071–1078, 1959
57 Tillmann, U., R. Adler, W. A. Fuchs: Pain in peripheral arteriography – a comparison of a low osmolality contrast medium with a conventional compound. Brit. J. Radiol. 52: 102–104, 1979
58 Van Waes, P.: New low osmolality water-soluble contrast compounds in selective arteriography of the peripheral limbs. Diagn. imaging 48: 209–215, 1979
59 Wagner, F. B.: Complications following arteriography of peripheral vessels. J. Amer. med. Ass. 125: 958, 1944
60 Waldron, R. L., R. B. Bridenbaugh, E. W. Dempsey: Effect of angiographic contrast media on the cellular level in the brain – hypertonic vs. chemical action. Amer. J. Roentgenol. 122: 469–476, 1974
61 Wolff, B. B., J. L. Potter, W. L. Vermeet, C. W. McEwen: Quantitative measure of deep somatic pain: preliminary study with hypertonic saline. Clin. Sci. 20: 345–350, 1961
62 Wolff, H. G.: Headache and Other Head Pain. Oxford University Press, New York 1963 (1st Ed. 1948)
63 Young, S. W.: Computed tomography after the intraarterial and intravenous administration of contrast media. In Felix, R., E. Kazner, O. H. Wegener: Contrast Media in Computed Tomography. Excerpta Medica, Amsterdam 1981 (pp. 262–268)
64 Zachrisson, B. F., R. Johannson, L. Björk: Two new contrast media in peripheral arteriography. A double blind study in patients with arterial insufficiency in the legs. Fortschr. Röntgenstr. 132: 208–211, 1980
65 Zinner, G., R. Gottlob: Die gefäßschädigende Wirkung verschiedener Röntgenkontrastmittel, vergleichende Untersuchungen. Fortschr. Röntgenstr. 91: 507, 1959

# Increased Pain Reactions as Hang-over Phenomena after Intra-arterial Injections of Contrast Media in Rats

B. Hagen, H. M. Siefert, W. Mützel and U. Speck

## Summary

In an intra-individual comparison of ioxaglate and iohexol in peripheral arteriography it was observed that iohexol caused more pain when it was injected after ioxaglate than when it was administered as the first contrast medium.
Systematic studies of the painfulness of contrast media were then performed in rats to describe this hang-over effect in greater detail. Injection of the contrast media meglumine diatrizoate and sodium meglumine ioxaglate acted in the rat for at least 15 minutes in such a way that the second injection of the same contrast medium or the subsequent injection of iohexol was found to be relatively more painful. When given as the first injection, the non-ionic substance iohexol caused no recognizable hang-over effects. The non-ionic substance iopromide was not painful even when it was injected after ioxaglate. Therefore no synergism regarding pain should be existing with the non-ionic contrast media at least up to the second injection.

## Zusammenfassung

Bei einem intraindividuellen Vergleich von Ioxaglat und Iohexol in der peripheren Arteriographie war aufgefallen, daß Iohexol, wenn es nach Ioxaglat injiziert wurde, schmerzhafter war als wenn es als erstes Kontrastmittel verabreicht wurde. Systematische Untersuchungen der Schmerzhaftigkeit von Kontrastmitteln wurden an Ratten durchgeführt, um den zufällig entdeckten Überhangeffekt näher zu beschreiben. Die Injektion der Kontrastmittel Meglumin Diatrizoat und Natrium-Meglumin Ioxaglat bewirkten bei der Ratte für mindestens 15 Minuten, daß die 2. Injektion des gleichen Kontrastmittels oder die nachfolgende Injektion von Iohexol als relativ schmerzhafter empfunden wurde. Die Erstinjektion des nicht-ionischen Iohexol verursachte keine erkennbaren Überhangeffekte. Das nicht-ionische Iopromid war selbst nach Vorinjektion von Ioxaglat nicht schmerzhaft. Ein Synergismus im Hinblick auf die Schmerzhaftigkeit dürfte daher bei den nicht-ionischen Kontrastmitteln zumindest bei der zweiten Injektion noch nicht ausgeprägt sein.

## Introduction

During the clinical investigation of iohexol (5) it was observed that this contrast medium was considerably more painful than ioxaglate when it was administered intra-arterially as the second injection a few minutes after administration of ioxaglate, whereas it was tolerated with virtually no pain when administered alone.
These observations prompted us to perform animal studies to seek answers to the following questions:

1. Can an increasing vascular pain effect be demonstrated in an animal model (vascular pain study in the rat) after repeated administration of contrast media?
2. Can any hang-over effects which do occur be avoided by extending the time interval between the individual contrast medium injections?

We hoped to establish from the animal experiments whether:

a) certain modalities must be observed in the design of intra-individual clinical trials of contrast media in order to eliminate hang-over phenomena;

b) certain contrast media in peripheral arteriography have the disadvantage of causing pain when administered as a necessary second injection into the same vascular region, although they are tolerated with virtually no pain on the first injection.

## Material and Methods

### Contrast Media

The study was conducted with meglumine amidotrizoate (Angiografin, Schering AG), iohexol (Nyegaard, Oslo; in Germany: Schering AG), iopromide (Schering AG) and meglumine sodium ioxaglate (Hexabrix, Guerbet, France; in Germany: Byk Gulden).
The substance meglumine amidotrizoate is an ionic contrast agent with an iodine content of 306 mg/ml, an osmolality of 1530 mosmol/kg $H_2O$ and a viscosity of 4.9 mpa · s (at 37°C).
Iohexol as used in the present study design is a nonionic contrast medium with an iodine content of 320 mg/ml, an osmolality of 770 mosmol/kg $H_2O$ and a viscosity of 8.1 mpa · s (at 37°C).

Iopromide is likewise a non-ionic contrast medium with an iodine content of 320 mg/ml (in the present study), an osmolality of 670 mosmol/kg $H_2O$ and a viscosity of 6.2 mpa · s (at 37 °C).

Ioxaglate is a monoacid, dimeric ionic contrast medium with an iodine content of 320 mg/ml. Its osmolality is 600 mosmol/kg $H_2O$ and its viscosity 7.5 mpa · s (at 37 °C).

## Study Protocol

The laboratory animals used were non-anaesthetized, free-moving rats (Sprague-Dawley, male: female = 50 : 50) with a bodyweight of 140–180 g. The injections were given at a rate of 0.05 ml/second via a catheter which had been inserted beforehand into the left femoral artery, and the behaviour of the animals during the injection was observed. The method has been described in detail by Speck et al. (11).

A total of 3 study series was carried out.

The first series was performed to establish whether the repeated injection of meglumine amidotrizoate in two different dosages at intervals of 30 and 60 minutes leads to an increase of the pain reactions of the animals (Table 1). The object of the second series was to determine whether the pain reactions are greater after a quick sequence of injections of the virtually painless contrast media with lower osmotic pressure than after a single injection and whether there are any differences in this respect between different less hypertonic contrast media (Table 2). The last series was conducted to determine how long the animals remained sensitized after injection of ioxaglate (Table 3).

## Results

### Repeated Injection of Meglumine Amidotrizoate

The administration of meglumine amidotrizoate 4 times at intervals of 30 minutes led under both the lower and the higher dose to an increased vascular pain effect of the contrast agent, as determined by the larger number of animals displaying pain reactions after the later injections. Virtually no increase of the vascular pain effect of the contrast agent was observed, however, when the interval between the injections has extended to 60 minutes (Table 1).

### Hang-over Effects after Injection of Contrast Media with Reduced Osmotic Pressure

Whereas first injections with meglumine sodium ioxaglate and iohexol caused virtually no vascular pain, a repeat injection of meglumine sodium ioxaglate itself and the administration of iohexol 1 minute after ioxaglate led to markedly greater vascular pain in the rat compared to the first injection (Table 2).

In contrast, the reaction of the animals to an injection of iopromide given after meglumine sodium ioxaglate was virtually no greater than that to the first injection. Thus, iopromide was not

Table 1 Pain reactions in rats after injection of meglumine diatrizoate into the femoral artery

| Experiment | Meglumine diatrizoate 306 mg I/ml | Dose and injection sequence | Number of animals with distinct pain reactions/total number of animals |
|---|---|---|---|
| 1 | 1st injection<br>2nd injection<br>3rd injection<br>4th injection | 4 × 0.3 ml/animal<br>at intervals of 30 mins. | 1/10<br>2/10<br>3/10<br>3/10 |
| 2 | 1st injection<br>2nd injection<br>3rd injection<br>4th injection | 4 × 0.6 ml/animal<br>at interval of 30 mins. | 5/10<br>8/10<br>10/10<br>10/10 |
| 3 | 1st injection<br>2nd injection<br>3rd injection | 3 × 0.3 ml/animal<br>at intervals of 60 mins. | 0/8<br>2/8<br>1/8 |
| 4 | 1st injection<br>2nd injection<br>3rd injection | 3 × 0.6 ml/animal<br>at intervals of 60 mins. | 3/6<br>3/6<br>2/6 |

Table 2  Pain reactions in rats after the first and second injection of different contrast media with reduced osmotic pressure into the femoral artery

| Experiment | Contrast medium 320 mg I/ml | Dose and injection sequence | Number of animals with distinct pain reactions/total number of animals |
|---|---|---|---|
| 1 | Ioxaglate<br>1st injection<br>2nd injection | 2 × 1.5 ml/animal<br>at intervals of 1 min. | 0/10<br>5/10 |
| 2 | Ioxaglate then iohexol<br>1st injection<br>2nd injection | 1.5 ml of each/animal<br>at interval of 1 min. | 1/10<br>6/10 |
| 3 | Ioxaglate then iopromide<br>1st injection<br>2nd injection | 1.5 ml of each/animal<br>at interval of 1 min. | 0/10<br>1/10 |
| 4 | Iohexol<br>1st injection<br>2nd injection | 2 × 1.5 ml/animal<br>at interval of 10 mins. | 0/10<br>0/10 |
| 5 | Iohexol then ioxaglate<br>1st injection<br>2nd injection | 1.5 ml of each/animal<br>at interval of 1 min. | 0/10<br>0/10 |

considered to be painful even after prior injection of ioxaglate.

An injection of meglumine sodium ioxaglate given after administration of iohexol was also tolerated by the rats without pain.

## Duration of the Hang-over Effect of an Ioxaglate Injection

When sodium meglumine ioxaglate was administered twice at an interval of 1 minute, the second injection was distinctly more painful than the first. Even when the interval between the two injections was extended to 5 minutes and 15 minutes, the animals still displayed more pain reactions after the second injection than after the first. The hang-over effect had disappeared completely 1 hour after the first injection (Table 3).

## Discussion of the Results

It has been well documented in numerous animal-experimental and clinical studies that contrast media are not inert substances. The intravascular administration of contrast media can lead not only to symptoms resembling IgE-induced phenomena, but also to symptoms of a non-idiosyncratic nature which – depending on the dose – are apparently attributable to the chemotoxicity and high osmolality of ionic contrast medium substances in particu-

Table 3  Pain reactions in rats after an initial injection of sodium meglumine ioxaglate and after a second injection of the same contrast medium into the femoral artery at different intervals

| Experiment | Sodium meglumine ioxaglate 320 mg I/ml | Dose and injection sequence | Number of animals with distinct pain reactions/total number of animals |
|---|---|---|---|
| 1 | 1st injection<br>2nd injection | 2 × 1.5 ml/animal<br>at interval of 1 min. | 0/10<br>5/10 |
| 2 | 1st injection<br>2nd injection | 2 × 1.5 ml/animal<br>at interval of 5 min. | 0/10<br>3/10 |
| 3 | 1st injection<br>2nd injection | 2 × 1.5 ml/animal<br>at interval of 15 mins. | 0/10<br>2/10 |
| 4 | 1st injection<br>2nd injection | 2 × 1.5 ml/animal<br>at interval of 60 mins. | 0/8<br>0/8 |

lar. The symptoms include sensations of pain and heat as troubling and unpleasant concomitant symptoms of contrast medium injections. The surprising result of a clinical study (5) of ioxaglate and iohexol carried out as an intraindividual double-blind design prompted us to take a closer look at these hang-over effects in animal studies.

Hang-over effects after double injections may be either potentiating or attenuating. The first case involves a synergism (or sensitization), the second a tachyphylaxis. They can be simple or crossed, depending on whether the same or different substances are involved.

The reactions which may be caused by the second injection can be classified as follows (CM = contrast medium):

| | |
|---|---|
| $CM_1 = CM_1$ | (indifferent type) |
| $CM_1 < CM_1$ | (autosynergism; psychological phenomena) |
| $CM_1 > CM_1$ | (tachyphylaxis; psychological phenomena) |
| $CM_1 = CM_2$ $CM_2 = CM_1$ | (indifferent type) |
| $CM_1 < CM_2$ $CM_2 < CM_1$ | (cross-synergism; psychological phenomena) |
| $CM_1 > CM_2$ $CM_2 > CM_1$ | (cross-tachyphylaxis; psychological phenomena) |

Different kinds of hang-over effects in respect of painfulness in blood vessels have been described both for pharmacological substances and for contrast media:

1. If several intra-arterial injections of bradykinin or serotonine are given at intervals of a few minutes, many receptors (including nociceptors) respond with more or less pronounced, dose-dependent tachyphylaxis (1, 2). Between different substances, however, there is no cross-tachyphylaxis, but rather a synergistic effect. This is true both for bradykinin and serotonine, and for both substances with prostaglandins of the E group (6).
2. The tachyphylaxis observed after repeated injections of adrenergic substances, e.g. ephedrine, results not from a direct effect of the substance on the receptors (vasoconstrictors), but from emptying of the noradrenalin stores by increased liberation of this substance (7).
3. It is known from comparative, intraindividual studies of contrast media that the first injection can influence the second. There have been several reports (3, 9, 12) that ionic hyperosmolar contrast media are considered by the patient to be very much more painful when administered as the second injection after a first injection with a non-ionic contrast medium than the other way round. Apparently, the first injection with a low-osmolar contrast medium lowers the tolerance limit or the expectation potential of the patient to the second injection with a higher osmolar contrast medium. It is extremely doubtful whether a pharmacologically relevant cross-synergism is present here – rather, it seems that psychological phenomena are playing a greater rôle.

However, the above-mentioned authors have also observed a slight but not statistically significant synergistic effect under low-osmolar contrast media when the ionic, sodium meglumine salt of ioxaglate acid was injected as the first substance before administration of non-ionic preparations (e.g. iopamidol). Skutta (10) observed statistically significant differences in intraindividual double-blind studies of iopromide and ioxaglate (substances of almost equal osmolality) as regards the reported sensations of heat. The injection of iopromide after a preceding injection of ioxaglate was considered by the patient to create much more heat than when iopromide was injected as the first substance. The author attributed this phenomenon to a hang-over effect of ioxaglate, suggesting that the release of histamine is sustained for a longer time under ioxaglate. The simultaneously recorded sensation of pain was identical under both substances, regardless of the sequence of the injections.

The results of our own clinical and animal studies lead us to the following conclusions: an increased vascular pain effect must be expected when ionic contrast media are injected repeatedly at intervals of less than 30 minutes. These phenomena are independent of the osmotic pressure of the contrast media administered, as the first study series (high-osmolar contrast media) and the third series (low-osmolar contrast media) clearly demonstrate. The synergistic effect, as documented by the intensity of the reactions in the laboratory animals, subsides almost completely within 60 minutes. As the study with iohexol and iopromide has shown, this increase of the vascular pain effect is not or is still not present with non-ionic contrast media on the second injection. The observed phenomena are found to take the form of simple synergism with ionic contrast agents (e.g. diatrizoate and ioxaglate), and also of cross-synergism with double injections of ionic dimers and non-ionic contrast media. According to available studies, however, the latter applies only when the ionic contrast medium is given as the first injection, and even then only when iohexol is given as the second injection. This effect was not observed when iopromide was given as the second injection.

It is conceivable that an effect of the anionic or cationic component of the contrast medium leads to sensitization of the receptors responsible for vascular pain (4). Whether such apparently substance-specific sensitization phenomena lead to a reduction of the stimulus threshold of nociceptive end-organs because of the electrical potential of the contrast medium itself, as a result of ion shifts or changes in the ion concentration or through the mediation of mediator substances requires further clarification.

Another aspect of potential importance in the screening of newly synthesized contrast media concerns the experimental possibility of differentiating two substances which do not differ clearly as regards their vascular pain effect by priming, i. e. injecting an ionic contrast medium beforehand. It can be assumed that the first injection with an ionic contrast medium will shift the "pain stimulus threshold" for the second injection into a range which is more favourable for the differentiation.

Observing long waiting times between the individual injections in order to avoid hang-over effects is probably impracticable in a comparative, intra-individual, clinical study of different contrast medium substances. An interval of at least 15 minutes between the first and second injection would seem, however, to be an acceptable recommendation. Any hangover phenomena could be detected by exact statistical analysis of the data.

## References

1 Beck, P. W., H. C. Handwerker: Bradykinin and serotonine effects on various types of cutaneous nerve fibres. Pflügers Arch. 347: 209–222, 1974
2 Guzman, F., C. Braun, R. K. S. Lim: Visceral pain and the pseudo-affective response to intra-arterial injection of bradykinin and other algesic agents. Arch. int. Pharmacodyn. 136: 353–384, 1962
3 Hagen, B.: Iopamidol, ein neues nicht-ionisches Röntgenkontrastmittel. Radiologe 22: 581–585, 1982
4 Hagen, B.: Contrast media and pain. Hypotheses on the genesis of pain occurring on intra-arterial administration of contrast media. In Taenzer, V., E. Zeitler: Contrast media. Fortschr. Röntgenstr., Erg.-Bd. 118. Thieme, Stuttgart 1983
5 Hagen, B.: Iohexol and iopromide – two new non-ionic water-soluble radiographic contrast media: Randomized, intraindividual double-blind study versus ioxaglate in peripheral angiography. In Taenzer, V., E. Zeitler: Contrast media. Fortschr. Röntgenstr., Erg.-Bd. 118. Thieme, Stuttgart 1983
6 Handwerker, H. O.: Influences of algogenic substances and prostaglandins on the discharges of unmyelinated cutaneous nerve fibres identified as nociceptors. In Bonica, J. J., D. Albe-Fessarel: Advances in Pain Research and Therapy. Vol. I. Raven Press, New York 1976

7 Kuschinsky, G., H. Lüllmann: Kurzes Lehrbuch der Pharmakologie, 1. Aufl. Thieme, Stuttgart 1964 (S. 24, 26); 9. Aufl. 1981
8 Lasser, E. C., G. Elizondo-Martel, R. C. Granke: The roentgen contrast media potentiation of pentobarbital anaesthesia in rats. Amer. J. Roentgenol. 91: 453, 1964
9 Mathias, K., P. Billmann, E. Schmiedel: Painless Angiography with New Contrast Media. Contrast Media in Radiology, 1st European Workshop, Lyon, 17.–19. Sept. 1981
10 Skutta, Th.: Erste klinische Erfahrungen mit dem neuen nicht-ionischen Röntgenkontrastmittel Iopromid. 15. Internationaler Kongreß für Radiologie, Brüssel, 24. 6.–1. 7. 1981
11 Speck, U., H. M. Siefert, G. Klink: Contrast media and pain in peripheral arteriography. Invest. Radiol. 15: 335–339, 1980
12 Zeitler, E., H. G. Kinski, H. Mader, E. J. Richter, W. Seyferth, I. M. Tønnesen-Georgi: Angiography in lower extremities with new contrast media: Review of double blind studies. Contrast Media in Radiology, 1st European Workshop, Lyon, 17.–19. Sept. 1981

# Effects of Ionic and Non-ionic Contrast Media after Selective Peripheral and Cerebral Arterial Injections in Rats

W. Mützel and U. Speck

## Summary

Experiments were conducted on non-anaesthetized, unrestrained rats to determine the effect of carotid and femoral artery injections of iopromide and other contrast media of low and high osmolality.

It was demonstrated that iopromide and metrizamide elicited only behavioural anomalies of the animals after intracarotid injections of dosages up to 3 g iodine per kg, while meglumine ioglicate and meglumine ioxithalamate from 1.5 g iodine per kg rat onwards caused severe postural anomalies, cramps and death. Severest pain to the animals was observed after femoral injection of meglumine sodium ioglicate at 350 mg I/ml. Iopromide and iopamidol were tolerated painlessly in concentrations up to 300 mg I/ml. Iopromide, iopamidol and iohexol caused pain to a certain extent at concentrations of more than 320 mg I/ml, which apparently is related to the hypertonicity of the solutions. Iopromide solutions, yielding at 400 mg I/ml lower osmolality than iopamidol and iohexol, caused less pain than the latter. Improved clinical tolerance of iopromide in arteriography is discussed.

## Zusammenfassung

An wachen Ratten wurde die Wirkung von Iopromid und anderen Kontrastmitteln mit niedriger und hoher Osmolalität nach Injektion in die A. carotis communis bzw. A. femoralis untersucht.

Iopromid und Metrizamid verursachten lediglich Haltungsanomalien der Tiere nach intracarotidealer Gabe von bis zu 3 g I/kg, während Ioglicinat und Ioxithalamat nach Dosierungen von 1,5 g I/kg an zu schweren Haltungsanomalien, Krämpfen und Tod führten. Heftiger Schmerz wurde nach Injektion von Meglumin-Natrium-Ioglicinat in einer Konzentration von 350 mg I/ml in die A. femoralis von Ratten beobachtet. Iopromid und Iopamidol wurden bis zu einer Konzentration der Lösungen von 300 mg I/ml schmerzlos vertragen, Metrizamid bis zu einer Konzentration von 370 mg I/ml. Bis zu einem gewissen Ausmaß verursachten Lösungen von Iopromid, Iopamidol und Iohexol mit mehr als 320 mg I/ml Schmerz, was offensichtlich auf die Hypertonizität der Lösungen zurückzuführen ist. Iopromid-Lösungen mit 400 mg I/ml, welche eine geringere Hypertonizität aufweisen als entsprechende Lösungen von Iopamidol und Iohexol verursachen weniger Gefäßschmerz als diese. Die verbesserte klinische Verträglichkeit von Iopromid in der Arteriographie wird diskutiert.

## Introduction

Vascular pain is one of the most frequent side effects in peripheral arteriography and also in cerebral arteriography, where some other side effects like headache may occur as well. Apparently, the majority of side effects in arteriography is attributable primarily to the high osmotic pressure of contrast media solutions rather than to their chemotoxicity, as was confirmed in test animals (3, 5) and in man (1, 4, 6). The introduction of low-osmolality contrast media for arteriography was a considerable advance, since the frequency of side effects has been reduced significantly.

The purpose of this study was to assess the tolerance of iopromide and other contrast media of low and high osmolality after cerebral and femoral arteriography in the rat as an animal model. Iopromide is a new non-ionic, low-osmolality contrast medium developed by Schering for vascular radiography.

## Material and Methods

### Common Carotid Artery

Non-anaesthetized, male and female SPF rats (strain: Wistar-Han-Schering-78) with a body weight of 95–105 g, in which a catheter had previously been inserted into the left common carotid artery, were given a single administration of (a) meglumine ioglicate (Rayvist 300, Schering) and meglumine ioxithalamate (Telebrix 300, Byk-Gulden, Konstanz) solutions containing 300 mg I/ml at 6 dose levels (0.9–3.3 g I/kg), and (b) iopromide (new from Schering, Berlin) and metrizamide (Amipaque, Schering, Berlin) solutions containing 370 mg I/ml at 4 dose levels (1.9–3.0 g I/kg). At the dosage of 3.0 g I/kg metrizamide containing 300 mg I/ml was also used. 10 animals per dose were employed. The injections were given at a speed of 0.05 ml per second. The animals' behaviour was observed over 24 hours. The tolerance was evaluated by scoring the unrestrained animals according to the following grades: 0 = no effect; 1 = slight ataxia; 2 = general tenseness, vocalisation; 3 = unequivocal postural abnormalities; 4 = cramped posture, rare convulsions of short duration; 5 = clonic-tonic or tonic convulsions, coma; 6 = death.

## Femoral Artery

Non-anaesthetized, unrestrained male and female rats (strain: Sprague-Dawley, bred by Willi Gassner) with a body weight of 140 to 150 g, in which a catheter had been previously inserted into the left femoral artery, as described by Speck et al. (5), received 10 ml/kg of the following contrast media at an injection rate of 0.05 ml/sec

a) iopromide (new from Schering, Berlin), iopamidol (Solutrast, Byk-Gulden, Konstanz), metrizamide (Amipaque, Schering, Berlin) and iohexol (new from Nyegaard, Oslo, and Schering, Berlin) solutions containing 370 mg I/ml, meglumine sodium (66 : 11) ioglicate (Rayvist 350, Schering, Berlin) containing 350 mg I/ml and NaCl 0.9% as control solution;
b) iopromide (new from Schering, Berlin), meglumine/sodium (2 : 1) ioxaglate (Hexabrix, Byk-Gulden, Konstanz), iopamidol (Amipaque, Schering, Berlin) and iohexol (new from Nyegaard, Oslo, and Schering, Berlin) solutions containing 320 mg I/ml.

10 animals per dosage were used. The animals' behaviour was observed during the injection for definite signs of painful reactions, which were scored (5).

In another investigation the vascular pain caused by a) iopromide and iopamidol and b) iopromide and iohexol was observed by injecting 10 ml/kg in concentrations of 300, 350 and 400 mg I/ml into a rat's femoral artery (n = 12 per concentration). The two pairs were tested by intra-individual comparison, i. e., each animal of six received each compound first and 1 hour later the second one. According to other studies (2), hangover phenomena can be precluded by this time interval. Finally, evident painful reactions were summed up for each compound.

## Results and Discussion

### Cerebral Arteriography

After injection of two ionic, hypertonic (~ 1800 mosm) contrast media, meglumine ioglicate and meglumine ioxithalamate, at dosages from about 1.8 g iodine/kg onwards severe postural abnormalities, cramps and lethality (scores 3–6) of the rats were observed. The effects are dose-related and very similar for the two contrast agents (Fig 1).

The intracarotid injection of iopromide and metrizamide, which yield only slightly hypertonic (~ 600 mosm) solutions of 300 mg I/ml, elicited only behavioural anomalies even in dosages up to 3 g iodine per kg, but no cramps, convulsions or death (Fig 2). A considerable extent of the reactions can be related to the volume injected, as is demonstrable from saline injections in the same study.

From the two investigations it is concluded that in the rat non-ionic contrast media cause distinctly less severe effects with regard to acute local and neurofunctional tolerance than ionic contrast media currently employed for cerebral angiography.

Iopromide has in this context very much the quality of metrizamide, which was described to be superior to metrizoate (ionic) in carotid arteriography in man with regard to side effects (4).

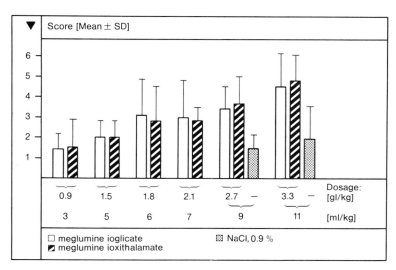

Fig 1 Mean scores (see methods) and standard deviations of neurotoxic effects observed following a single intracarotid injection of two ionic, monomeric contrast media in rats (n = 10 per dose)

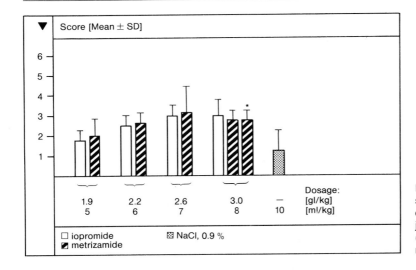

Fig 2 Mean scores (see methods) and standard deviations of neurotoxic effects observed following a single intracarotid injection of iopromide and metrizamide in rats (n = 10 per dose) *solution contained 300 mg I/ml

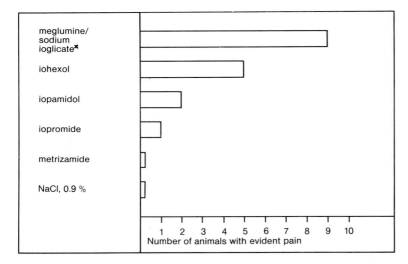

Fig 3 Effects of arterial injection of 10 ml/kg solutions of different contrast media containing 370 mg iodine per ml (or 350 mg I/ml) in rats (n = 10 or *9 per group)

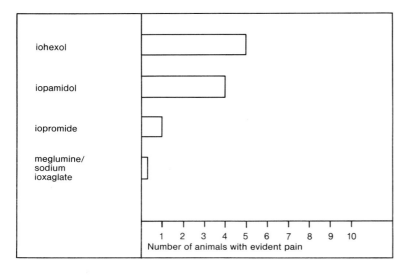

Fig 4 Vascular pain after injection into the femoral artery of rats: solutions containing 320 mg iodine per ml; dose 10 ml/kg, 12 animals per group

## Peripheral Arteriography

Evident vascular pain was observed in all rats after the injection of meglumine/sodium ioglicate, which is highly hypertonic at 350 mg I/ml (~ 2240 mosm). In the group of non-ionic contrast media of high concentration (370 mg I/ml) iohexol was found to be painful in 5 of 10 rats, while iopromide and iopamidol were painful only in one or two of 10 animals. After femoral arterial injection of metrizamide no pain was observed, as after injections of sodium chloride (Fig 3). The reactivity to the non-ionic contrast media solution is apparently mainly related to their osmolalities, which differ in high concentrations depending on the degree of association of the molecules in water: iohexol, being less associated, has an osmolality at 37°C of 1 mol/kg $H_2O$, iopamidol of 0.83, iopromide of 0.75 mol/kg $H_2O$ and metrizamide 0.6 mol/kg $H_2O$.

After injections into a rat's femoral artery, of iohexol, iopamidol and iopromide at 320 mg I/ml which corresponds to the commercial concentration of meglumine/sodium ioxaglate, again iopromide was somewhat less painful than iopamidol and iohexol, while ioxaglate did not reveal any pain reaction (Fig 4).

Changing the animal model to intraindividual comparisons (described under methods) by injecting iopromide and iopamidol at three different concentrations, the two contrast media were tolerated painlessly at concentrations of 300 mg I/ml. When injecting the solutions containing 350 mg I/ml, iopamidol generated pain in one third of the ani-

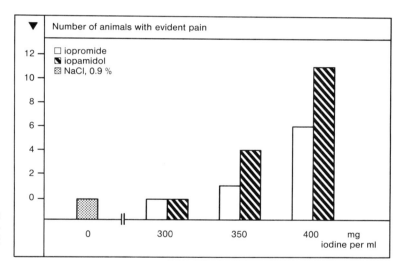

Fig 5 Vascular pain caused by iopromide and iopamidol injected in different concentrations into a rat's femoral artery (n = 12 per group, dose = 10 ml/kg)

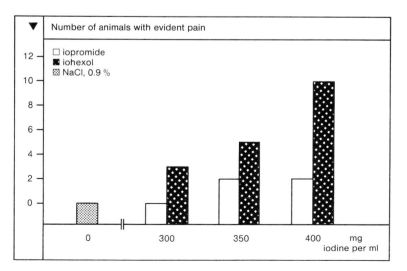

Fig 6 Vascular pain caused by iopromide and iohexol injected in different concentrations into a rat's femoral artery (n = 12 per group, dose = 10 ml/kg)

mals tested and iopromide in about one tenth. 11 out of 12 animals showed evident pain when exposed to iopamidol solution containing 400 mg I/ml (~ 1.1 mol/kg $H_2O$), while iopromide (~ 0.83 mol/kg $H_2O$) at the same concentration caused pain in 6 of 12 animals only (Fig 5). Again, the differences are supposed to be related to the different osmolalities of the two formulations.

Another study with iopromide was conducted for intra-individual comparison with iohexol at the three different concentrations mentioned above. Vascular pain occurred more rarely with iopromide than with iohexol in all three concentrations tested, probably due to iohexol's higher osmolality in aqueous solutions (Fig 6).

## Conclusions

1. Commonly used ionic contrast media, which yield high osmolalities at high iodine concentrations, obviously cause more neural and local disturbances in the rat when injected into the carotid artery than the new non-ionic contrast media of low osmolality do, even when applied in very high concentrations.

2. Vascular pain in rats is clearly related predominantly to the osmolality of a contrast agent. Osmolalities of $\geq 0.6$ mol/kg $H_2O$ are supposed to induce local vascular pain, disregarding the contrast medium employed. Evident pain, as was reconfirmed for hypertonic ionic agents, can also be observed after arterial injection of non-ionic, monomeric contrast media solutions containing more than 320–350 mg I/ml.

3. The individual tendency of different non-ionic, monomeric contrast compounds to be associated with water at high concentrations results in different osmolalities, which then cause more or less pain in arteriography.

4. Iopromide, a new, non-ionic contrast medium for vascular use, is tolerated well after intracarotid injections in rats, like metrizamide, and far better than ioglicate and ioxithalamate. After injection into the femoral artery of the rat, iopromide consistently caused less pain than the two ionic momoners, but also than iopamidol and iohexol at concentrations of $> 320$ mg I/ml. Improved clinical tolerance for iopromide in selective peripheral and cerebral arteriography may be inferred.

## References

1 Grainger, R. G.: A clinical trial of a new osmolality contrast medium; sodium and meglumine ioxaglate (Hexabrix) compared with meglumine iothalamate (Conray) for carotid arteriography. Brit. J. Radiol. 52: 781, 1979
2 Hagen, B., H.-M. Siefert, W. Mützel, U. Speck: This volume, p. 57
3 Siefert, H.-J., W.-R. Press, U. Speck: Tolerance to iohexol after intracisternal, intracerebral and intraarterial injection in the rat. Acta radiol. (Stockh.) Suppl. 362: 77, 1980
4 Skalpe, I. O., A. Lundervold, K. Tjörstad: Cerebral angiography with nonionic (metrizamide) and ionic (meglumine metrizoate) watersoluble contrast media. A. comparative study with double blind technic. Neuroradiology 14: 15, 1977
5 Speck, U., H.-M. Siefert, G. Klink: Contrast media and pain in peripheral arteriography. Invest. Radiol. 15: 335, 1980
6 Wilmink, J. T., W. van den Burg, H.-J. Kramer, L. Penning: Comparative evaluation of metrizamide and meglumine ioxithalamate in angiography of the vessels of the head. Neuroradiology 15: 267, 1978

# Haemodynamics

## Reduced Side Effects of Low Osmolality Non-ionic Contrast Media in Coronary Arteriography
### Comparative Experimental Study in Dogs*

R. Schräder, D. Baller, A. Hoeft, H. Korb, H. G. Wolpers and G. Hellige

## Summary

Acute cardiac side effects during coronary angiography with contrast media of low osmolality – iopamidol, iohexol, iopromide, and ioxaglate – were compared. As a reference, an ionic compound of high osmolality, diatrizoate, as well as Ringer's solution were included. Experiments were performed on anaesthetized closed-chest mongrel dogs (n = 10) with mean left ventricular weight of 163 g in cardiac catheterization techniques.

After intracoronary injection of 8 ml contrast medium various effects were demonstrable on haemodynamics, ECG, and physicochemical properties in coronary sinus blood such as osmolality, cationic content and pH. Ionic compounds – ioxaglate and diatrizoate – initially induced negative inotropic effects. In contrast, non-ionic contrast media – iopamidol, iohexol, and iopromide – only acted in a positive inotropic way. Correspondingly, the ratio between sodium and ionized calcium ($Na^+/Ca^{++}$) in coronary sinus blood increased after injection of cardiodepressive agents compared to control status, whereas the non-ionic contrast media slightly decreased this quotient. Diatrizoate produced strongest side effects. Ioxaglate had smaller effects compared to diatrizoate but stronger ones in comparison with non-ionic compounds. Overall, no significant differences were seen between non-ionic contrast media.

We conclude that 1) under clinical conditions no significant differences should be expected between iopamidol, iohexol, and iopromide with regard to parameters examined, 2) these new contrast media may offer reduction of acute cardiac side effects during coronary-angiography and, 3) physicochemical properties of contrast media are mainly causal for haemodynamic reactions.

## Zusammenfassung

Die akuten kardialen Nebenwirkungen von Koronarangiographien mit niederosmolaren Röntgenkontrastmitteln – Iopamidol, Iohexol, Iopromid und Ioxaglat – wurden verglichen. Als Referenzsubstanzen wurden ein konventionelles, hochosmolares Kontrastmittel – Diatrizoat – sowie Ringerlösung einbezogen. Als Versuchstiere dienten anästhesierte große Bastardhunde (n = 10) mit einem mittleren linksventrikulären Gewicht von 163 g. Die Experimente wurden in Herzkathetertechnik ausgeführt.

Nach intrakoronarer Injektion von 8 ml Kontrastmittel konnten unterschiedliche Auswirkungen auf Hämodynamik, EKG und physikochemische Größen des koronarvenösen Blutes – Osmolalität, Kationengehalt und pH – nachgewiesen werden. Die ionischen Präparate, Ioxaglat und Diatrizoat, verursachten primär negativ inotrope Reaktionen. Im Gegensatz dazu wirkten die nichtionischen Substanzen, Iopamidol, Iohexol und Iopromid ausschließlich positiv inotrop. Dementsprechend stieg das Verhältnis von Natrium zu ionisiertem Kalzium im koronarvenösen Blut nach Injektion der kardiodepressiv wirkenden Kontrastmitteln im Vergleich zu den Kontrollbedingungen an, wohingegen die nichtionischen Präparate diesen Quotienten leicht senkten. Diatrizoat verursachte die stärksten Nebenwirkungen. Ioxaglat hatte geringere Effekte im Vergleich zu Diatrizoat aber ausgeprägtere im Vergleich zu den nichtionischen Röntgenkontrastmitteln. Insgesamt waren zwischen den nichtionischen Präparaten keine signifikanten Unterschiede nachweisbar.

Daraus ist zu folgern, daß 1. unter klinischen Bedingungen keine signifikanten Unterschiede zwischen Iopamidol, Iohexol und Iopromid im Hinblick auf die untersuchten Parameter erwartet werden sollten, 2. diese neuen Röntgenkontrastmittel eine Verminderung akuter kardialer Nebenwirkungen im Rahmen einer Koronarangiographie mit sich bringen werden und 3. physikochemische Eigenschaften der Kontrastmittel die Hauptursache für deren hämodynamische Effekte darstellen.

---

* Supported in part by the Deutsche Forschungsgemeinschaft, SFB 89, Kardiologie Göttingen.

*Acknowledgement:* We would like to express our thank to Mrs. D. Horst and Mrs. M. Hummes for technical assistance, Mrs. M. Rubbert for the preparation of figures and Mrs. A. Hartmann for typing the manuscript.

## Introduction

Acute cardiac side effects caused during coronary arteriography by common ionic contrast media of high osmolality are thoroughly investigated. They produce disturbed impulse formation and delayed conduction. This may induce bradycardia, premature beats and, sometimes, ventricular fibrillation (4, 11, 12, 15). Characteristically, a fall in systemic arterial pressure and peak velocity of pressure rise occurs, followed by a delayed positive inotropic effect and long-lasting increase of coronary blood flow combined with reduced coronary vascular resistance (8, 9). These effects depend on specific physicochemical properties of the contrast media: hyperosmolality, acidosis after mixing with blood, calcium chelation, and cation composition in particular content of sodium (8, 9, 17, 25).

Theoretical considerations led to the development of new contrast media with markedly reduced osmolality. Since 1973, metrizamide a nonionic compound for myelography has been used under experimental and clinical conditions. Despite less marked haemodynamic effects following intracoronary application compared to commonly used contrast materials its routine use in clinical angiocardiography seems unlikely because of relatively high cost and the necessity of prior mixing (1, 27).

These disadvantages led to an intensive search for other compounds of low osmolality: Ioxaglate is a dimer with six iodine atoms but only one anionic functional group. Other new contrast media, such as iopamidol, iohexol and iopromide, are nonionic compounds and are available in stable solution (3, 7, 16, 19, 20, 21). Ioxaglate as well as iopamidol have been already used in clinical trials. (2, 14, 26). Thus, a number of substances is available with different chemical constitutions on the one hand but comparable physicochemical properties on the other (see table 1). The question arises whether these various contrast media produce different or similar effects after intracoronary administration. The purpose of our study was 1) to quantify the influence of these new contrast media with low osmolality on cardiac function and on physicochemical properties in coronary venous blood unter standardized conditions. 2) to compare intraindividually the effects of the different agents by repeated intracoronary application, 3) to determine the reduction of side effects compared to conventional contrast materials and, 4) to assess the mechanisms by which contrast media may alter the parameters of cardiac function.

## Material and Methods

### Animal Preparation and Catheter Arrangement

Experiments were carried out on 10 closed-chest mongrel dogs of either sex. 30 min after premedication with 0.5 mg atropine and 2 mg/kg bw piritramide (Dipidolor, Janssen GmbH, Düsseldorf, W.-Germany) i. m., general anaesthesia was induced with 5 mg/kg bw sodium thiopental (Trapanal, Byk Gulden, Konstanz, W.-Germany) i. v. and maintained by infusion of 2 mg/kg · h piritramide (13). Animals were mechanically ventilated (Engström respirator system 300 ER 311, LKB Medical AG, Bromma, Sweden) with $N_2O : O_2$ at a ratio of 70 : 30 and respiration was adjusted to an endexspiratory $CO_2$-content at about 5 Vol% (Uras, Hartmann und Braun AG, Frankfurt, W.-Germany). All dogs were heparinized (100 IE/kg · h) (Thrombophob, Nordmark Werke GmbH, Hamburg). Arterial blood-gas status was measured repeatedly to assure adequacy of ventilation and acid-base balance.

Catheters were placed in the left ventricle, ascending aorta, left coronary artery, and coronary sinus under fluoroscopic control. For coronary angiography a 7F Judkins catheter was used. The positions of coronary sinus and coronary artery catheters were checked by test injection of contrast medium.

### Haemodynamic Recordings

Haemodynamic parameters were continuously monitored on a ten-channel recorder (Hellige, GmbH, Freiburg, W.-Germany): ECG (extremity lead II); myocardial blood flow (pressuredifference coronary sinus catheter (10)); aortic pressure (Pressure transducer, Statham P 23 ID, Gould Inc., Oxnard, California, USA); left ventricular pressure (Catheter tip pressure transducer PC 350, Millar Instruments, Inc., Houston Texas, USA). Left ventricular signal was recorded at low and high gain to determine left ventricular ($P_{LV}$) and left ventricular end-diastolic pressure ($P_{LVED}$), as well as differentiated (differentiating amplifier FN 1367, August Fischer KG, Göttingen, W.-Germany) for measurement of peak velocity of left ventricular pressure rise ($dP/dt_{max}$).

### Experimental Protocol

The following contrast media were investigated: 1) Sodium meglumine diatrizoate (Urografin 76, Schering AG, Berlin/Bergkamen, W.-Germany), 2) Iohexol (Nyegaard & Co., Oslo, Norway), 3)

Iopamidol (Solutrast, Byk Gulden, Konstanz, W.-Germany, 4) Iopromide (Schering AG, Berlin/Bergkamen, W.-Germany), and 5) Ioxaglate (Hexabrix, Byk Gulden, Konstanz, W.-Germany). In each experiment two injections of each tested contrast medium and one of Ringer's solution were prepared for randomization. Each injection was performed only on the premises that the basic haemodynamic parameters were closely comparable to control conditions at the beginning of each experiment (range ± 10%).

In intervals of 30 min we injected an effective volume of 8 ml subselectively into the left anterior descending artery (LAD). Contrast injections were made under fluoroscopic control by hand to ensure good filling of the LAD with minimum reflux into the aortic root. The average flow rate was between 1 and 1.5 ml per second.

For estimation of physicochemical parameters blood was sampled from coronary sinus. Two control samples of 5 ml were withdrawn just before each contrast injection. After starting contrast injection, three further samples were taken during the time interval from 10–20 s (1st sample), 20–30 s (2nd sample) and 30–40 s (3rd sample) p. i. For examination of electrophysiological side effects ECG (extremity lead I, II, III) was recorded on a six-channel recorder (Hellige GmbH, Freiburg, W.-Germany) during the interval from 10 s before beginning the injection to 60 s after the end of injection at a paper speed of 50 mm per second.

Changes of peak systolic aortic pressure ($P_{AO}$), peak velocity of left ventricular pressure-rise ($dP/dt_{max}$), left ventricular end-diastolic pressure ($P_{LVED}$) and coronary sinus blood flow ($V_{cor}$) were determined from continuous haemodynamic recordings. Heart rate (HR), PQ-, QRS- and QT-intervals, the height of $R_{II}$ as well as the direction of R- and T-wave vectors were taken from the ECG recordings.

## Physicochemical Estimations

Blood from coronary sinus was assayed for the following parameters: plasma osmolality, measured by freezing point depression (Osmometer Typ 4b, Roebling, Berlin, W.-Germany) and plasma content of sodium, potassium, and ionized calcium by using specific ion electrodes (Nova 1 and 2, respectively, Nova Biomedical, Newton, Massachusetts, USA). Total calcium was analyzed by the fluorometric method using EGTA as calcium chelating agent (Corning Calcium Analyzer 940, Corning Ltd., Halstead, Essex, England). Moreover, pH-values were determined (Blood-Gas-Analyzer 1302, Instrumentation Laboratory, Inc., Lexington, Massachusetts, USA). From these data we calculated the hydrogen ionic concentration. Furthermore, the ratio between sodium and ionized calcium ($Na^+/Ca^{++}$), between sodium and total calcium ($Na^+/Ca$) as well as the fraction of ionized calcium ($Ca^{++}/Ca$) was determined.

## Data Assessment

The maximal changes of haemodynamic and electrocardiographic parameters and the physicochemical data were calculated in per cent of the corresponding control values. Mean values and standard deviation were calculated for each measured parameter.

To determine the statistical significance of the changes in haemodynamic and physicochemical parameters compared to control values as well as for comparison of the various contrast media, Student's t-test for paired values was used.

## Results

Data result from 10 dogs weighing from 27 to 40 kg. Averaged weight of left ventricles was 163 g. Overall, 12 injections of both, iopamidol and ioxaglate, 11 injections of iohexol and iopromide, 10 injections of diatrizoate and 7 injections of Ringer's solution were performed. First, data from coronary sinus blood due to contrast injection are presented in Table 2 and Figures 1–3, respectively. Hemodynamic effects and ECG changes are demonstrated by Table 3 and Figures 4–8 and Table 4, respectively.

### Data from Coronary Sinus Blood

All contrast media tested caused changes of physicochemical parameters in coronary sinus blood in a significant manner. Strongest effects were always seen in the 1st sample following injection. The 2nd sample showed less marked changes and values from 3rd sample nearly reached control status.

*Osmolality (Fig 1):* Following injection of each contrast agent osmolality in coronary sinus blood increased significantly ($p < 0.001$). Diatrizoate led to significant ($p < 0.01$) higher increase of osmolality compared to all other contrast media. Only small differences were found between the contrast media of low osmolality. Nevertheless, these differences were partially significant. Ioxaglate produced lowest increase of this parameter. The difference between ioxaglate and iopamidol was on a significant level ($p < 0.01$) in the 1st and 2nd

Tab. 1 Physicochemical properties of the contrast media tested in this study. Data are obtained from (3, 7, 16)

| Characterization | iopamidol | iohexol | iopromide | ioxaglate | diatrizoate |
|---|---|---|---|---|---|
| | non-ionic, low osmolality | | | ionic, low osmolality | ionic, high osmolality |
| Iodine content (mg/ml) | 370 | 370 | 370 | 320 | 370 |
| Osmolality (mosmol/kg) | 799 | 980 | 810 | 580 | 1949 |
| Viscosity 37° C (mPa · s) | 9.5 | 13.5 | 10.4 | 7.5 | 8.5 |
| Sodium content (mmol/l) | 0 | 0 | 0 | 157 | 157 |

Table 2  Changes of physicochemical parameters in coronary sinus blood 10–20 s (1st sample) after starting injection. Data are calculated in percent of correspondent control values. Mean control values result from averaged control values of the 10 dogs and data are given in mmol/l (Ca, $Ca^{++}$, $Na^+$, $K^+$, $H^+$) and mosmol/l (osmolality), respectively

| | | mean control | iopamidol | iohexol | iopromide | ioxaglate | diatrizoate | ringer |
|---|---|---|---|---|---|---|---|---|
| | | absolute | changes in percent of control values | | | | | |
| $\dfrac{Na^+}{Ca^{++}}$ | n | 10 | 12 | 10 | 11 | 11 | 10 | 7 |
| | x̄ | 106.9 | 93.9 | 96.1 | 97.1 | 108.8 | 112.8 | 93.9 |
| | sx | 3.2 | 4.5 | 5.2 | 4.7 | 8.1 | 19.3 | 3.4 |
| $\dfrac{Na^+}{Ca}$ | n | 10 | 8 | 7 | 7 | 8 | 7 | 7 |
| | x̄ | 64.1 | 116.3 | 119.4 | 111.6 | 124.2 | 130.3 | 98.2 |
| | sx | 2.3 | 17.0 | 14.5 | 15.1 | 19.8 | 27.9 | 3.7 |
| $\dfrac{Ca^{++}}{Ca}$ | n | 10 | 8 | 6 | 7 | 7 | 6 | 7 |
| | x̄ | 0.59 | 123.9 | 123.2 | 113.3 | 115.1 | 102.7 | 104.7 |
| | sx | 0.01 | 22.9 | 17.7 | 18.5 | 13.6 | 10.6 | 5.5 |
| Ca | n | 10 | 8 | 7 | 7 | 8 | 6 | 7 |
| | x̄ | 2.33 | 76.3 | 74.6 | 79.4 | 78.6 | 69.6 | 101.7 |
| | sx | 0.06 | 18.7 | 16.3 | 17.5 | 13.9 | 20.3 | 5.4 |
| $Ca^{++}$ | n | 10 | 12 | 11 | 11 | 12 | 10 | 7 |
| | x̄ | 1.37 | 92.0 | 91.4 | 89.7 | 87.6 | 77.6 | 106.3 |
| | sx | 0.04 | 6.9 | 9.4 | 6.0 | 6.6 | 18.2 | 3.6 |
| $Na^+$ | n | 10 | 12 | 11 | 11 | 12 | 10 | 7 |
| | x̄ | 146.4 | 86.5 | 88.2 | 87.1 | 95.0 | 84.5 | 99.7 |
| | sx | 1.0 | 8.6 | 8.4 | 6.9 | 2.7 | 9.7 | 2.2 |
| $K^+$ | n | 10 | 12 | 11 | 11 | 11 | 10 | 7 |
| | x̄ | 3.31 | 88.9 | 90.2 | 89.3 | 91.1 | 81.5 | 100.6 |
| | sx | 0.06 | 7.1 | 7.2 | 6.0 | 7.4 | 13.6 | 2.7 |
| Osm | n | 10 | 12 | 11 | 11 | 12 | 10 | 7 |
| | x̄ | 304 | 114.7 | 110.8 | 113.1 | 109.3 | 122.4 | 99.0 |
| | sx | 2.81 | 8.3 | 6.6 | 6.4 | 4.7 | 13.2 | 1.0 |
| $H^+$ | n | 10 | 12 | 10 | 11 | 12 | 10 | 7 |
| | x̄ | $4.48 \cdot 10^{-8}$ | 124.2 | 120.8 | 118.6 | 120.8 | 150.3 | 104.7 |
| | sx | $5.72 \cdot 10^{-10}$ | 20.5 | 15.6 | 10.0 | 12.9 | 35.9 | 3.8 |

Table 3  Maximum changes of haemodynamics after contrast injection. Data are calculated in percent of correspondent control values. Mean control values result from averaged control values of the 10 dogs and data are given in mm Hg ($P_{AO}$, $P_{LVED}$), mm Hg/sec ($dP/dt_{max}$), and ml/min ($V_{cor}$). ./. = changes of control values < 1%

|  |  | mean control | iopamidol | iohexol | iopromide | ioxaglate | diatrizoate | ringer |
|---|---|---|---|---|---|---|---|---|
|  |  | absolute | changes in percent of control values | | | | | |
| $P_{AO}$ (Phase 1) | n | 10 | 12 | 11 | 11 | 12 | 9 | 7 |
|  | x̄ | 124.6 | ./. | ./. | ./. | 87.1 | 89.0 | ./. |
|  | sx | 2.5 | ./. | ./. | ./. | 6.0 | 4.3 | ./. |
| $dP/dt_{max}$ (Phase 1) | n | 10 | 12 | 11 | 11 | 12 | 9 | 7 |
|  | x̄ | 1712 | ./. | ./. | ./. | 76.4 | 78.2 | ./. |
|  | sx | 112 | ./. | ./. | ./. | 4.0 | 7.6 | ./. |
| $P_{LVED}$ (Phase 1) | n | 10 | 12 | 11 | 11 | 12 | 9 | 7 |
|  | x̄ | 8.3 | ./. | ./. | ./. | 152.6 | 146.2 | ./. |
|  | sx | 0.7 | ./. | ./. | ./. | 35.9 | 26.6 | ./. |
| $P_{AO}$ (Phase 2) | n | 10 | 12 | 11 | 11 | 12 | 9 | 7 |
|  | x̄ | 124.6 | 109.2 | 111.4 | 109.7 | 105.6 | 106.8 | 104.6 |
|  | sx | 2.5 | 3.8 | 3.9 | 6.0 | 3.0 | 3.7 | 5.2 |
| $dP/dt_{max}$ (Phase 2) | n | 10 | 12 | 11 | 11 | 12 | 9 | 7 |
|  | x̄ | 1712 | 179.0 | 179.6 | 170.1 | 128.9 | 161.3 | 111.2 |
|  | sx | 112 | 33.0 | 30.3 | 21.0 | 14.4 | 25.2 | 9.1 |
| $P_{LVED}$ (Phase 2) | n | 10 | 12 | 11 | 11 | 12 | 9 | 7 |
|  | x̄ | 8.3 | 62.2 | 64.1 | 68.8 | 83.2 | 78.3 | ./. |
|  | sx | 0.7 | 16.9 | 19.5 | 20.8 | 13.5 | 16.5 | ./. |
| $V_{cor}$ | n | 10 | 12 | 11 | 11 | 12 | 9 | 7 |
|  | x̄ | 67.8 | 264.3 | 263.2 | 253.7 | 267.6 | 296.2 | 190.4 |
|  | sx | 6.4 | 74.5 | 56.3 | 57.9 | 74.9 | 98.8 | 50.6 |

Table 4  Maximum changes of ECG-parameters after contrast injection. Data are calculated in percent of correspondent control values. Mean control values result from averaged control values of the 10 dogs. Changes of PQ- and OT-intervals are related to heart rate. Data are given in 1/min (HR), s (PQ, QRS, QT), and mV ($R_{II}$). ./. = changes of control, values < 1%

|  |  | mean control | iopamidol | iohexol | iopromide | ioxaglate | diatrizoate | ringer |
|---|---|---|---|---|---|---|---|---|
|  |  | absolute | changes in percent of control values | | | | | |
| HR | n | 10 | 8 | 8 | 7 | 8 | 6 | 7 |
|  | x̄ | 78 | ./. | ./. | 101.9 | 108.4 | 104.1 | ./. |
|  | sx | 3.9 | ./. | ./. | 3.3 | 9.4 | 5 | ./. |
| QT | n | 10 | 8 | 8 | 7 | 8 | 6 | 7 |
|  | x̄ | 0.32 | 127.5 | 125.6 | 125.7 | 135.6 | 142.2 | ./. |
|  | sx | 0.01 | 7.2 | 12.4 | 7.2 | 12.4 | 14.9 | ./. |
| QRS | n | 10 | 8 | 8 | 7 | 8 | 6 | 7 |
|  | x̄ | 0.08 | 121.9 | 111.0 | 103.6 | 112.2 | 129.2 | ./. |
|  | sx | 0.01 | 16.2 | 15.4 | 9.4 | 19.4 | 24.6 | ./. |
| PQ | n | 10 | 8 | 8 | 7 | 8 | 6 | 7 |
|  | x̄ | 0.14 | ./. | ./. | ./. | ./. | ./. | ./. |
|  | sx | 0.01 | ./. | ./. | ./. | ./. | ./. | ./. |
| $R_{II}$ | n | 10 | 8 | 8 | 7 | 8 | 6 | 7 |
|  | x̄ | 1.95 | 164.0 | 181.0 | 183.8 | 177.2 | 149.0 | ./. |
|  | sx | 0.01 | 30.5 | 25.2 | 32.3 | 23.5 | 36.5 | ./. |

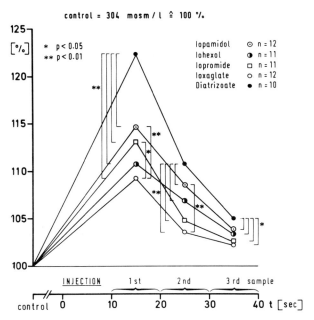

Fig 1 Changes of osmolality in coronary sinus blood after contrast injection. Data are calculated in per cent of corresponding control values. 100% value results from average control values of the 10 dogs

sample, respectively. Difference between ioxaglate and iopromide was significant in the 1st sample ($p < 0.05$). Ringers's solution led to slight but significant ($p < 0,05$) decrease of osmolality in coronary sinus blood.

*Hydrogen-ionic content (Fig 2):* All contrast media led to acidosis after mixing with blood. Correspondingly, significant ($p < 0.01$) increase of hydrogen-ionic concentration was found in all samples after each contrast injection. Diatrizoate caused the most marked effects with significant difference to all other contrast media tested. Between the latter ones no distinction was found. Ringer's solution produced acidosis, too.

*Sodium, potassium, and calcium:* Significant decrease of concentration of sodium, potassium and both, total and ionized calcium in coronary sinus blood occurred after each contrast injection. The degree of these changes was different due to the various injectates. Potassium and total calcium levels were significantly ($p < 0.01$) lower following injection of diatrizoate compared to all other media. Ioxaglate altered sodium values less than diatrizoate, iohexol, iopamidol, and iopromide ($p < 0.01$). Between those nonionic substances there were no significant differences in electrolyte

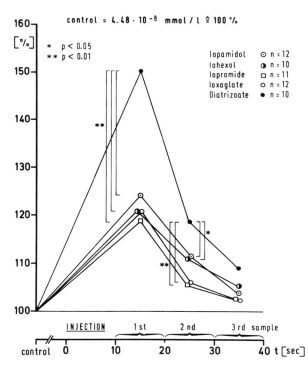

Fig 2 Changes of hydrogen ionic concentration in coronary sinus blood after contrast injection. Data are calculated in per cent of corresponding control values. 100% value results average control value of the 10 dogs

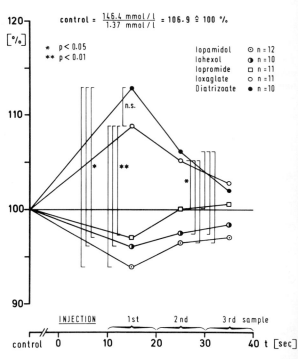

Fig 3 Changes of $Na^+/Ca^{++}$ ratio in coronary sinus blood after contrast injection. Data are calculated in per cent of corresponding control values. 100% value results from average control value of the 10 dogs

Fig 4 Haemodynamic recordings following intracoronary injection of iopamidol ▶

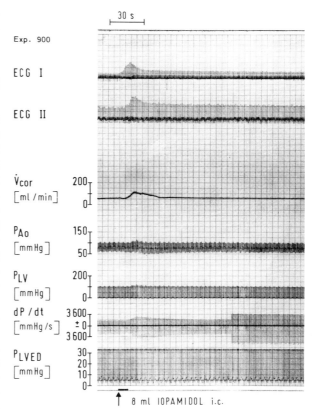

shifts. Ringer's solution caused a slight increase of ionized calcium but did not alter other cations.

*Fraction of ionized calcium ($Ca^{++}/Ca$), ratio between sodium and both total and ionized calcium ($Na^+/Ca$, $Na^+/Ca^{++}$) (Fig 3):* While all agents of low osmolality led to a lower decrease of ionized calicum compared to total calcium, as shown by an increase of the ionized calcium fraction, this fraction was on the average not influenced by diatrizoate. The complex effects of the various contrast media on the electrolyte balance in blood can be shown by means of the $Na^+/Ca^{++}$ ratio. Following non-ionic compounds ionized calcium decrease was of lower degree compared to sodium consequently leading to a slight decrease of $Na^+/Ca^{++}$ ratio. In contrast diatrizoate and ioxaglate led to an increase of this ratio compared to control values, due to a stronger reduction of ionized calcium related to sodium. Differences reached significant levels ($p < 0.05$, $p < 0.01$) in the 1st and 2nd sample respectively. Between diatrizoate and ioxaglate there was no significant distinction as well as between iohexol, iopamidol, and iopromide.

## Haemodynamics

Typical changes of haemodynamic parameters due to low osmolality contrast injection into the LAD are demonstrated in Fig 4–7. Complete data are presented in Table 3 and Fig 8. Ionic compounds, diatrizoate and ioxaglate, influenced haemodynamic parameters in a characteristic biphasic way with primary negative inotropic reaction (phase 1) followed by positive inotropic changes (phase 2). In contrast, following injection of non-ionic contrast media, no negative inotropic reaction was seen and only positive inotropic effects occurred. Negative inotropic reaction lasted from 5th to 10th second after starting injection with maximum degree of changes after 7–8 seconds on an average. Positive inotropic effects appeared 10 seconds after starting injection. The maximum of changes was attained at about the 15th second, and changes disappeared within the first minute.

*Peak velocity of pressure rise ($dP/dt_{max}$) (Fig 8):* Both ioxaglate and diatrizoate caused similar falls

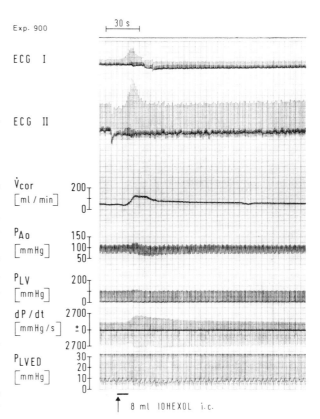

Fig 5 Haemodynamic recordings following intracoronary injection of iohexol ▶

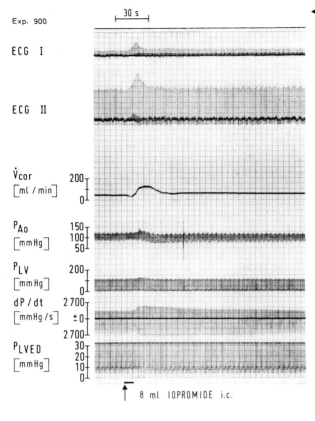

Fig 6 Haemodynamic recordings following intracoronary injection of iopromide

of $dP/dt_{max}$. There was no significant difference between these ionic compounds. After non-ionic contrast media no decrease in $dP/dt_{max}$ was seen. Only peak velocity of pressure fall ($dP/dt_{min}$) was slightly diminished, but this effect did not appear in every case. Increase of $dP/dt_{max}$ following ioxaglate was lower ($p < 0.001$) compared to all non-ionic compounds as well as to diatrizoate ($p < 0.01$). Between iopamidol, iohexol, and iopromide no significant differences were found. Effects caused by diatrizoate were smaller compared to non-ionic contrast media but the difference did not attain significant levels. Ringer's solution also produced an increase of $dP/dt_{max}$.

*Peak systolic aortic pressure ($P_{AO}$):* Initially, changes of aortic pressure paralleled those of $dP/dt_{max}$. Subsequently a fall in aortic pressure was seen due to the peripheral vasodilatative action of all contrast media. Non-ionic compounds produced higher increases of $P_{AO}$ than ioxaglate ($p < 0.05$). Differences between iohexol and diatrizoate reached significant levels as well ($p < 0.05$). Increase of systolic pressure occurred also following injection of Ringer's solution.

*Left ventricular end-diastolic pressure ($P_{LVED}$):* During "phase 1", following ioxaglate and diatrizoate, increase of $P_{LVED}$ was always seen. Fall of $P_{LVED}$ during "phase 2" paralleled the extend of concomitant changes of $dP/dt_{max}$. Ioxaglate produced a less marked fall of $P_{LVED}$ compared to all other agents ($p < 0.05$). Ringer's solution did not change $P_{LVED}$.

*Myocardial blood flow ($\dot{V}_{cor}$):* All contrast media tested led to an increase of coronary blood flow. This effect did last for 1–5 minutes following injections. Strongest effects were seen after diatrizoate but the differences compared to agents of low osmolality did not reach significant levels. Ringer's solution increased $\dot{V}_{cor}$ only a small degree ($p < 0.05$) and this effect disappeared on an average 30 seconds after injection.

## ECG

Changes of ECG parameters are shown in Table 4. All contrast media produced changes in ECG of

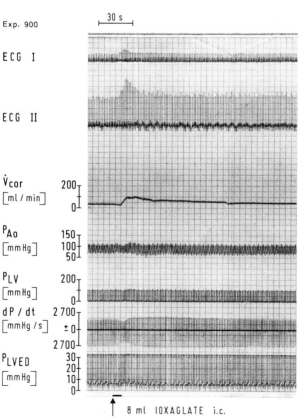

Fig 7 Haemodynamic recordings following intracoronary injection of ioxaglate

the same kind. Maximum effects were commonly seen about 10 seconds after starting contrast injection. Ringer's solution did not alter ECG parameters.

*Heart rate (HR):* HR remained unchanged following injection of iopamidol and iohexol whereas iopromide, ioxaglate, and diatrizoate let to slight acceleration. Difference between ioxaglate and both iopamidol and iohexol was significant (p < 0.05).

*PQ, QRS, and QT intervals:* PQ interval was not influenced by contrast injections on an average, QRS interval was prolonged. Diatrizoate had strongest effects but no significant differences were seen. Ioxaglate and diatrizoate increased QT duration to a greater degree than non-ionic compounds (p < 0.05).

*Height of $R_{II}$:* All agents caused hypervoltage as well as shifting of R and T vectors.

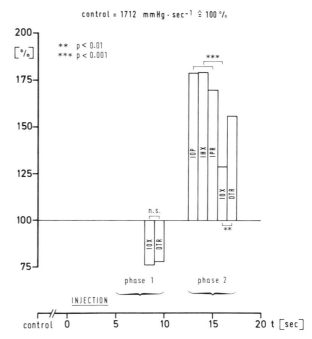

Fig 8 Changes of dP/dt$_{max}$ (left ventricle) during phase 1 and phase 2 after contrast injection. Data are calculated in per cent of corresponding control values. 100% value results from average control value of the 10 dogs. DTR = diatrizoate, IHX = iohexol, IOP = iopamidol, IOX = ioxaglate, IPR = iopromide

## Discussion

Previous investigators have repeatedly pointed out the importance of osmolality and cation content in respect of acute cardiac side effects of contrast media. (6, 18, 25, 27) Consequently, isofonicity in relation to plasma and absence of disturbance of the physiological electrolyte balance in blood should be required of 'ideal' contrast materials. Low-osmolality compounds tested in this study represent marked progress with regard to conventional substances but, depending on the required iodine content, they are still strongly hypertonic compared to blood.

In our experimental model iopamidol, iohexol, and iopromide caused a new type of haemodynamic reaction acting only in a positive inotropic way, different from the alterations after injection of diatrizoate. In contrast, the low osmolality but ionic contrast medium, ioxaglate, initially had a cardiodepressive effect comparable to diatrizoate. These different haemodynamic side effects can be explained by different alterations of physicochemical parameters in blood due to the various contrast media. Contrast injection leads to complex electrolyte shifts due to the dilution of the plasma ions by contrast media themselves, from water shift caused by hyperosmolality, from sodium content, and from calcium chelation of contrast medium. Additionally the fraction of ionized calcium may be altered by acidosis due to hydrogen ionic shifts from red blood cells into the plasma (8, 9, 24). Nevertheless, it must be considered that calibration of the specific ion electrode is influenced by hyperosmolality of blood-contrast mixture. Under in-vitro conditions, this effect can be quantified as an overestimation of ionized calcium values of about 5%. However, under in-vivo conditions, this overestimation cannot be rectified with certainty (unpublished results).

First of all, the imbalance between sodium and calcium ions seems to be a cause of cardiodepressive side effects. The degree of increase of this ratio correlates well with negative inotropic reactions following intracoronary injection of contrast media (8, 9, 23). Due to its sodium content ioxaglate led to an enhanced $Na^+/Ca^{++}$ ratio and produced cardiodepressive effects. Correspondingly, non-ionic low osmolality compounds slightly decreased this quotient and no negative inotropic effects were seen. Non-ionic compounds only led to positive inotropic reactions. This effect seems to be related to a temporary increase in calcium concentration in the heart muscle cells due to osmotic dehydration. This may improve excitation contraction coupling of the heart. The phase-2 positive inotropic reactions after ioxaglate and diatrizoate are based on the same mechanism but are smaller compared to non-ionic contrast media because of initial superposition of cardiodepression (8). In spite of their different chemical constitution the haemodynamic reactions following iopamidol, iohexol, and iopromide were closely comparable. Correspondingly, no significant differences were found with regard to physicochemical properties in coronary sinus blood.

This new type of haemodynamic reactions caused by the intracoronary administration of non-ionic contrast media demonstrates that a reduction of unfavourable properties does not necessarily lead to a reduction of undesirable side effects. Positive inotropism causes increased oxygen demand of the heart. This effect has been discussed as being deleterious under ischemic conditions (16). On the other hand, cardiodepression action reduces coronary perfusion pressure by decreasing the aortic pressure as well as by increasing the left ventricular end-diastolic pressure. This effect may be relevant for post-stenotic areas of the myocardium to a higher degree than an increased oxygen demand due to positive inotropism.

To answer the question whether these experimental findings are applicable to clinical conditions, some aspects of the experimental model have to be discussed. The left ventricular weight of the dogs was strongly comparable to human conditions including the catheterization techniques and the possibility of subselective coronary angiography as well as the injection volume. Furthermore, this experimental model allows estimation of a great number of parameters which cannot be assessed under clinical conditions. In the dog, the area of the myocardium supplied by the LAD closely corresponds to the area drained by the vena cordis magna (5). It can therefore be assumed that alterations of physicochemical properties in the blood were ascertained quantitatively. Repeated injections performed on the same animal are necessary for comparison of contrast media independent of anatomic and functional differences between the various individuals. Premature beats occurred inconsistently after contrast injection. Non-ionic compounds seemed to provoke supraventricular and ventricular extrasystoles a little more frequently than ionic contrast media, but the number of injections was too small for statistical analysis. Premature beats should not only be referred to electrophysiological disturbances. Under these experimental conditions they may also be due to mechanical triggering, e. g. by the tip catheter during reduction of the ventricular volume caused by positive inotropism.

Nevertheless, there is one deviation from clinical experience: After contrast injection, no bradycardia was seen. Previous investigators demonstrated the role of reflectory depression of the sinus node due to hyperosmolality (22). This reflectory bradycardia seems to be suppressed in the anaesthetized organism, in particular under piritramide anaesthesia, which, on the other hand, produces a very stable haemodynamic steady state. Clinical experience has shown that low-osmolality compounds such as metrizamide, ioxaglate, and iopamidol cause bradycardia during coronary angiography, too, but to a lower degree compared to diatrizoate (1, 2, 14, 26, 27). Parallel to this, a slight cardiac depression is seen after these contrast media. This effect seems to be due to a negative-frequency inotropism caused by bradycardia (27). Because no significant differences were seen between iopamidol, iohexol, and iopromide under experimental conditions, it can be assumed that iohexol as well as iopromide will act in the same way as other non-ionic, low-osmolality compounds during clinical coronary angiography.

In view of these considerations it can be concluded that all tested non-ionic compounds should offer a marked reduction of acute cardiac side effects after coronary arteriography in man, compared to commonly used contrast media.

## References

1 Cumberland, D. C.: Amipaque in coronary angiography and left ventriculography. Brit. J. Radiol. 54: 203–206, 1981
2 Cumberland, D. C.: Hexabrix – a new contrast medium in angiocardiography. Brit. Heart J. 45: 698–702, 1981
3 Felder, E. D. Pitrè, P. Tirone: Radiopaque contrast media. XLIV. Pre-clinical studies with a new nonionic contrast agent. Farmaco, Ed. sci. 32: 835–844, 1977
4 Fischer, H. W., K. R. Thomson: Contrast media in coronary arteriography: A review. Invest. Radiol. 13: 450–459, 1978
5 Friesinger, G. C., J. Schaefer, R. A. Gaertner, R. S. Ross: Coronary sinus drainage and measurement of left coronary artery flow in dogs. Amer. J. Physiol. 206: 57–62, 1964
6 Grainger, R. G.: Formulation and clinical introduction of low-osmolality contrast media. Radiologe 21: 261–267, 1981
7 Haavaldsen, J.: Iohexol. Acta radiol. (Stockh.) Suppl. 362: 9–11, 1980
8 Hellige, G.: Elektrolytverschiebungen durch Röntgenkontrastmittel und ihre Rückwirkungen auf die Funktion des Herzens. In Weikl, A., E. Lang: Kontrastmittel in der Kardiologie. Steinkopff, Darmstadt 1981 (S. 35–51)

# References

9 Hellige, G., D. Baller, A. Hoeft, H. Korb, H. G. Wolpers, J. Zipfel: The importance of electrolyte shifts and calcium binding on cardiotoxicity of contrast media. In Amiel, M., J. F. Moreau: Contrast Media in Radiology – Estimate and Future. Springer, Berlin (S. 80–83) 1982

10 Hensel, I., H. J. Bretschneider: Pitot-Rohr-Katheter für die fortlaufende Messung der Koronar- und Nierendurchblutung im Tierexperiment. Arch. Kreisl.-Forsch. 62: 249–292, 1970

11 Higgins, C. B.: Overview and methods used for the study of the cardiovascular actions of contrast materials. Invest. Radiol. 15: 188–193, 1980

12 Higgins, C. B., W. Schmidt: Direct and reflex myocardial effects of intracoronary administered contrast materials in the anaesthetized and conscious dog: Comparison of standard and newer contrast materials. Invest. Radiol. 13: 205–216, 1978

13 Kettler, D., V. Braun, L. A. Cott, H. W. Heiss, I. Hensel, J. Martel, K. Paschen, H. J. Bretschneider: Kombination von Piritramid und $N_2O$ – ein neues Narkoseverfahren. Teil I: Tierexperimentelle Untersuchungen. Z. prakt. Anästh. Wiederbeleb. 6: 329–336, 1971

14 Partridge, J. B., P. J. Robinson, C. M. Turnbull, J. B. Stroker, R. M. Boyle, G. W. Morrison: Clinical cardiovascular experiences with iopamidol: An new non-ionic contrast medium. Clin. Radiol. 32: 451–455, 1981

15 Prennschütz-Schützenau, H., H. Sigmund-Duchanova, G. Hellige: Analysis of physicochemical parameters on cardiac effects of contrast media. Pflügers Arch. ges. Physiol. Suppl. R 19: 1978

16 Speck, V., G. Mannesmann, W. Mützel, G. Schröder: Preliminary evaluation of new non-ionic contrast media. In Donner, M. W., F. H. W. Heuck: Radiology Today. Springer, Berlin 1981 (pp. 45–49)

17 Thomson, K. R., M. R. Violante, T. Kenyon, H. W. Fischer: Reduction in ventricular fibrillation using calcium-enriched Renografin 76. Invest. Radiol. 13: 238–240, 1978

18 Thomson, K. R., C. A. Evill, J. Fritzsche, G. T. Benness: Comparison of iopamidol, ioxaglate and diatrizoate during coronary arteriography in dogs. Invest. Radiol. 15: 234–241, 1980

19 Trägardh, B.: Coronary angiography with iohexol and other contrast media in the dog. I. Electrocardiographic alteration. Acta radiol. (Stockh.) Suppl. 362: 17–20, 1980

20 Trägardh, B.: Coronary angiography with iohexol and other contrast media in the dog. II. Left ventricular contractility and work. Acta radiol. (Stockh.) Suppl. 362: 21–24, 1980

21 Träghardh, B., C. G. Cederlund: Coronary angiography with iohexol and other contrast media in the dog. III. Contractility of the left ventricle. Acta radiol (Stockh.) Suppl. 362: 25–27, 1980

22 Vogt, A., K. L. Neuhaus, H. dal Ri, G. Schmidt, H. Kreuzer: Reflektorische Kardiodepression durch Röntgenkontrastmittel. In Weikl, A., E. Lang: Kontrastmittel in der Kardiologie. Steinkopff, Darmstadt 1981 (S. 172–176)

23 Wolpers, H. G., D. Baller, F. B. M. Ensink, W. Schröter, J. Zipfel, G. Hellige: Influences of arteriographic contrast media on the $Na^+/Ca^{++}$-ratio in blood. Cardiovasc. Intervent. Radiol. 4: 8–13, 1981

24 Wolpers, H. G., D. Baller, F. B. M. Ensink, A. Hoeft, H. Korb, G. Hellige: Einfluß von Röntgenkontrastmitteln auf das Membranpotential am schlagenden Herzen. Z. Kardiol. 71: 82–86, 1982

25 Zipfel, J., D. Baller, H. Blanke, K. R. Karsch, P. Rentrop, G. Hellige: Decrease in cardiotoxicity of contrast media in coronary angiography by addition of calcium ions: A combined experimental and clinical study. Clin. Cardiol. 3: 178–183, 1980

26 Zipfel, J., D. Baller, H. Blanke, K. R. Karsch, H. G. Wolpers, G. Hellige, P. Rentrop: Koronarangiographie im chronischen und akuten Stadium der koronaren Herzkrankheit. Vorteile eines niederosmolaren Kontrastmittels. Z. Kardiol. 71: 576–580, 1982

27 Zipfel, J., D. Baller, H. Blanke, K. R. Karsch, P. Rentrop, V. W. Wiegand, H. G. Wolpers, G. Hellige: Reduktion kardialer Nebenwirkungen von Röntgenkontrastmitteln in der Angiokardiographie durch Zusatz von Kalzium und Verwendung eines nichtionischen Kontrastmittels. Klin. Wschr. 58: 1339–1346, 1980

# Haemodynamic Side Effects of Meglumine Ioglicate, Meglumine Sodium Ioxaglate and Iohexol in Aortofemoral Angiography: Comparison of a High-osmolar and Two Low-osmolar Radiological Contrast Media

V. Wiebe and H. Straub

## Summary

The haemodynamic side effects of the high-osmolar ionic contrast medium ioglicate, the low-osmolar ionic ioxaglate and the low-osmolar non-ionic iohexol were compared in 60 aortofemoral angiographies. Ioxaglate and iohexol do not differ regarding their haemodynamic side effects. Their hypotensive effect is significantly lower than that of ioglicate, and they cause a rise of blood pressure in some patients. They also increase the heart rate to a lesser extent, and even lower it in some cases, although the difference from ioglicate is not significant.

Overall, the low-osmolar substances are better tolerated haemodynamically, but even they may cause considerable side effects in pre-existing cardiovascular disease.

## Zusammenfassung

Anhand von 60 Beckenbeinangiographien wurden die hämodynamischen Nebenwirkungen des hochosmolaren ionischen Röntgenkontrastmittels Ioglicinat, des niederosmolaren ionischen Ioxaglats und des niederosmolaren nicht-ionischen Iohexols miteinander verglichen. Ioxaglat und Iohexol unterscheiden sich untereinander hinsichtlich ihrer hämodynamischen Nebenwirkungen nicht. Sie haben eine signifikant geringere blutdrucksenkende Wirkung als Ioglicinat und verursachen bei einem Teil der Patienten eine Blutdrucksteigerung. Sie bewirken weiterhin eine geringere Steigerung der Herzfrequenz, teilweise sogar eine Frequenzsenkung. Dieser Unterschied gegenüber Ioglicinat ist jedoch nicht signifikant. Insgesamt erweisen sich die niederosmolaren Substanzen als hämodynamisch besser verträglich. Bei vorbestehenden kardiovaskulären Erkrankungen können aber auch sie erhebliche Nebenwirkungen haben.

## Introduction

Owing to the production of non-toxic, water-soluble but high-osmolar tri-iodinated contrast media, which are now regarded as classical, angiography of all regions of the body developed into routine clinical procedures. Aortofemoral angiography is a particularly common examination. If classical contrast media are used for this procedure, intensive vascular pain is the most unpleasant immediate side effect, which can only be reduced by the addition of a local anaesthetic or eliminated by general anaesthesia. However, it is the concomitant haemodynamic effects of classical contrast media, which place the patient at risk, particularly because most of the patients are elderly and liable to have additional cardiac and vascular disease beside the aortofemoral region. Over the last 10 years, low-osmolar substances, which are chemically very similar to the classical contrast media, have been developed with the object of reducing the side effects. Under conditions of routine clinical aortofemoral angiography, we compared firstly the haemodynamic side effects of the high-osmolar compound meglumine ioglicate (Rayvist, Schering) with those of the low-osmolar substance meglumine sodium ioxaglate (Hexabrix, Guerbet) and, secondly, the haemodynamic side effects of meglumine sodium ioxaglate with those of the low-osmolar compound iohexol (Nyegaard/Schering/Winthrop) to establish, whether the tolerance of low-osmolar contrast media is better from a haemodynamic standpoint. A local anaesthetic was added to meglumine ioglicate to reduce the pain.

## Patients and Methods

We studied 30 non-premedicated patients with a mean age of 64 years, who were suffering from arterial occlusive disease of the lower extremities. Each patient underwent aortofemoral angiography twice at an interval of 15 to 25 minutes, the only difference in the two examinations being the contrast medium used (paired trial design).

The following contrast media were used in a random sequence unknown to either the patient or the examiner (double-blind procedure):

a) Meglumine ioglicate (total amount 80 ml including 5 ml lidocaine 2%, iodine content 280 mg/ml, osmolality 1.69 osm/kg H$_2$O)
b) Meglumine sodium ioxaglate (total amount 80 ml, iodine content 320 mg/ml, osmolality 0.60 osm/kg H$_2$O)
c) Iohexol (total amount 80 ml, iodine content 300 mg/ml, osmolality 0.69 osm/kg H$_2$O)

The chemical structures of the contrast media studied are shown in Fig 1.

A total of 60 aortofemoral angiograms with the following distribution were obtained: 30 with ioglicate and ioxaglate in 15 patients (first paired group), and 30 with iohexol and ioxaglate in 15 patients (second paired group).

After local anaesthesia of the inguinal region, the tip of a pigtail catheter was placed 3 cm proximal of the aortic bifurcation using Seldinger's method. The contrast medium was injected mechanically through the catheter at a rate of 10 ml/second. The arterial blood pressure was recorded continuously via the angiography catheter with the exception of 15 seconds immediately before, during and after the injection. The heart rate was recorded by continuous electrocardiography.

There was no significant difference between the mean initial systolic blood pressures of the two groups. The individual maximum changes of the systolic blood pressure and heart rate after contrast medium injection, calculated as percentage of the respective initial values of each patient, were classified in steps of 10%. The changes of blood pressure and heart rate occurring within the paired groups after injection of the one and then the other contrast medium were then compared.

The mean percental changes of the haemodynamic parameters of the two groups werde described in their temporal course from the end of the injection to 120 seconds after the end of the injection and tested for statistically significant differences using the Wilcoxon test for paired differences with 2-sided questioning. Since one of the three contrast media studied (meglumine sodium ioxaglate) was used in both groups, comparison of all three substances was possible.

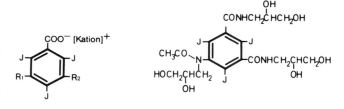

Fig 1 Chemical structure of the contrast media used. Top left: Basic structure of high-osmolar contrast media (ioglicate R$_1$ = –NH–CO–CH$_3$  R$_2$ = CO–NH–CH$_2$–CO–NH–CH$_3$). Top right: Iohexol. Bottom: Ioxaglate

## Results

### First Paired Group: Meglumine Ioglicate and Meglumine Sodium Ioxaglate

The systolic blood pressure fell in all patients after injection of ioglicate. Classification of the individual blood pressure changes showed, that the pressure fell by 8% in one patient, by 10–19% in 8 patients, by 20–29% in 3 patients and by 30–39% in 3 patients. After injection of ioxaglate, the blood pressure fell in 8 patients, remainded the same in one and increased in 6 patients. Individually, the blood pressure rose by 14% in one patient and by 1–10% in 5 patientes. It fell by 1–9% in 5 patients and by 10–19% in 3. Fig 2 shows this distribution of

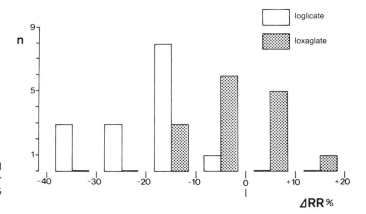

Fig 2 Individual maximum changes in the blood pressure as a percentage of the initial values after paired injection of ioglicate and ioxaglate in n = 15 patients

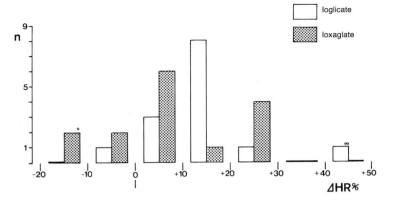

Fig 3  Individual maximum changes in the heart rate as a percentage of the initial values after paired injection of ioglicate and ioxaglate in n = 15 patients.
0 = 2nd degree AV Block/frequent ventricular extrasystoles
00 = absolute arrhythmia

the individual maximum changes of systolic blood pressure as a percentage of the initial values after injection of ioglicate and ioxaglate.

After injection of ioglicate, the heart rate remained the same in one case and increased in all the others: it rose by 1–10% in 4 patients, by 11–20% in 8 and by 22% in one patient. In another patient with absolute arrhythmia, the increase was 41%. After ioxaglate, the heart rate fell by 19% in one patient with an atrioventricular block, by 10% in a patient with frequent supraventricular extrasystoles and by 3% in a patient without cardiac symptoms. There was no change of heart rate in one patient. It increased by 1–10% in 6 patients, by 11–20% in one and by 21–30% in 4. Fig 3 shows this distribution of the individual maximum changes of heart rate as a percentage of the initial values after injection of ioglicate and ioxaglate. After injection of ioglicate, the mean systolic blood pressure of the first paired group fell within 30 seconds to a minimum of 79% of the initial value, before increasing again to 94% of the initial pressure after 120 seconds. During the same period, the heart rate increased to a maximum of 11% above the initial rate after 30 seconds before falling again, although it was still 6% above the initial value after 120 seconds. After ioxaglate, the mean blood pressure increased by 3% after 15 seconds, but had reached the initial pressure again after only 30 seconds. The heart rate after ioxaglate reached a maximum of 13% above the initial value after 60 seconds before falling again. However, the increase was still 7% after 120 seconds. The difference between the mean changes of systolic blood pressure after ioglicate and ioxaglate is statistically significant ($p < 0.05$), but the difference between the changes in the heart rate is not. Fig 4 shows the course of the mean percental changes of heart rate and systolic blood pressure in the first paired group after the end of the injection of ioglicate and ioxaglate.

## Second Paired Group: Meglumine Sodium Ioxaglate and Iohexol

The extent and distribution of the individual maximum blood pressure changes after ioxaglate were similar to those observed in the first paired group: 4 patients displayed an increase of 1–10%, 8 patients a decrease of 1–9% and 3 patients a decrease of 10–19%. After iohexol, the blood pressure increased in 7 patients, remained the same in one and fell in 7 patients. The increase was 11–20% in 2 patients and 1–10% in 5, while the decrease was up to 9% in 6 patients and 12% in one. Fig 5 shows this

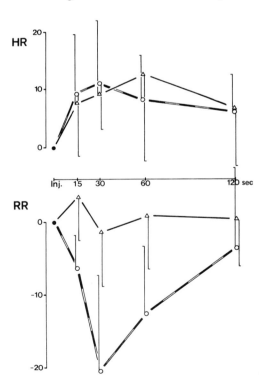

Fig 4  Mean percental changes of the heart rate (HR) and systolic blood pressure (RR) after paired injection of ioglicate (0———0) and ioxaglate (△———△) in n = 15 patients

distribution of the individual maximum changes of blood pressure as a percentage of the initial values after injection of ioxaglate and iohexol. The change of the heart rate after ioxaglate was equal in the second and in the first group too. The rate increased by 29% in one patient; in 5 cases it increased by 11–20% and in another 5 by 1–10%. The heart rate fell by 1–9% in 3 patients. One patient with contrast medium-induced nausea had a 23% decrease of the heart rate. After iohexol, 3 patients had a decrease of the heart rate of up to 9%. The rate remained the same in one patient, while it increased by 1–10% in 8 patients, by 11% in one and by 21–30% in 2. Fig 6 shows the distribution of the individual percental changes in the heart rate after ioxaglate and iohexol. In the second group, the mean blood pressure after ioxaglate fell to a minimum of 97% in 30 seconds and had reached the initial value again after 120 seconds. No mean change in the blood pressure could be determined after iohexol. After ioxaglate, the mean rate increased to a maximum of 9% in 30 seconds, and then fell again to the range of the initial value. The change in the rate after iohexol was almost identical: It increased to a maximum of 8% in 30 seconds, and then fell again to the initial range. The course of the mean percental changes of the systolic blood pressure and heart rate in the second paired group after the end of the injection of ioxaglate and iohexol is shown in Fig 7.

The differences between the changes of blood pressure and heart rate after ioxaglate and iohexol are not statistically significant.

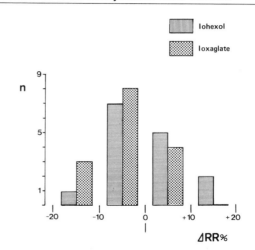

Fig 5   Individual maximum changes in the blood pressure as a percentage of the initial values after paired injection of ioxaglate and iohexol in n = 15 patients

## Discussion

The osmolality of the so-called classical water-soluble contrast media in concentrations used for angiography is at least 5 times that of human blood. The marked vasodilatory effect of these agents on the arteries of the extremeties and skeletal muscles is in direct proportion to their osmolality (9). This vasodilatory effect can be measured both experimentally and clinically by the increase of blood flow, which they cause. Using venous occlusion plethysmography under clinical conditions, Delius

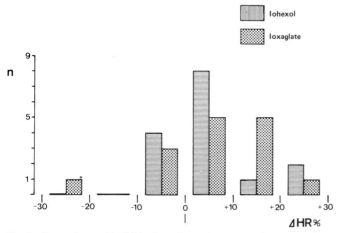

Fig 6   Percentage of individual maximum heart rate changes, calculated on the initial values after paired injection of ioxaglate and iohexol in n = 15 patients.
0 = contrast agent reaction

Fig 7   Average percentage change in heart rate (HR) and systolic ▶ blood pressure (RR) after paired injection of ioxaglate (△———△) and iohexol (□———□) in n = 15 patients

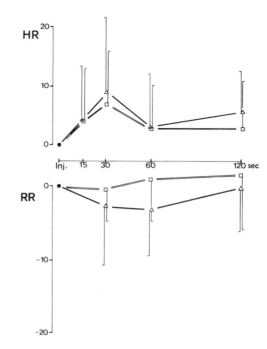

and Erikson (2) studied the changes of the arterial blood flow, which high-osmolar contrast media cause in the lower extremities during aortofemoral angiography. On injection of 30 ml contrast medium in 1.5 seconds, they observed, that the blood flow was increased by the factor 2. The increase began about 30 seconds after the injection, reached its maximum after 60 seconds and ended after 120 seconds. Boijsen et al. (1) observed a similar increase in the blood flow under almost identical conditions. It was less pronounced and lasted longer in extremities with occlusion of the main artery. Hence, classical contrast media exert their vasodilatory effect under the clinical conditions of aortofemoral angiography in man as well. Parallel in time to the increase of blood flow, the patients in the study of Delius and Erikson (2) showed a 25% mean decrease of systolic and a 13% mean decrease of diastolic blood pressure, while the heart rate increased by 20%. As several other studies demonstrate (1, 7, 17), a decrease in blood pressure of this magnitude invariably occurs during aortofemoral angiography with high-osmolar contrast media.

It is generally regarded as a consequence of the decrease in peripheral resistance caused by contrast medium-induced vasodilation (5).

Even without simultaneous flow measurements, the systemic blood pressure is therefore regarded as a parameter for the vasodilatory side effect of contrast media, while the extent of the decrease also depends on the initial pressure (17). In turn, a simultaneous increase of heart rate is usually interpreted as a baroreceptor-controlled reflectory effect of the fall in the blood pressure.

After injection of ioglicate in high dose and low injection rate and with the addition of lidocaine to reduce the pain, our patients showed a decrease of systolic blood pressure, the extent and temporal course of which agreed exactly with the data for other high-osmolar contrast media reported in the literature. This means, that ioglicate, too, has the usual, clinically relevant vasodilatory effect of classical contrast media and can therefore be used as a reference substance for the study of low-osmolar contrast media. The hypotensive effect of ioglicate with lidocaine does not correlate with the angiographic pain or with the sensation of heat (15), as suggested by some authors for high-osmolar contrast media (5). Basing on experimental injections in models and animal studies, Schröder et al. (14) divided the haemodynamic effects of classical contrast media into three phases: During the first phase, which covers the period of the injection, the transmission of kinetic energy from the contrast medium to the contents of the vessel leads to an increase of flow and pressure, when catheters with a hole at the tip are used. However, the increase is much less pronounced with side-hole catheters as used by us. During the second phase, a decrease in the rate of flow occurs. It has its maximum about 5–10 seconds after the start of the injection and is caused by the viscosity of the contrast medium bolus, which is higher than that of the blood. We were unable to record this phase of the haemodynamic side effects of the contrast media because of the design of our study, but it had been previously demonstrated by Delius and Erikson (2) and by Boijsen et al. (1) in some of their patients. The third phase is that of the previously described dilatation-induced increase of flow.

Low-osmolar contrast media have a slight vasodilatory effect in animal studies (11). The osmolality of meglumine sodium ioxaglate and iohexol is twice and two and two thirds that of blood respectively. In our studies, neither ioxaglate nor iohexol, when administered in aortofemoral angiography, brought about a mean change of blood pressure, which exceeded the physiological range of fluctuation. The hypotensive effect of the low-osmolar compound ioxaglate is significantly less than that of the high-osmolar substance ioglicate. Iohexol, another low-osmolar compound, reduces blood pressure just as little. As was to be expected, low-osmolar contrast media have an only slight effect on the blood pressure. Holm and Praestholm (7), Zachrisson et al. (18), Walter et al. (16) and Dewitz et al. (4) obtained similar results in aortofemoral angiography with low-osmolar substances.

The individual maximum blood pressure changes after ioxaglate and iohexol in a third of the patients consisted of a 1–20% increase of pressure. We consider it possible, that the injection led to other direct contrast medium effects as a result of the abolition of peripheral vasodilation: Firstly, Mann and Zeitler have demonstrated transient hyperosmolality of the blood during angiography with larger amounts of contrast medium (10), a reaction, which must lead to hypervolaemia. Secondly, an increase of cardiac output has been observed by Jehle et al. (8) after intracardial injection of contrast material in animal experiments, and by Denkhaus et al. (3) after intra-aortic injection in man.

We observed a mean increase in the heart rate of 11% following aortofemoral angiography with ioglicate plus lidocaine. This increase is less than the 20% reported by Delius and Erikson (2) for other high-osmolar contrast media without a local anaesthetic. We are unable to offer an explanation for this difference in the results. At the dose at which it is added to the contrast agent, lidocaine is unlikely to reduce the heart rate (12). It is also improbable, that ioglicate directly lowers the heart rate: Hahn et al. (6) failed to observe any effect on the heart rate after intracardial injection of ioglicate in animal experiments.

After injection of the low-osmolar compounds ioxaglate and iohexol, the heart rate in our patients increased by an average of 13 respectively 9% and of 8%. The difference between ioxaglate and the high-osmolar substance ioglicate is not significant. The two low-osmolar substances equally increased the heart rate and more so than observed by other authors (7, 16). According to Holm and Praestholm (7), the increase brought about by ioxaglate is significantly lower than that caused by a high-osmolar contrast medium. Our study still shows that ioxaglate and iohexol – unlike ioglicate – mostly caused a less than 10% maximal increase of heart rate, and that it remained the same or fell slightly in some. Summarizing our results, therefore, shows that the tolerance of low-osmolar contrast media in aortofemoral angiography is clearly better than that of high-osmolar substances regarding their effect on the blood pressure, but to a lesser degree regarding their effect on the heart rate.

Overall, the haemodynamic tolerance of low-osmolar contrast media in aortofemoral angiography is definitely better than that of high-osmolar substances. In individual cases, however, the side effects of both high- and low-osmolar contrast media can accentuate the symptoms of pre-existing cardiovascular diseases in an unpredictable manner. In our study, the injection of ioglicate in a patient with absolute arrhythmia brought about an increase of the heart rate of 41%, compared to 25% after ioxaglate. In another patient with a 2nd degree atrioventricular block, ioxaglate caused a 19% decrease in the heart rate, while ioglicate led to a 28% decrease in the blood pressure. In yet another patient with frequent supraventricular extrasystoles, the blood pressure fell by 18% after both ioglicate and ioxaglate, while the heart rate increased by 10% after ioglicate and fell by 10% after ioxaglate. High-risk patients, therefore, still require careful supervision even if low-osmolar contrast media are used for aortofemoral angiography.

## References

1 Boijsen, E., J. Dahm, T. Hallböök: Hemodynamic effect of contrast medium in arteriography of legs. Acta radiol. (Stockh.) 11: 295–309, 1971
2 Delius, W., U. Erikson: Effect of contrast medium on blood flow and blood pressure in lower extremities. Amer. J. Roentgenol. 152: 869–876, 1969
3 Denkhaus, H., G. Pohlen, J. Timmermann, E. Löhr, V. Sadony, M. David: Veränderungen hämodynamischer Parameter bei peripherer Angiographie. In Müller-Wiefel, H., J.-P. Barras, H. Ehringer, M. Krüger: Mikrozirkulation und Blutrheologie. Therapie der peripheren arteriellen Verschlußkrankheit. Witzstrock, Baden-Baden 1980 (S. 498–503)
4 Von Dewitz, H., M. Langer, R. Langer, W. Th. Glöckler: Verträglichkeit des Kontrastmittels Joxaglinsäure bei angiographischen Untersuchungen. Eine klinische Studie. Röntgen-Bl. 33: 525–528, 1980
5 Grainger, R. G.: Osmolality of intravascular radiological contrast media. Brit. J. Radiol. 53: 739–746, 1980
6 Hahn, N., B. Raqué, J. Schuppert, J. Schmidt, J. Mählmann, N. Logemann, E. Potthoff, R. Pantenburg, D. Stiemert, T. Siering, V. Steinijans, E. Diletti, R. Felix: Contrast media-induced side effects on excitation and conduction of electrical activity in the heart on intracardial application. Investigations in anaesthetized dogs. Europ. J. Radiol. 1: 270–277, 1981
7 Holm, M., J. Praestholm: Ioxaglate, a new low osmolar contrast medium used in femoral angiography. Brit. J. Radiol. 52: 169–172, 1979
8 Jehle, J., J. Köhler, K. L. Neuhaus, R. Pehle, H. Rose, P. Spiller, F. K. Schmiel; Tierexperimentelle Untersuchungen zur Hämodynamik des linken Ventrikels vor, während und nach Kontrastmittelinjektion. In Weikl, A., E. Lang: Kontrastmittel in der Kardiologie. Steinkopff, Darmstadt, 1981 (S. 101–107)
9 Lindgren, P.: Hemodynamic responses to contrast media Invest. Radiol. 5: 424–435, 1970
10 Mann, S., E. Zeitler: Verhalten der Serumosmolarität bei hohen Kontrastmitteldosen im Rahmen der Angiographie. Fortschr. Röntgenstr. 122: 135–137, 1975
11 Nymann, U., T. Almen, M. Landtman: Effect of contrast media on femoral blood flow. Comparison between nonionic and ionic monomeric and monoacidic dimeric contrast media in the dog. Acta radiol. (Stockh.) Suppl. 362: 43–48, 1980
12 Runge, M.: Lidocain als antiarrhythmische Substanz. Med. Welt 23: 928–930, 1972
13 Schmidt, K. R., K. J. Pfeifer, H. Welter, H. Ingrisch, G. Heyde; Untersuchungen zur Schmerzverminderung bei der Extremitätenangiographie. Fortschr. Röntgenstr. 130: 200–204, 1979
14 Schröder, J., H. Keller, B. Terwey, U. Mittmann: Hämodynamische Effekte der intraarteriellen Kontrastmittelinjektion. Fortschr. Röntgenstr. 135: 143–151, 1981
15 Straub, H., V. Wiebe: Verminderung von Nebenwirkungen bei der Beckenbeinangiographie: Niederosmolares Kontrastmittel im Vergleich mit konventionellem Kontrastmittel plus Lokalanästhetikum. Röntgen-Bl. 34: 139–142, 1981

16 Walter, E., K.-J. Wolf, R. Hippeli, P. Ostendorf: Metrizamid und Megluminamidotrizoat zur retrograden Beinarteriographie. Eine klinisch-radiologisch-laborchemische Vergleichsstudie. In Frommhold, W., H. Hacker, H. E. Schmitt, H. Vogelsang: Amipaque Workshop. Excerpta Media, Amsterdam 1978 (pp. 144–150)

17 Wenz, W.: Abdominale Angiographie. Springer, Berlin 1972 (S. 22)

18 Zachrisson, B.-F., R. Johansson, L. Björk: Two new contrast media in peripheral arteriography. A double blind study in patients with arterial insufficiency in the legs. Fortschr. Röntgenstr. 132: 208–211, 1980

# Pharmacokinetics

## Pharmacokinetics of Iopromide in Rat and Dog

W. Mützel, U. Speck and H.-J. Weinmann

## Summary

After oral or intraduodenal administration of $^{125}$I-labelled iopromide to rats less than 2 per cent of the dose is absorbed. The distribution and excretion of iopromide in the rat after intravenous injection is independent of the dose given, about 90 per cent of the dose being excreted via the kidneys with a half-life of 20 min. No metabolism occurred in the rat.

In dogs the compound is distributed in the extravascular space with a half-life of only about 8 min, the elimination half-life being about 45 min. 94 ± 6 per cent of the dose was found in urine and 2 ± 1 per cent in faeces within seven days after intravenous injection. Iopromide is apparently not metabolized in the dog either. The pharmacokinetic characteristics of iopromide in laboratory animals are very similar to those of other non-ionic contrast media, i. e., metrizamide and iopamidol.

## Zusammenfassung

Iopromid wird nach peroraler bzw. intraduodenaler Verabreichung an Ratten zu weniger als 2% resorbiert. Verteilung und Ausscheidung von Iopromid sind nach intravenöser Injektion an Ratten dosisunabhängig, wobei jeweils etwa 90% der Dosis mit einer Halbwertszeit von etwa 20 min renal ausgeschieden werden. Eine Metabolisierung von Iopromid war bei Ratten nicht nachzuweisen.

Bei Hunden verteilt sich die Verbindung mit einer Halbwertszeit von 8 min ausschließlich extravaskulär. Die Eliminationshalbwertszeit liegt bei 45 min. Im Urin sind bis sieben Tage nach intravenöser Injektion 94 ± 6% und in den Faeces 2 ± 1% der verabreichten Dosis wiedergefunden worden. Iopromid wird offenbar auch vom Hund nicht metabolisiert. Die pharmakokinetische Charakteristik von Iopromid bei Versuchstieren ist sehr ähnlich derjenigen anderer nichtionischer Röntgenkontrastmittel wie Metrizamid und Iopamidol.

## Introduction

Iopromide is a non-ionic water-soluble contrast agent recently developed by Schering, Berlin, mainly for vascular radiography. The compound exhibits very good tolerance in test animals (8, 12). With reference to the majority of pharmacological-toxicological experiments conducted in rats and dogs, studies on the pharmacokinetics in these species are of basic interest to clarify the fate of the compound in the living organism.

Rats were exposed to $^{125}$I-labelled iopromide by intravenous, intraduodenal and oral administration in order to establish the main route of excretion, the extent of absorption and possible dose-dependent organ affinity. Blood level and excretion rates were also investigated in dogs after single intravenous injection of $^{125}$I-iopromide. Studies on potential metabolism of iopromide in the two species were included.

## Material and Methods

### Experiments in the Rat

$^{125}$I-labelled iopromide (Schering, Berlin) was injected once into a tail vein in male rats (90–170 g, SPF Wistar strain) at a dose of 60 mg I/kg body weight in the form of an aqueous solution containing 12 mg I/ml (specific activity: 5.6 kBq/mg I). The blood level of $^{125}$I was monitored at 5 min and 30 min after injection (5 animals), and biliary and urinary excretion were monitored up to 3 h after injection (10 animals respectively, acute biliary fistula in one group).

Another group of 10 animals received an aqueous solution of $^{125}$I-labelled iopromide orally at the same dose level. The absorption of the compound was analysed by measuring the $^{125}$I urinary excretion rates up to 4 h after administration.

Biliary excretion rates were evaluated in another group of 10 animals for 4 h after intraduodenal administration of an aqueous solution of $^{125}$I-labelled iopromide.

Urinary and faecal excretion rates were determined after intravenous injection of 60 mg I/kg body weight (24 h, 10 rats), 1 and 10 g I/kg body weight (7 days, 5 and 3 rats per dosage). The radioactive dose per animal was about 30–100 kBq as $^{125}$I-labelled iopromide. The animals were anaesthetized and sacrificed by exsanguination from the vena cava 24 h and 7 days after the injection, respectively.

$^{125}$I-activity was determined in the blood, liver, kidney, muscle, thyroid gland, pancreas, gastrointestinal tract and the remaining parts of the body using an Auto-Gamma-Scintillation spectrometer Model 5285 (Packard Instr., Ill.). Aliquots of the injected solutions were used as references for all determinations and calculations. The data were evaluated by the computer system Honeywell-Bull CHB 66/40.

Biotransformation analysis in urine and bile (24-h pool) after intravenous injection of 60 mg I/kg into female rats (140–160 g, n = 3, acute biliary fistulae) was conducted by thin-layer chromatography (TLC) and high-pressure liquid chromatography (HPLC). The $^{125}$I-labelled compound (spec. activity 20 kBq/mg I) was purified before injection in the rat only for this experiment by means of HPLC.

TLC was performed by applying 20 to 50 µl of unpurified fresh urine in streaks 3.5 cm wide to TLC plates precoated with silica gel 60 $F_{254}$ (Merck). Samples of the solution injected were also applied for reference. The plates were developed in two solvent systems:

System I:   dioxane/water/ammonia 25%
            80 : 7.5 : 1.0 (v/v/v)
System II:  n-butanol/ethanol/ammonia 25%/water
            11 : 1 : 2 : 1 (v/v/v/v)

Activity measurements on TLC plates were made directly using the Thin-Layer Scanner II (Berthold und Friesecke, Wildbad), equipped with a windowless 2-pi Geiger detector.

HPLC was conducted by applying 5 to 20 µl of untreated, fresh urine and of the solution injected (as reference) to reversedphase HPLC columns (precolumn: length 2 cm, internal diameter 4.7 mm, LiChrosorb RP 2, Merck; analytical column: length 50 cm, internal diameter 4.7 mm, LiChrosorb RP 8,5 µm, Merck) using methanol/water 15 : 100 (v/v) as eluant (flow rate 1.0 ml/min; pump: FR-30, Knauer, Berlin). UV absorbance of the constituents separated was continuously monitored at 238 nm (UV spectrophotometer by Knauer, Berlin, connected to a Hewlett Packard 3380 A integrator). In addition, 0.5-min fractions of the eluant were measured for activity by gamma scintillation counting.

## Experiments in the Dog

Three female beagle dogs (weight 8.6–9.6 kg) received single intravenous doses of 600 mg I/kg body weight of $^{125}$I-labelled iopromide in aqueous solution (specific activity: 140–690 Bq/mg I). Plasma levels of $^{125}$I were monitored for seven days after injection. In order to examine the excretion rates urine and faeces were quantitatively collected (metabolic cages) for seven days after injection ($^{125}$I-measurements as mentioned). Samples of urine (15–30 min and 60–90 min after injection) were analysed for radioactive constituents by means of TLC and HPLC in order to obtain information on the metabolic fate of iopromide. The computer system Honeywell Bull CHB 66/40 and its special pharmacokinetic programmes for open two-compartment models were used to evaluate the data.

Table 1  Blood level and excretion after intravenous, oral and intraduodenal injection in male rats. 60 mg I/kg body weight. Data given in per cent of dose administered in total blood volume or in fractions collected (mean value ± SD)

| no. of animals | | 5 | 10 | 10 | 10 | 10 |
|---|---|---|---|---|---|---|
| weight | | 160 | 100 | 150 | 100 | 150 |
| administration | | intravenous | intravenous | intravenous | oral | intraduodenal |
| measurement | | blood | urine | bile | urine | bile |
| – | 5 min | 13.37±0.92 | | | | |
| – | 30 min | 4.79±1.02 | 64.05±7.04 | 1.70±1.23 | | 0.01±0.01 |
| 1 h | – | | 10.68±3.40 | 1.87±0.90 | | 0.09±0.09 |
| 2 h | – | | 5.48±1.35 | 1.74±0.52 | | 0.31±0.24 |
| 3 h | – | | 1.39±0.35 | 0.59±0.12 | | 0.23±0.18 |
| 4 h | – | | | | 1.28±0.22 | |
| total | | | 81.60±3.41 | 5.90±2.54 | 1.28±0.22 | 0.79±0.52 |
| half-life (min) | | 17.0±5.5 | 16.0±3.2 | | | |

# Results

## Experiments in the Rat

About 82 per cent of the dose of $^{125}$I-labelled iopromide was excreted via the kidneys within 3 h after intravenous injection of 60 mg I/kg body weight into male rats. The elimination half-life (in blood and urine) was about 17 min. Intestinal absorption was found to be 1.3 per cent of the dose (Table 1).

In urine, 84.1 ± 3.4 per cent of $^{125}$I-labelled iopromide was found 24 h after intravenous injection, and 9.7 ± 1.6 per cent in faeces. The remaining activity in the body was 2.1 ± 0.4 per cent. Leaving aside the thyroid gland, the highest tissue concentration of $^{125}$I was found in the kidneys (2.1 ± 0.2 µg iodine per g wet tissue; Table 2).

The amounts of active material recovered seven days after intravenous injection of $^{125}$I-labelled iopromide in dosages equivalent to 1.0 and 10.0 g I/

Table 2  Excretion and distribution of $^{125}$I-labelled iopromide after intravenous injection in 10 male rats (100 g body weight). 60 mg I/kg. Data given in per cent of dose administered per fraction collected or per organ and in µg I/g wet tissue (mean value ± SD)

| time after injection (hours) | Excretion (per cent of dose given) | | Organ | Tissue distribution (24 h after injection) | |
|---|---|---|---|---|---|
| | urine | faeces | | per cent of dose given | µ I/g wet tissue |
| 0.5 | 64.05±7.04 | | blood | 0.22±0.03 | 1.96±0.27 |
| 1 | 10.68±3.40 | | liver | 0.04±0.01 | 0.42±0.11 |
| 2 | 5.48±1.35 | | kidneys | 0.03±0.01 | 2.09±0.22 |
| 3 | 1.39±0.35 | | gastrointestinal tract | 0.37±0.31 | 1.99±1.83 |
| 24 | 2.54±0.22 | 9.69±1.57 | muscle | 0.01±0.01 | 0.45±0.05 |
| | | | thyroid gland | 0.05±0.01 | 193±36 |
| | | | pancreas | 0.01±0.01 | 1.14±0.21 |
| | | | body (remaining parts) | 1.45±0.11 | 1.18±0.12 |
| Total | 84.14±3.41 | 9.69±1.57 | | 2.08±0.39 | |

Total activity recovered (per animal): 96.0±2.4 per cent of dose given

Table 3  Recovery of $^{125}$I-labelled iopromide in urine, faeces and organs after intravenous injection of 1 g I/kg body weight in 5 male rats (100 g body weight)

| time after injection | | Excretion (per cent of dose given) | | Organ | Tissue distribution (7 days after injection) | |
|---|---|---|---|---|---|---|
| hours | days | urine | faeces | | per mil of dose given | µ I/g wet tissue |
| 0.5 | – | 55.6 ±9.3 | | blood | 0.01±0.01 | 0.18 ±0.13 |
| 1 | – | 18.5 ±5.3 | | liver | 0.02±0.00 | 0.26 ±0.02 |
| 2 | – | 10.4 ±3.2 | | kidney | 0.08±0.01 | 7.02 ±1.27 |
| 3 | – | 2.34±0.72 | | gastrointestinal tract | 0.18±0.02 | 0.87 ±0.05 |
| 5 | – | 1.32±0.43 | | muscle | 0.01±0.01 | 0.38 ±0.36 |
| 8 | – | 0.68±0.59 | | thyroid gland | 0.05±0.01 | 300 ±63 |
| – | 1 | 0.69±0.59 | 8.35±1.68 | pancreas | 0.01±0.00 | 0.001±0.00 |
| – | 2 | 0.15±0.05 | 0.88±0.80 | adrenal gland | 0.01±0.00 | 0.001±0.00 |
| – | 3 | 0.05±0.00 | 0.07±0.02 | body (remaining parts) | 1.52±0.22 | 1.65 ±0.23 |
| – | 4 | 0.04±0.01 | 0.06±0.01 | | | |
| – | 5 | 0.01±0.00 | 0.04±0.00 | | | |
| – | 6 | 0.02±0.01 | 0.05±0.02 | | | |
| – | 7 | 0.05±0.01 | 0.06±0.02 | | | |
| total | | 90.0±2.1 | 9.50±1.75 | | 0.19±0.02 | |

Total activity recovered (per animal): 100.62±2.11 per cent of dose given

Table 4  Recovery of $^{125}$I-labelled iopromide in urine, faeces and organs after intravenous injection of 10 g I/kg body weight in 3 male rats (100 g body weight)

| time after injection | | Excretion (per cent of dose given) | | Organ | Tissue distribution (7 days after injection) | |
|---|---|---|---|---|---|---|
| hours | days | urine | faeces | | per mil of dose given | µ l/g wet tissue |
| 0.5 | – | 25.5 ±9.0 | | blood | 0.01±0.00 | 0.000.00 |
| 1 | – | 20.4 ±5.9 | | liver | 0.44±0.22 | 53.44±26.29 |
| 2 | – | 12.0 ±7.0 | | kidney | 0.12±0.02 | 101.51±21.16 |
| 3 | – | 11.7 ±6.2 | | gastrointestinal tract | 0.06±0.04 | 2.81± 2.45 |
| 5 | – | 14.5 ±1.2 | | muscle | 0.01±0.01 | 4.08± 3.54 |
| 8 | – | 3.65±1.49 | | thyroid gland | 0.01±0.01 | 74 ±32 |
| – | 1 | 3.63±1.49 | 8.70±0.55 | pancreas | 0.01±0.00 | 0.00± 0.00 |
| – | 2 | 0.56±0.13 | 1.20±1.03 | adrenal gland | 0.01±0.00 | 0.00± 0.00 |
| – | 3 | 0.14±0.06 | 0.23±0.10 | body (remaining parts) | 1.29±0.22 | 12.39± 1.62 |
| – | 4 | 0.05±0.04 | 0.11±0.04 | | | |
| – | 5 | 0.00±0.00 | 0.00±0.00 | | | |
| – | 6 | 0.01±0.02 | 0.00±0.00 | | | |
| – | 7 | 0.08±0.03 | 0.15±0.08 | | | |
| total | | 92.2±1.8 | 10.4±1.7 | | 0.19±0.01 | |

Total recovered activity (per animal): 103±1 per cent of dose given

kg body weight were found to be about the same: 90 per cent of the doses administered was recovered in urine and 10 per cent of the doses administered was recovered in urine and 10 per cent in faeces (Tables 3,4). The total recoveries were 100 ± 2 per cent and 103 ± 1 per cent, respectively. No specific accumulation in the organs examined was indicated. Only $^{125}$I-concentration in the thyroid gland was found to be high, as may be expected after administration of any contrast medium due to the permissible content of free iodide.

No difference was found between distribution of urinary or biliary activity (24-h pool, representing 85 per cent or 10 per cent of the dose injected) on the TLC plates and that of the labelled compound from the solution injected, nor did HPLC analysis reveal any difference between the active constituents in the urine and the administered compound.

## Experiments in the Dog

Five minutes after injection, 20 per cent of the dose of 600 mg I/kg body weight was found in total plasma volume. This is equal to a plasma concentration of 2.75 mg I/ml plasma. The apparent distribution volume $V_D$ of iopromide was calculated to be 1580 ± 370 ml. After a brief distribution phase (alpha) with a halflife of 8 ± 6 min, a disposition and elimination phase (beta) with a half-life of 46 ± 3 min commenced (Fig 1). Total clearance from plasma was calculated to be 3.7 ± 2.0 ml/min$^{-1}$/kg$^{-1}$.

Table 5  Recovery of $^{125}$I-labelled iopromide in urine and faeces after intravenous injection of 600 mg I/kg body weight in female dogs (n = 3). Values are given as mean ± SD

| time after injection | | Excretion (per cent of dose given) | |
|---|---|---|---|
| hours | days | urine | faeces |
| 0–0.25 | | 11.57±12.77 | |
| 0.5 | | 17.80± 2.27 | |
| 0.75 | | 15.40± 2.72 | |
| 1 | | 9.92± 4.46 | |
| 1.5 | | 9.81± 3.20 | |
| 2 | | 7.41± 2.00 | |
| 3 | | 7.84± 0.59 | |
| 4 | | 4.64± 1.86 | |
| 5 | | 2.60± 1.12 | |
| 6 | | 1.56± 0.87 | |
| | 1 | 4.29± 4.58 | |
| | 2 | 0.40± 0.11 | |
| | 3 | 0.18± 0.06 | 1.69±1.21 |
| | 4–7 | 0.16± 0.03 | 0.29±0.14 |
| total | 0–7 | 93.57± 5.74 | 1.94±1.03 |

Total recovery in urine and faeces, day 0 to 7, 95.5±5.7 per cent of dose given.

During the 3 hours following injection, 80 ± 9 per cent of the dose administered was excreted via the kidneys. The half-life of this excretion was 50 ± 10 min. Total excretion via the kidneys during the seven days after injection was 94 ± 6 per cent of the dose administered and total faecal excretion 2 ± 1 per cent (Table 5; Fig 2). The renal clearance was found to be 2.5 ± 0.7 ml/min$^{-1}$/kg$^{-1}$.

TLC and HPLC analysis of undiluted urine did not indicate that iopromide excreted via the kidneys is in a metabolized form. As in the rat, only the unchanged material was detectable.

## Discussion

Due to the hydrophilic substituents attached to the tri-iodinated benzene ring, iopromide is an extremely hydrophilic molecule with a very low apparent partition coefficient (13). The hydrophilicity prevents iopromide from crossing cell membranes, i. e., iopromide is unable to enter the intracellular lumen. Therefore, like diatrizoate and metrizamide, iopromide is not absorbed after oral administration (2, 3, 6).

After intravenous injection iopromide is rapidly distributed, almost exclusively in the extracellular space. This was demonstrated by the distribution volume of 1.6 litres in the dog, which is equivalent to about 15–20 per cent of the body weight.

On the basis of a two-compartment open model, the alpha-phase of distribution is followed by the beta-phase of disposition and elimination. The biological half-life of iopromide in the rat was found to be 20 min and in the dog 50 min. The half-lives determined for iopromide are in the order of magnitude of those published for diatrizoate, iothalamate and metrizamide (2, 3, 7, 10, 11).

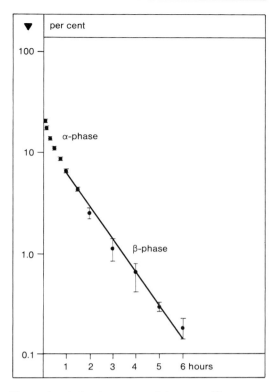

Fig 1 Plasma level after intravenous injection of $^{125}$I-labelled iopromide in 3 dogs (600 mg I/kg). Plasma concentration in per cent of dose given/total plasma volume; semilogarithmic plot. Alpha-phase (distribution): Half-life 8 ± 6 min. Beta-phase (elimination): Half-life 46 ± 3 min (calculated by computer analysis, open two-compartment model)

The total clearance of iopromide from plasma and the renal excretion rates indicate that iopromide is excreted without tubular reabsorption or secretion, mainly by glomerular filtration. The excretion mechanism of iopromide is very much the same as

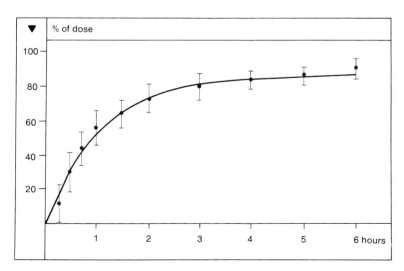

Fig 2 Urinary excretion after intravenous injection of $^{125}$I-labelled iopromide in 3 dogs (600 mg I/kg). Cumulated excretion in per cent of the given dose

that described for diatrizoate and inulin in the dog (7), and for iopamidol (9).

In rats, about 90 per cent of the dose was recovered from urine and 10 per cent from faeces, irrespective of the dose administered. In the dog the ratio of urinary to faecal excretion was about 97 to 3. Similar ratios of urinary/faecal excretion in the rat were reported for metrizamide (3) and in the dog for iopamidol (9).

Leaving aside the thyroid gland, no special preference for any organ or tissue is evident at different dose levels from 0.06 to 10 grams iodine per kg in the rat. The concentration of radioactive constituents is by far the highest in the thyroid gland, which should be considered as a target tissue. Inorganic iodide contaminating the solution injected may cause the specific thyroidal uptake observed, which is comparable to that found by Golman (4) in rats after injection of metrizamide. If iopromide is used in patients, a transient thyroid blockade should be considered as for any other iodinated contrast agent.

Iopromide is not metabolized after intravenous injection, as can be concluded from our results analysing bile and urine of rats and the urine of dogs. Other non-ionic contrast media, like metrizamide and iopamidol, did not exhibit biotransformation in laboratory animals either (1, 5, 9). The absence of biotransformation was also shown for several ionic urographic contrast media in man (14).

Iopromide revealed after intravenous injection in rats and dogs pharmacokinetic characteristics demonstrating it to be highly suitable for use as a contrast agent for angiography, computerassisted tomography and urography.

## References

1 Frey, K.: Thin-layer chromatography of $^{125}$I-labelled metrizamide in urine from laboratory animals. Acta radiol (Stockh.) Suppl. 335: 286, 1973

2 Golman, K.: Excretion of metrizamide. I. Comparison with diatrizoate and iothalamate after intravenous administration in rabbits. Acta radiol. (Stockh.) Suppl. 335: 253, 1973

3 Golman, K.: Excretion of metrizamide. II. An experimental investigation in rabbit, rat and cat after intravenous, suboccipital and peroral administration of $^{125}$I-labelled metrizamide. Acta radiol. (Stockh.) Suppl. 335: 258, 1973

4 Golman, K.: Distribution and retention of $^{125}$I-labelled metrizamide after intravenous and suboccipital injection in rabbit, rat and cat. Acta radiol. (Stockh.) Suppl. 335: 300, 1973

5 Golman, K.: Column gel chromatography of $^{125}$I-labelled metrizamide. Acta radiol. (Stockh.) Suppl. 335: 292, 1973

6 Langecker, H., A. Harwart, K. Junkmann: 3,5-Diacetylamino-2,4,6-triiodbenzosäure als Röntgenkontrastmittel. Arch. exp. Path. Pharmakol. 22: 584, 1954

7 McChesney, E. W., J. O. Hoppe: Studies on the tissue distribution and excretion of sodium diatrizoate in laboratory animals. Amer. J. Roentgenol. 78: 137, 1957

8 Mützel, W., U. Speck: This volume, p. 11

9 Pitrè, D., P. Tirone: Radiopaque contrast media XLVI: Preliminary studies of the metabolism of iopamidol in the dog, the rabbit and man. Farmaco, Ed. sci. 35: 826–835, 1980

10 Schlungbaum, W.: Verteilung, Ausscheidung und Resorption nierengängiger, mit $I^{131}$-markierter Röntgenkontrastmittel. Fortschr. Röntgenstr. 95: 795, 1962

11 Schlungbaum, W., H. Billion: Untersuchung der Verteilung von radioaktivem Urografin im menschlichen Organismus. Klin. Wschr. 34: 45, 1956

12 Schräder, R., D. Baller, A. Hoeft, H. Korb, H. G. Wolpers, G. Hellige: This volume, p. 67

13 Speck, U., W. Mützel, H.-J. Weinmann: This volume, p. 2

14 Speck, U., R. Nagel, W. Leistenschneider, W. Mützel: Pharmakokinetik und Biotransformation neuer Röntgenkontrastmittel für die Uro- und Angiographie beim Patienten. Fortschr. Röntgenstr. 127: 270, 1977

# Clinical Application

# Angiography

## Anaesthesia Problems in Angiography with Special Reference to Modern Contrast Media

W. Wenz, K. Wiemers, D. Schlürmann, W.-D. Reinbold and P. Anger

## Summary

The problem of anaesthesia in angiography is as old as the first examination of a patient with intravascular contrast medium. Developments in recent years have shown that modification of the contrast material in respect of its osmolality has been an extremely important step towards eliminating the pain generated on injection of contrast media. When used in association with premedication and a well-applied local anaesthetic, we believe it is now no longer necessary to mix analgesic anaesthetics with the contrast medium. General anaesthesia, epidural and spinal anaesthesia and conduction anaesthesia still have their indications – particularly in high – risk patients, restless patients and infants. Over and above this, epidural anaesthesia is again gaining in importance via the modern procedure of interventional angiography (Fig 1).

## Zusammenfassung

Das Problem der Anästhesie bei der Angiographie ist so alt wie die erste intravasale Kontrastmitteluntersuchung am Patienten.

Die Entwicklung der letzten Jahre hat gezeigt, daß durch Änderung des Kontrastmittels im Hinblick auf seine Osmolalität ein außerordentlich wichtiger Schritt getan werden konnte, die Kontrastmittelinjektion weitgehend schmerzarm zu halten. Im Zusammenhang mit einer Prämedikation und einer gut applizierten Lokalanästhesie ist es heute unseres Erachtens nicht mehr notwendig, dem Kontrastmittel schmerzhemmende Anästhetika beizumischen. Narkose, Epidural- und Spinalanästhesie sowie die Leitungsanästhesie haben nach wie vor ihre Indikationen besonders beim Risikopatienten, beim unruhigen Kranken und beim Kleinkind. Darüber hinaus gewinnt die Epiduralanästhesie bei den modernen Verfahren der interventionellen Angiographie wieder zunehmend an Bedeutung (Abb. 1).

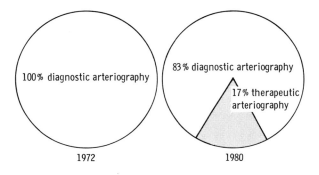

Fig 1  Diagnostic and therapeutic arteriographies at the University of Freiburg 1972 and 1980

## Introduction

Angiography – for many years an indispensable part of clinical diagnosis – is an invasive procedure. Vascular puncture and administration of the contrast material are considered highly unpleasant by some patients, which is why special efforts have been made from the very start of angiography to eliminate the pain generated during this procedure.

This paper, which drew upon the patients of the University Hospital of Freiburg, provides a survey of the present problems of anaesthesia in angiography and suggests possible solutions. The study relates to the development of angiography to date and discusses the pertinent literature.

## Historical Background

In 1923, after innumerable experiments, the pathologist Berberich and the internal specialist Hirsch of Frankfurt am Main succeeded in demonstrating vessels in vivo using strontium bromide (6). These experiments resulted in the first publication of arteriographs and venographs, which were made possible only by the use of water-soluble halogenized salts (cf [4] for literature).

To gain the time required for qualitatively perfect x-ray films, the same authors recommended the injection of highly viscous contrast media. The one they used was the oily substance lipiodol, with which Carnett and Greenbaum had gained their first experience in angiography of the extremities in 1927 (9). The paper by these latter authors provides the first detailed description of the exposure of the femoral artery at its bifurcation for the purpose of contrast medium injection, and also states that local anaesthesia is required for this procedure.

A little later, local anaesthesia proved to be necessary in the first attempts to catheterize arm veins for probing the right heart. Forssmann (14) writes: "I performed a venesection in my left elbow under local anaesthesia, since venepuncture with a thick needle on my own body proved to be technically difficult, and inserted the whole length of the catheter – 65 cm – without any resistance. Insertion and removal of the catheter were completely painless". This publication by the later Nobel prize winner is a significant pointer to the future of selective catheter angiography and angiocardiography.

Almost all the publications at the end of the 20's contain complaints about the painfulness of contrast medium injections; in most cases the medium concerned was sodium iodide. As Charbonell and Masse wrote in 1929, the administration is particularly unpleasant in chronic arteritis of the extremities (10).

At about the same time, in 1929, Oka recommended a contrast medium on a completely new basis which could be injected painlessly and was particularly well tolerated (30). The preparation concerned was a thorium dioxide sol, which was notable for a particularly vivid contrast.

As we now know, the euphoria over the "ideal contrast medium" was disastrously misplaced. The radioactivity of the thorium with its intensive alpha radiation as well as the sequelae of the degradation products and, not least, the foreign body reaction around the contrast depots in the reticulo-endothelial system led to fibrous changes of the depot organs, to the formation of tumours and to leukaemias. The contrast medium was withdrawn at the beginning of the 40's.

The introduction of cerebral arteriography (26) and lumbar aortography (34) considerably extended the field of radiological contrast examinations. The number of published epoch-making angiographs increased – but so did the number of reports on painful side effects and the realisation that "systematic" anaesthesia was required.

Moniz, for example, recommended that 0.3 g Luminal be given as premedication on the evening and morning before the examination and that a Novocain blister be set at the puncture site. He also stated that bathyanaesthesia is unnecessary if Thorotrast is used as contrast medium.

The choice of contrast medium also appears to dictate the form of anaesthesia which must be chosen. In 1941, for instance, Klostermeyer wrote that, of the diiodinated contrast substances, arteriography with Perobrodil is so painful that it must be performed under a general anaesthetic (15).

The first indications of anaesthesia problems in pulmangiography were published by Löffler (20), who injected 30–60 ml of a virtually non-irritant contrast medium within 2–4 seconds at body temperature and a pressure of 25–30 mm HG under bathyanaesthesia. Reason: to avoid shock, which is a disturbing factor.

The early literature also points out the need for general anaesthesia in restless patients. In 1932 Löhr and Jacobi reported that, in agreement with Moniz, they would always perform cerebral arteriography under a local anaesthetic (21). In restless patients or in longer investigations such as combined encephalo-arteriography, however, premedication with Pantopon should be followed by anaesthesia with Avertin.

In 1952, Pässler summarized his experience with anaesthesia in contrast angiography as follows (31):

"Percutaneous vasography can always be performed with local anaesthesia of the puncture site. However, the pain caused by vasodilation due to the pressure of the injection cannot be avoided even by the addition of Novocain to the contrast medium and frequently makes more extensive anaesthesia advisable. Because of this we almost invariably perform arteriography and aortography of the abdominal organs and lower extremities under a peridural anaesthetic. We occasionally examine anxious patients under Evipan anaesthesia – either alone or additionally".

Seldinger's ingenious idea (39) of puncturing arteries percutaneously and of inserting the catheter with the aid of a guidewire without exposing the vessel marks the start of the true era of angiography. The main effort was no longer directed at eliminating the pain during exposure of the vessel, but rather at inserting the catheter or puncture needle with as little discomfort to the patient as possible and at administering the contrast medium painlessly.

The main angiographic techniques are shown in Table 1.

Table 1   Modern angiography techniques

Catheter aortography/arteriography (femoral/axillary)
Counterflow arteriography (brachial/femoral)
Puncture arteriography: Carotid
　　　　　　　　　　　　Brachial
　　　　　　　　　　　　Abdominal aorta
Phlebography/cavography
Lymphography
Angiocardiography/pulmangiography

While the technical performance of the individual examinations has been largely standardized, there has been no agreement at all in past years about the choice of the anaesthetic procedure. Hence, discussion of the pro and contra of the different methods of anaesthesia seems appropriate (Table 2).

Table 2   Anaesthesia in angiography

1. Complete freedom from pain
2. Amnesia
3. Central and vegetative depression
4. Muscle relaxation

The advantages for the patient, and hence for the radiologist, can be deduced from this: elimination of pain, anxiety, restlessness and defensive reactions; no movement artifacts and virtually no severe contrast medium reactions (32). Furthermore, hypotensive reactions and disturbances of rhythm are sometimes easier to manage and treat (16).

In cerebral angiography, inhalation anaesthesia also permits differentiation between normal and tumour vessels because the former contract at low $CO_2$ tension, i. e. on hyperventilation, while the latter do not.

Viehweger and Plötz (46) point out another big advantage of anaesthesia which applies in particular to the demonstration of arteries of the upper extremities: apart from organic, pathological changes of the vascular system, a number of etiologically different functional disorders of the circulation also exist which we know as Raynaud's disease (Fig 2).

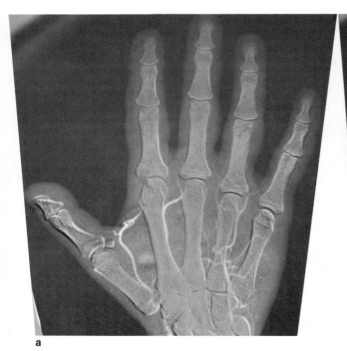
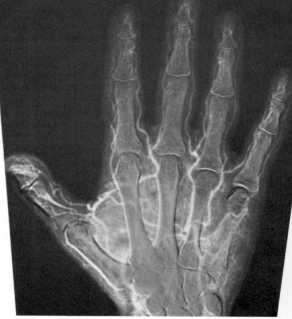

Fig 2   Raynaud's disease
a) Angiography of the hand with a local anaesthetic and a 60% conventional contrast medium
b) Excellent peripheral filling after conduction anaesthesia

It involves increased vegetative excitability leading to vasoconstriction which can intensify in attacks. Angiography then frequently fails to depict the end-arteries if only a local anaesthetic or the so-called double injection after Sgalitzer (41) is employed. General anaesthesia and conduction anaesthesia bring about a reduction in the peripheral vascular resistance and, hence, acceleration of the circulation in the arterial and venous limb, resulting in improved angiographic demonstration of the vascular periphery. The effect can be achieved with the anaesthetics thiopental, ketamine hydrochloride and halothane, but not with the use of nitrous oxide alone.

Birkner and Oldenburg (7) stress the fact that general anaesthesia permits not only a completely undisturbed examination of the vessels, but also repetition of an abortive series without causing the patient any discomfort. An experienced anaesthetist can manage complications such as severe contrast medium incidents much better than the radiologist. Incidentally, both authors recommend that all angiographic examinations involving a large amount of contrast material should be performed under a general anaesthetic.

Table 3 General anaesthesia in angiography Counter-arguments

| |
|---|
| Higher risk in cardiovascular and pulmonary disease |
| Additional, methodological incidents |
| Contrast medium incidents cannot be suppressed |

As far as the risk posed by general anaesthesia in angiography is concerned, Barth and Bräutigam (5) believe that it can outweigh the benefits in the case of relatively minor procedures. Laxenaire et al. (19) disagree with the opinion that severe contrast medium reactions can be avoided by general anaesthesia. They believe that histamine can be released independently of the contrast medium. Their study shows that, although contrast medium reactions were observed in 35% of cases examined without a general anaesthetic, they were still seen in 17% of cases examined under a general anaesthetic.

The special status of cerebral angiography is emphasized by a report on more than 3000 examinations conducted under Trapanal anaesthesia (24). The advantages claimed are: prevention of critical incidents, avoidance of constrictions, venous congestion, maintenance of a stable circulatory situation and elimination of mental stress on the patient.

In our own patient population at the Surgical Clinic of the University of Heidelberg we conducted a total of 1,556 arteriographic examinations with contrast media under general anaesthesia. The majority of complications observed in the patients – most of them elderly and high-risk – involved the cardiovascular system and the respiratory organs. A 71-year old man died 45 minutes after lumbar aortography with signs of cardiovascular failure. A severe inflammatory florid arteriosclerosis with parietal thrombi and numerous peripheral embolisms was found at autopsy, but no direct association between death and the anaesthetic procedure or the arteriographic examination could be demonstrated (23).

Carrying out anaesthesia within an x-ray department has, of course, its own problems.

Table 4 Difficulties facing the anaesthetist in an x-ray department

1. Poor visibility in semi-dark rooms
2. Small, often poorly ventilated rooms
3. Obstacles presented by x-ray equipment and radiation protection
4. Interference with monitoring equipment from high tension
5. Special positioning of the patient

Semi-dark rooms with poor visibility, restricted freedom of movement due to the x-ray equipment and the indispensable radiation protection, the narrow confines of the rooms and the special positioning of the patients, e. g. the abdominal position for lumbar aortography, can severely impair the work of the anaesthetist. Over and above this, the anaesthetist must also expect to deal with the peculiarities of contrast medium reactions, which can range from acidosis to myocardiac infarction.

## Epidural and Spinal Anaesthesia

Epidural or spinal anaesthesia is, without any doubt, of great assistance to the examining radiologist at aorto-arteriography.

Table 5 Advantages of epidural and spinal anaesthesia

1. Complete elimination of pain
2. Absolute relaxation
3. Vasodilation due to sympathetic blockade
4. If catheter are used, the anaesthesia can be prolonged for subsequent surgery
5. No need of central anaesthetics as premedication

Spigos et al. (43) injected 12–16 ml bupivacain = Marcaine 0.5% into the epidural space in 77 patients – in 6 cases via a catheter. 70 of them experienced no pain at all during the aorto-arteriographic examination, 2 patients suffered considerable discomfort because of technical errors in the performance of the anaesthesia, while the other 5 still experienced moderate heat and sensations of pain.

In the study population of Miller et al. (25), 59 patients were given strong premedication (Diazepam 5–10 mg, Meperidine 50–100 mg and Atropin 0.4–0.6 mg i. m.) 60 minutes before the examination and 8–12 ml of a local anaesthetic. Complete elimination of pain was achieved in 8 cases only, the patients experiencing slight heat. However, demonstration of the distal small vessels was very good thanks to the marked vasodilation.

Disadvantages are that the examination takes longer because of the application of the epidural block by the anaesthetist and that the costs are higher compared to the so-called angiographic standard (25).

An example of a negative aspect of angiography carried out under these conditions seems appropriate here: the patient – a 64-year old doctor – informed us at follow-up on the day after the examination that he had experienced no pain at all during the examination. However, when the anaesthesia and the motor paralysis lasted longer than the 5 hours predicted by the anaesthetist he became highly excited for fear of permanent paralysis – a condition which he would have willingly swopped for temporary pain and discomfort. Such unusual mental reactions are, by their very nature, difficult to predict.

## Intraarterial Administration of Local Anaesthetics

At the end of the 70's, several papers appeared which dealt with the elimination of pain in angiography by means of intraarterial injection of local anaesthetics. Some of these authors gave the impression that they had discovered something new.

In fact, first mention of this approach was made by Sgalitzer in 1932, and Pässler (31) attempted on a wide scale to reduce the pain of contrast medium injections by the admixture of Novocain. We ourselves have administered local anaesthetics since the beginning of the 60's as a routine measure in femoral arteriography and catheter aorto/arteriography of the lower extremities.

Papers by Schmidt et al. (35, 36, 37) are quoted here as "pars pro toto": the addition of 1 mg lidocaine/ml contrast medium in 95 patients resulted in a highly significant reduction of pain in comparison to 87 patients who received only the contrast medium with 10% saline solution. The additional administration of diazepam as premedication reduced the pain and sensation of heat even further, but was accompanied by hypotension. The authors later reported that slightly better examination results were obtained when higher lidocaine dosages were administered and intravenous Valium was given as premedication, but the side effects rate was also higher. In another, double – blind study in which lidocaine was combined with an ionic and a non-ionic contrast medium, no difference was found as regards the sensation of pain.

Diametrically opposed to this are the results of a double-blind study by Eisenberg et al. (12). More than half their patients experienced more pain after the addition of lidocaine than without a local anaesthetic.

Reports on several thousand aorto-arteriographic examinations conducted with the addition of a local anaesthetic show that opinions are, in fact, divided. We tried various modifications: mixing a local anaesthetic with the contrast medium, intraarterial injection 10,5 or 1 minute before administration of the contrast medium, varying the amount of local anaesthetic (5–15 ml). We used Novocain 0.5% initially, but later changed to Xylocain 0.5% (47).

It has unfortunately never been possible to predict reliably freedom from pain in the individual case. We are unable to explain why one patient responds very well to the additional administration of a local anaesthetic, while another responds only poorly or not at all. We do, however, doubt the theory that the pain is generated merely by irritation of peripheral nerve endings or by the provocation of local muscular contractions.

Fortunately, there are very recent signs of a possible solution to this problem, in that growing importance is being attached both experimentally and clinically to the osmolality of the contrast media used (cf. [29] for bibliography).

Table 6 Pain after intraarterial administration of contrast media

1. Chemical irritation
2. Muscular contractions
3. Vasodilation
4. Osmolality

Vascular pain can be provoked by various noxae, for example by mechanical force, inflammation, ischaemia, alteration of the pH value and osmotic pressure and by histamine and plasma kinins. Intraarterial injections of chemical agents such as hypertonic salts, acids, alkalis, certain cations (potassium, sodium) and organic anions have led to pain reactions in animal experiments.

Table 7  Side effects of contrast media

> Disturbances of electrolyte and fluid exchange
> Endothelial lesions
> Clotting disorders
> Histamine release

From what has already been said, we know that there are several ways of combating pain:

1. General anaesthesia, which has its own mortality and morbidity as a disadvantage.
2. Massive premedication, the disadvantages of which are unreliable control of pain, respiratory depression and hypotension. For high-risk patients it constitutes poor anaesthesia with all its risks.
3. Epidural and spinal anaesthesia; both procedures are almost 100% reliable in the suppression of pain, but cannot be used in clotting disorders or myelopathy or after laminectomy and inflammatory changes of the back.
4. Conduction anaesthesia, which is particularly effective in Raynaud's disease.
5. Intraarterial administration of local anaesthetics, the effect of which is unpredictable and has apparently not been confirmed statistically.

A new explanation for the generation of pain in the extremities is provided by Lange (17), who draws attention to the direct effect of the contrast medium molecule on nociceptive tissue receptors: different contrast medium compounds having the same concentration and osmolality bring about pain reactions of different severity.

Furthermore, ionic, monomeric contrast media reduce total perfusion of the legs by 30% in healthy subjects and by an average of 45% in occlusion patients. Hyperosmolar contrast media attract water from the interstitial space into the capillaries and, as a sort of osmotic plug, could temporarily block the flow of blood. Although this exchange of flow is hardly likely to occur so quickly, it is conceivable that this is the reason why dimeric and non-ionic contrast media of low osmolality cause less pain in angiography of the extremities.

It follows from this that the injection parameters must be chosen in such a way that the contrast is as high as necessary while the pain is kept as low as possible. Since contrast media and their composition apparently play a decisive role in the generation of pain, this problem must be investigated more thoroughly (cf. B. Hagen: page 48).

## Low Osmolality Contrast Media

The basic skeleton of modern angiographic agents is the tri-iodinated benzoic acid molecule.
In its ionic form, it is present as a sodium salt or methyl glucamine salt.
The osmolality and viscosity can be reduced on the one hand by coupling the benzoic acid molecule with a second triiodinated benzene ring – in which case we speak of a dimeric contrast medium – or, on the other, by suitably modifying the molecule configuration so that the substance dissolves neutrally, i. e. without the concomitant cation. The result in this case is a non-ionic contrast medium.
First experiences with the use of low osmolality contrast media were published by Björk et al. (8), who reported on a dimer of metrizoate, and by Almen and Tragardh (2), who studied the non-ionic compound metrizamide.
Until then, water-soluble substances with an osmolality of 1.5–2.5 mosm/kg had been used for angiography, the osmolality of human serum being 0.3 mosm/kg. According to Almen et al. (3), such contrast media are therefore extremely hypertonic in comparison to plasma, and the result is marked vasodilation. In the patient, the low osmolality contrast medium – in this case Amipaque – leads to a smaller increase of blood flow in the plethysmogram and had been injected in 20 patients without any pain reactions.
In the meantime, dozens of papers have appeared on the favourable effects of modern low-osmolality and non-ionic contrast media, although it must be said that it is often extremely difficult to distinguish between those written as true critical comparisons and those written as a favour.

## Personal Methods and Experience

This historical survey and the comparison of the advantages and disadvantages of individual anaesthetic procedures are necessary to show just where and how we stand. The theoretical reflections on how pain is generated on injection of contrast

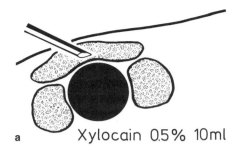

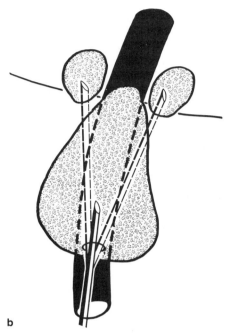

Fig 3 Applikation of the local anaesthetic in preparation for vascular puncture and catheter insertion
a) Cross-section
b) View with the distribution of the local anaesthetic in the vicinity of the artery

media have important implications for the methodological procedure in angiographic examinations. These remarks are necessary if the preparation of the patient is to be seen in the correct light.

Snowdon (42) claims that it is here, with the preparation of the patient, that the inadequacies begin. In contrast to preparation for surgery, the patient "is only being x-rayed". He has, perhaps, just arrived at the hospital and the angiographic examination is his first experience of what is to him a completely strange environment. It can be assumed that the mass of equipment will make him highly apprehensive from the very start.

This is where we believe the first line of defence against pain should be. Before he enters the angiography room, the patient should be prepared gently but openly for the examination. He must be told what is to happen to him and that a clear-cut diagnosis cannot be made without these investigations. The possible complications must be explained to him as gently as possible.

Once in the angiography room, we find it particularly helpful to let the patient participate in his own examination by watching the monitor. The radiologist who warns the patient early enough that "it will now get a little warm" and that this feeling will disappear again within 8–10 seconds will rarely see an unpleasant reaction from the patient.

30 minutes before the examination we administer intramuscular premedication, which consists at present of an ampoule of Psyquil 10 mg. On the occasions when the injection was forgotten, however, no reactions were reported or observed other than those experienced by patients with premedication. In fact, there is no study which proves the value of premedication in angiography beyond all doubt. We nevertheless have the impression that patients with premedication face the examination with greater equanimity and regard such a "tranquilizing injection" as pleasant.

The local anaesthetic is administered after the patient has been positioned. At present we use an average of 10 ml xylocain 0.5%, which is injected first of all in the form of a weal, then dorsal to the vascular bed and above the later puncture site laterally and medially of the artery so that it is surrounded by a belt of local anaesthetic.

We also inject local anaesthetics – about 5 ml – for examinations under general anaesthesia, the aim being to prevent spasms of the puncture vessel. The local anaesthetic should be placed in the immediate vicinity of the vessel – particularly in the region of the axillary artery – to avoid prolonged devitalization of the nerves on accidental intraneural injection.

Puncture of the brachial artery immediately above the elbow requires about 6 ml Xylocain 0.5%, and similarly small amounts are required for carotid arteriography.

For reasons of cost, however, we use the considerably less expensive, conventional contrast media for thoracic aortography and for abdominal angiography – particulary the selective procedures (coeliacography, mesentericography, renovasography) –, since these examinations are considered to be less painful, but always prefer the more expensive low-osmolality contrast media or nonionic contrast media for the periphery and the cerebral vessels.

It is extremely rare for our patients to report pain with this procedure. A sensation of heat is certainly

present, but it is surprising how much patients who have previously undergone peripheral angiography with one of the conventional contrast media notice the progress which has been made. There can be no doubt about the appreciation with which the new generation of contrast media has been received.
Our own experience has convinced us of the advantages of performing angiography under local anaesthesia (Fig 4).

Table 8  Angiography. Advantages of local anaesthesia

1. Quicker examination procedure
2. Out-patients can be examined
3. Desirable cooperation from the patient
4. No narcotic risk
5. Cost factor

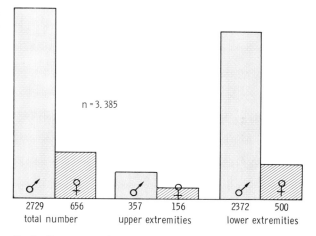

Fig 4  Frequency of peripheral arteriography at the Institute for Radiodiagnosis of the University of Freiburg 1973–1980

Up to 2 years ago we always performed lumbar aortography under general anaesthesia. Although the introduction of the axillary catheter technique initially reduced the frequency of lumbar aortography, it is now increasing again with the use of local anaesthetics.

General anaesthesia is still indicated in high-risk patients, in very restless patients (the mentally ill) and in infants (Fig 5).

That the collaboration of the anaesthesiologist will still be required in the future is shown by a very recent extension of angiography in the direction of interventional angiography – especially in embolization of renal arteries. The ischaemic pain here is so intense that the examination must be performed under general anaesthesia or under epidural or spinal anaesthesia. Fig 6 shows the frequency of embolization in our own patient population.

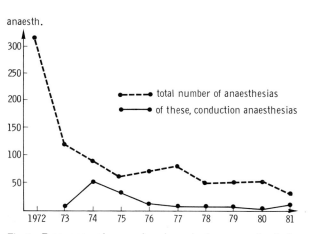

Fig 5  Frequency of general and conduction anaesthesia in angiographic examinations at the University of Freiburg 1972–1981

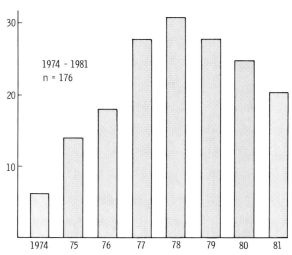

Fig 6  Frequency of therapeutic embolization at the Institute for Radiodiagnosis of the University of Freiburg 1974–1981

# References

1 Almen, T.: Cardiovascular effects of injection of metrizamide and other contrast media into the aortic bulb of cats. Acta radiol. (Stockh.) Suppl. 335: 209, 1973

2 Almen, T., B. Tragardh: Effects of non-ionic contrast media on the blood flow through the femoral artery of the dog. Acta radiol. Suppl. (Stockh.) 335: 197, 1973

3 Almen, T., E. Boijsen, S. E. Lindell: Metrizamide in angiography. Acta radiol. Diagn. 18: 33, 1977

4 Anger, P., W. Wenz: Aus der Pionierzeit der Arteriographie. Radiologe 21: 65, 1981

5 Barth, V., K. H. Bräutigam: Zum Risiko von Angiographien in lokaler und allgemeiner Narkose. Dtsch. med. Wschr. 104: 1549, 1979

6 Berberich, J., S. Hirsch: Die röntgenographische Darstellung der Arterien und Venen am lebenden Menschen. Klin. Wschr. 2: 2226, 1923

7 Birkner, R., K. Oldenburg: Ist die Angiographie mit hohen Kontrastmitteldosen ohne Vollnarkose noch zu verantworten? Münch. med. Wschr. 114: 1793, 1972

8 Björk, U., U. Erikson, B. Ingelmann: Clinical experiences with a new type of contrast medium in peripheral arteriography. Amer. J. Roentgenol. 106: 418, 1969

9 Carnett, J. B., S. S. Greenbaum: Sichtbarmachung der Blutgefäße. J. Amer. med. Ass. 89: 2039, 1927

10 Charbonnel, F., E. Masse: La valeur comparée des moyens employés pour l'étude de la circulation dans les artérites chroniques et la conduite actuelle de la chirurgie. J. Méd. Bordeaux 106: 431, 1929

11 Dimtza, A., W. Jaeger: Zur Technik der Arteriographie der unteren Extremitäten. Zbl. Chir. 65: 355, 1938

12 Eisenberg, R. L., R. L. Mani, M. W. Hedgcock: Pain associated with peripheral angiography: is Lidocaine effective? Radiology 127: 109, 1978

13 Fischer, H. G.: Anaesthesie in der Angiographie. In Loose, K. E.: Angiographie. Thieme, Stuttgart 1966, (S. 32)

14 Forssmann, W.: Die Sondierung des rechten Herzens. Klin. Wschr. 8: 2085, 1929

15 Klostermeyer, W.: Die arteriographische Diagnostik der peripheren arteriellen Durchblutungsstörungen. Fortschr. Röntgenstr. 66: 103, 1942

16 Koch, P., C. Müller, K. D. Schierholt: EKG- und Blutdruckveränderung während translumbaler Aortographie in Intubationsnarkose. Prakt. Anaesth. 9: 425, 1974

17 Lange, S.: Die lokale Schmerzreaktion bei der Extremitätenarteriographie und ihre Abhängigkeit von der Kontrastmittelkonzentration. Röntgen-Bl. 34: 231, 1981

18 Langecker, H., A. Harwart, K. Junkmann: 3,5-Diacetylamino-2, 4,6-trijodbenzoesäure als Röntgenkontrastmittel. Arch. exp. Path. Pharmakol. 222: 584, 1954

19 Laxenaire, M. C., J. Fays, A. Chastel: L'anesthésie générale protège-t-elle contre les accidents d'intolérance aux produits de contraste? Anesth. Analg. Réanim. 33: 1035, 1976

20 Löffler, L.: Füllungsbilder des Arteria pulmonalis-Systems bei akut entzündlichen Prozessen im Lungenparenchym am lebenden Menschen. Fortschr. Röntgenstr. 70: 178, 1945

21 Löhr, W., W. Jacobi: Die kombinierte Enzephalo-Arteriographie. Arch. klin. Chir. 173: 399, 1932

22 Löhr, W., W. Jacobi: Die kombinierte Enzephal-Arteriographie. Thieme, Leipzig 1933

23 Lutz, H., W. Wenz, J. Winkler, F. Heilmann: Röntgenkontrastdarstellung des Gefäßsystems in Allgemeinanaesthesie. Dtsch. med. Wschr. 93: 291, 1968

24 Maus, H., S. J. Loennecken: Zerebrale Angiographie und Narkose. Fortschr. Neurol. Psychiat. 30: 155, 1962

25 Miller, P. A., L. Fagraeus, I. S. Johnsrude, D. C. Jackson, S. R. Mills: Epidural anesthesia in aortofemoral arteriography. Ann. Surg. 192: 227, 1980

26 Moniz, E.: L'encéphalographie artérielle, son importance dans la localisation des tumeurs cérébrales. Rev. neurol. (Paris) 11: 73, 1927

27 Moniz, E.: Arteriogramme bei dem Symptomenkomplex der arteriosklerotischen, intrakraniellen Pseudohypertension. Encéphale 24: 337, 1929

28 Morris, T. W., A. N. King, H. W. Fischer: The effects of pentobarbital on systemic responses to intravenous contrast media. Invest. Radiol. 14: 383, 1979

29 Nyman, U.: Reduction of Vascular Effects and Pain in Aortofemoral Angiography. Diss., Malmö 1982

30 Oka, M.: Eine neue Methode zur röntgenologischen Darstellung der Milz (Lienographie). Fortschr. Röntgenstr. 40: 497, 1929

31 Pässler, H. W.: Die Angiographie zur Erkennung, Behandlung und Begutachtung peripherer Durchblutungsstörungen. Thieme, Stuttgart 1952

32 Penn, W., J. G. H. Vroomen: Der Wert der Anaesthesie für die Angiographie. In Loose, K. E.: Angiographie und ihre Fortschritte. Thieme, Stuttgart 1972 (S. 85)

33 Plötz, J.: Anaesthesiologische Aspekte bei der angiographischen Diagnostik. Folia angiol. 12: 194, 1974

34 Dos Santos, R., A. C. Lamas, J. P. Caldas: L'artériographie des membres de l'aorte et de ses branches abdominales Bull. Soc. nat. Chir. 55: 587, 1929

35 Schmidt, K. R., K. J. Pfeifer: Effektivität von intraarteriellem Lidocain in der Schmerzbekämpfung bei Arm- und Beinarteriographien. Münch. med. Wschr. 122: 1159, 1980

36 Schmidt, K. R., K. J. Pfeifer, R. Huber, H. Welter: Schmerzreduktion bei peripheren Arteriographien der oberen und unteren Extremität im Doppelblindversuch. Lidocain/Ioglicinat gegen Metrizamid. Röntgen-Bl. 33: 571, 1980

37 Schmidt, K. R., K. J. Pfeifer, H. Welter, H. Ingrisch, G. Heyde: Untersuchungen zur Schmerzverminderung bei Extremitätenangiographie. Fortschr. Röntgenstr. 130: 200, 1979

38 Schmitt, H. E., A. Da Silva: Zum Schmerzproblem bei der peripheren Arteriographie. Vasa 8: 295, 1979

39 Seldinger, S. I.: Catheter replacement of the needle in percutaneous arteriography: a new technique. Acta radiol. (Stockh.) 39: 368, 1953

40 Sgalitzer, M.: Über Kontrastfüllung der Gefäße. Sitzungsbericht der Wiener Gesellschaft für Röntgenkunde. Fortschr. Röntgenstr. 43: 103, 1931

41 Sgalitzer, M.: Unterscheidung funktioneller und organischer Erkrankungen der Extremitätenarterien durch die Röntgenuntersuchung. „Das Doppelinjektionsverfahren". Fortschr. Röntgenstr. 56: 385, 1937

42 Snowdon, S. L.: Anaesthesia for x-ray investigations. In T. C. Gray, J. F. Nunn, I. E. Utting: General Anaesthesia, Vol. II, 4th Ed. Butterworths, London 1980 (p. 1417–1429)

43 Spigos, D. G., S. Akkineni, W. Tan, G. Espinoza, D. P. Flanigan, A. Winnie: Epidural anesthesia. Analgesia in aortoiliofemoral arteriography. Amer. J. Roentgenol. 134: 335, 1980

44 Straub, H., V. Wiebe: Verminderung von Nebenwirkungen bei der Beckenangiographie: niederosmolares Kontrastmittel im Vergleich mit konventionellem Kontrastmittel plus Lokalanaesthetikum. Röntgen-Bl. 34: 139, 1081

45 Tillmann, U., R. Adler, W. A. Fuchs: Pain in peripheral arteriography – a comparison of a low osmolality contrast medium with a conventional compound. Brit. J. Radiol. 52: 102, 1979
46 Viehweger, G., J. Plötz: Vergleichende angiographische Untersuchungen in Lokal-, Regional- und Allgemeinanaesthesie an der oberen Extremität. Fortschr. Röntgenstr. 121: 303, 1974
47 Wenz, W., D. Beduhn: Extremitätenangiographie. Springer, Berlin 1976
48 Zeitler, E.: Risiko der Arteriographie in Lokalanaesthesie. Münch. med. Wschr. 120: 129, 1978

# Comparative Evaluation of Low Osmolar Contrast Media in (Femoral) Arteriography

K.-J. Wolf, B. Steidle, D. Banzer, W. Seyferth and R. Keysser

## Summary

A comparison of the low osmolar contrast media ioxaglate, iopromide and iopamidol reveals no difference between these preparations in regard to quality of contrast, sensations of warmth or pain, and involuntary movement or facial expressions. The ionic dimer ioxaglate is equivalent to the nonionic monomers. However, the nonionic substances are characterized by a significantly lower rate of side effects such as nausea, vomiting and dizziness. Severe reactions to contrast media did not occur. Premedication with analgesics was not necessary with any of the test substances.

## Zusammenfassung

Beim Vergleich der niederosmolaren Kontrastmittel Ioxaglat, Iopromid und Iopamidol ergeben sich keine Unterschiede zwischen diesen Präparaten bezüglich der Kontrastqualität, Schmerz- und Hitzeempfindung, Mimik und Motorik. Das ionische dimere Präparat Ioxaglat ist den nichtionischen monomeren Substanzen gleichwertig. Doch zeichnen sich die nichtionischen Präparate durch eine deutlich niedrigere Nebenwirkungsrate aus, wie z. B. Übelkeit, Erbrechen, Schwindel. Schwere unerwünschte Nebenwirkungen traten nicht auf. Bei keiner der geprüften Substanzen ist zur Durchführung einer peripheren Arteriographie eine analgesierende Prämedikation erforderlich.

## Introduction

Early clinical experience with the nonionic contrast medium metrizamide (1, 3, 13) provided impressive evidence of the significance of osmotic pressure in the appearance of side effects due to contrast media, especially in regard to vascular pain and unpleasant sensations of warmth at arteriography of the extremities (11). Favourable experience with this nonionic low osmolar medium paved the way for subsequent developments. Extremely high price and instability in solution rendered this well-tolerated contrast medium unsuitable for routine diagnostic studies. Introduction of the dimeric ionic contrast medium ioxaglate provided a substance with less than half the osmotic pressure of previously available contrast media and brought the advantages of a low osmolar contrast medium ready for application in clinical arteriographic studies (9). The advantages of nonionic contrast media in reducing side effects (2) were realized with the development of iopamidol (5), which became commercially available in October, 1981 (Solutrast). This contrast medium is also provided ready for use.
Iohexol is another substance of this group offered commercially under the name Omnipaque (7).
A similar contrast medium, iopromide, is currently in the clinical testing stage. This substance is a nonionic monomer in a solution ready for use (14, 15). The rapid development and introduction of these substances may be a source of uncertainty for clinical radiologists in selecting the appropriate contrast medium for a given study. For this reason

we performed a comparative evaluation of three different low osmolar contrast media in a group of patients with arteriographic studies of the extremities. Ioxaglate, iopromide and iopamidol were compared in these investigations (Fig 1).

## Material and Methods

We performed two series of studies. In the first group the ionic dimer ioxaglate (Hexabrix) was compared with the nonionic monomer iopromide (Schering AG). Hexabrix is the meglumine-sodium salt of ioxaglate and is a monoacidic dimer containing 320 mg iodine/ml in the commercially available solution. Osmolality is 600 mOsmol/kg $H_2O$ and viscosity is 7,5 mPa. s at 37°C. Iopromide, a new nonionic monomer with an iodine content of 300 mg/ml was used for purposes of comparison in this study. The latter substance has an osmolality of 580 mOsmol/kg $H_2O$ and a viscosity of 4.9 mPa.s at 37°C.

The second study compared ioxaglate, iopromide and iopamidol (Solutrast). The latter contains 300 mg iodine/ml, and has an osmolality of 616 mOsmol/kg $H_2O$ and a viscosity of 4.5 mPa. s at 37°C. The slight differences in iodine content among the three substances were not considered in the evaluation.

## Study I

This randomized double-blind multicentre study was performed by three investigators at 3 radiology departments. 141 patients received ioxaglate in arteriographic studies of the pelvis and leg, while 145 patients received iopromide. The contrast medium was administered by means of a pigtail-catheter placed in the distal abdominal aorta below the renal arteries. 80 ml of contrast medium were injected at a flow rate of 18 ml/sec. Premedication with analgesics was not administered, though light sedatives were provided in some cases. The protocol used for computer analysis contained usual personal data as well as information on previous reactions to contrast media, the indication for the current study, preparation for the study, quality of the results (good, adequate, unavailable), as well as detailed information on side effects and their treatment. Evaluations of pain and sensations of warmth were made by the patient themselves using visual analog scales (dolorimeter and calorimeter) (8, 10, 12). Each patient was able to make his own independent evaluation of subjective feelings of pain or heat on a scale. The starting point of the scale at O corresponded to freedom from pain, while the opposite extreme of the scale indicated unbearable pain, arbitrarily assigned a value of 100. This procedure allowed quantification of the subjective feelings of pain and warmth experienced by the patients. In addition, facial and motor reactions were recorded during the study and assigned to one of three categories (strong, slight, none). Heart rate and blood pressure measurements with standard blood pressure cuffs on the left arm were made before and at 5 and 20 minutes after injection of the contrast medium.

## Study II

This series of examinations was performed in a single radiology department (Radiology Department, University of Tübingen). Both, the procedure and evaluation, were identical to those in study I. Randomization was originally planned for 200 patients in this series. We performed a preliminary evaluation after 97 patients had been studied. This explains the difference in the number of patients in each group, as 37 patients received ioxaglate, 27 patients iopromide and 33 patients iopamidol.

## Results

### Study I

Presence of arteriosclerotic changes provided the indication for arteriography in almost all of the 286 cases. As a result, the sex distribution demonstrates a clear preponderance of males with 74%. The majority of patients was older than 50 years of age. Vascular tumours were found in 3 cases, while one patient had an arteriovenous shunt and another vascular dysplasia. 2% of patients were classified in stage I (Fontaine), 51% in stage II, 31% in stage III and 17% in stage IV. Stenoses were found in 76% of cases and single or multiple occlusions in 59%.

The results of this series are presented in Table 1. Quality of demonstration was classified as "good" in almost all cases with both contrast media. Evaluation of vascular pain and sensations of heat was performed using the point system described above. Each patient was assigned to 1 of 5 point groups (table I), with the result that over ⅔ of all patients reported less than 20 points, which means that these subjects experienced little or no pain. There were no differences between the 2 contrast media in the group of patients reporting a high number of points.

This is evident when mean values are considered. The mean number of points for vascular pain was

Table 1  Evaluation of study I

|  |  | ioxaglat n = 145 % | iopromid n = 141 % |
|---|---|---|---|
| quality of contrast | good | 95 | 92 |
|  | adequate | 5 | 7 |
|  | inadequate | 0 | 1 |
| pain | 0– 19 | 69 | 68 |
|  | 20– 39 | 16 | 16 |
|  | 40– 59 | 12 | 6 |
|  | 60– 79 | 3 | 9 |
|  | 80–100 | 1 | 1 |
| sensations of warmth | 0– 19 | 26 | 25 |
|  | 20– 39 | 28 | 27 |
|  | 40– 59 | 28 | 28 |
|  | 60– 79 | 13 | 14 |
|  | 80–100 | 6 | 6 |
| facial expressions | none | 83 | 83 |
|  | slight | 13 | 14 |
|  | pronounced | 4 | 4 |
| involuntary movement | none | 90 | 87 |
|  | slight | 9 | 11 |
|  | pronounced | 1 | 2 |
| other side effects |  | 13 | 4 |

Table 2  Evaluation of study II

|  |  | ioxaglat n = 37 % | iopromid n = 27 % | iopamidol n = 33 % |
|---|---|---|---|---|
| quality of contrast | good | 100 | 100 | 100 |
|  | adequate |  |  |  |
|  | inadequate |  |  |  |
| pain | 0– 19 | 100 | 100 | 100 |
|  | 20– 39 |  |  |  |
|  | 40– 59 |  |  |  |
|  | 60– 79 |  |  |  |
|  | 80–100 |  |  |  |
| sensations of warmth | 0– 19 | 35 | 48 | 39 |
|  | 20– 39 | 57 | 48 | 52 |
|  | 40– 59 | 11 | 4 | 9 |
|  | 60– 79 |  |  |  |
|  | 80–100 |  |  |  |
| facial expressions | none | 100 | 100 | 100 |
|  | slight |  |  |  |
|  | pronounced |  |  |  |
| involuntary movement | none | 100 | 100 | 100 |
|  | slight |  |  |  |
|  | pronounced |  |  |  |
| other side effects |  | 8 | – | – |

14.6 ± 20.6 (x ± S.D.) for ioxaglate, as compared to 16.2 ± 21.6 for iopromide.

Sensations of heat were more pronounced than was vascular pain with both contrast media. Mean values for ioxaglate were 36.4 ± 21.2 (x ± S.D.) and 38.6 ± 22.3 for iopromide. Totals above 60 points were attained in approximately 20% of cases. Once again, there was no difference between the 2 substances.

There was also no difference in the frequency of observed involuntary movements or facial expressions of pain during and after injection of the contrast media.

Heart rate and blood pressure measurements at defined time intervals did not vary significantly within individual groups nor among the 3 groups studied.

However, there was a significant difference in the frequency of other side effects such as nausea, vomiting, urticaria, cardiovascular reactions and dizziness. The side effects were observed in 13% of patients with ioxaglate, as compared to 4% with iopromide.

## Study II

Presence of arteriosclerotic changes was the indication for angiographic studies in almost all cases in this collective. 74% of patients were males, and the majority of patients was over 50 years of age. 3% were in stage I, 51% in stage II, 36% in stage III and 6% in stage IV (Fontaine).

Table 2 shows that quality of demonstration was generally considered good. All patients reported little or no pain with all 3 contrast media. Evaluation of unpleasant sensations of warmth attained 40 points in a few cases. Mean values were 22.3 ± 8.8 with ioxaglate, 20.2 ± 7.9 with iopromide and 21.9 ± with iopamidol. No involuntary movements or facial expressions were observed in these patients. Other side effects occurred only with ioxaglate, with 3 patients (8%) complaining of serious nausea. Heart rate and blood pressure determinations were made at the same predetermined intervals in this study. There were no significant differences in these parameters over time within the single group nor among the 3 groups.

## Discussion

Evaluation of the multicentre study (I) shows good quality of contrast in almost all cases, which is to be expected, since both substances contained almost identical quantities of iodine. There were no differences in sensations of pain or warmth with the 2 contrast media. More than ⅔ of all patients reported little or nor pain. A large number of studies has implicated high osmolality of the contrast medium as an essential factor in the development of vascular pain (9, 12, 13, and others). Speck et al. (11) called attention to a possible role of other factors such as the nature of the cation and the anion. Our results show that osmolality is clearly of primary importance.

Unpleasant sensations of heat may be very pronounced and are related of vasodilation (6). However, neither pain nor unpleasant sensations of heat seriously disrupted the angiographic studies, as the rare observation of involuntary motion or facial expression shows. As a result, analgesic medication was not necessary in a single case, although sedation may be necessary in some patients. We were unable to detect significant differences between ioxaglate and iopromide as regards quality of contrast, sensations of warmth or pain, and involuntary motion and facial expression in 286 patients.

Study II included iopamidol (Solutrast) for purposes of comparison, and a preliminary evaluation demonstrates no significant differences among the 3 in the parameters discussed above. This study was performed at one institution (Radiology Department, University of Tübingen). It is interesting to note the number of patients reporting little or no pain with all 3 preparations, since this group is larger than in study I. Unpleasant sensations of heat also appeared to be somewhat less common. We attribute this to different techniques of handling and questioning the patients. Although the visual analog scales permit objective and quantitative judgements of sensations of pain and heat, this type of questioning has obvious limits. Factors such as the observer's increasing familiarity with absence of pain as well as the physician's increasing familiarity with a new substance may play a role here. Direct measurements of blood pressure were not considered essential, since the total number of patients in the study was so large. The fact that no significant variation in heart rate and blood pressure was reported during the course of angiographic studies does not contradict results reported by Holm and Praestholm (9), who found variations in both parameters amounting to several percent immediately after injection of ioxaglate.

In contrast, there were differences between the ionic contrast medium ioxaglate and the nonionic substances iopromide and iopamidol in incidence of side effects. Although one must be cautious in interpreting differences in percentages in a study involving a total of 383 patients, the advantage of the nonionic contrast media is quite clear. No severe or threatening reactions to contrast media (4) were observed in any group. A decision favouring routine use of low osmolar contrast media in arteriographic studies of the extremities is very tempting.

## References

1. Almen, T.: Contrast agent design. J. theor. Bio. 24 216–226, 1969
2. Almen, T.: Experience from 10 years of development of water-soluble non-ionic contrast media. Invest. Radiol. 15: 283–288, 1980
3. Almen, T., E. Boisen, S. E. Lindell: Metrizamide in angiography. Acta radiol. Diagn. 18: 33–38, 1977
4. Ansell, G.: Adverse reactions to contrast media. Scope of problem. Invest. Radiol. 5: 374–384, 1970
5. Felder, E.: Preclinical Studies with a New Non-Ionic Contrast Agent. Second Congress of the European Society of Cardiovascular Radiology Uppsala, 1977, May 25–27
6. Guthaner, D. F., J. F. Silverman, W. G. Hayden, L. Wexler: Intraarterial analgesia in peripheral arteriography. Amer. J. Roentgenol. 128: 737–739, 1977
7. Haavaldsen, J.: Iohexol, Introduction. Acta radiol. (Stockh.) Suppl. 362: 9–11, 1980
8. Hagen, B., W. Clauss: Kontrastmittel und Schmerz. Radiologe (in press)
9. Holm, M., J. Praestholm: Ioxaglate, a new low osmolar contrast medium used in femoral angiography. Brit. J. Radiol. 52: 169–172, 1979
10. Ohnhaus, E. E., R. Adler: Methodological problems in the measurement of pain: a comparison between the verbal rating scale and the visual analogue scale. Pain 1: 379–384, 1975
11. Speck, U., H. M. Sieffert, G. Klink: Contrast media and pain in peripheral arteriography. Invest. Radiol. 21: 283–289, 1978
12. Tillman, M. D., R. Adler, W. A. Fuchs: Pain in peripheral arteriography – a comparison of a low osmolality contrast medium (ioxaglate) and a conventional compound. Brit. J. Radiol. 52: 102–104, 1979

13 Walter, E., K.-J. Wolf, R. Hippeli, P. Ostendorf: Metrizamid und Megluminamidotrizoat zur retrograden Beinarteriographie. Eine klinisch-radiologisch-laborchemische Vergleichsstudie. Amipaque Workshop Berlin 1978. Excerpta Medica, Amsterdam 1978 (S. 144–150)

14 Wolf, K.-J.: New Contrast Substances for Angiography. Radiology Today, Salzburg 1982. Springer, Berlin (in press)

15 Wolf, K.-J., B. Steidle, T. Skutta, W. Mützel: Iopromide – first clinical experience with a new non-ionic, renally excreted X-ray contrast medium. Acta radiol. (Stockh.) 1982

# Iohexol and Iopromide – Two New Non-ionic Water-soluble Radiographic Contrast Media: Randomized, Intraindividual Double-blind Study Versus Ioxaglate in Peripheral Angiography

B. Hagen

## Summary

Taking the frequency of idiosyncratic side effects as a basis, iohexol and iopromide – two new, non-ionic, monomeric, water-soluble contrast media of low osmolality – displayed distinctly better tolerance properties than the ionic, dimeric but likewise low-osmolar substance ioxaglate in an intra-individual double-blind study. As regards symptoms such as pain and heat encountered in angiography of the extremities, however, ioxaglate revealed a tendency to be better tolerated than iohexol and perhaps iopromide. When ioxaglate is injected as the first substance, a hang-over effect is demonstrable on administration of iohexol as the second substance ($p < 0.01$). Osmolality and chemotoxicity are discussed in detail as causal parameters of the observed side effects.

## Zusammenfassung

Iohexol und Iopromid, zwei neue, nicht-ionische, monomere wasserlösliche Röntgenkontrastmittel mit niedriger Osmolalität, zeigen im intraindividuellen Doppelblindversuch gegenüber dem ionischen, dimeren, ebenfalls niedrig osmolaren Ioxaglat deutlich bessere Toleranzeigenschaften – gemessen an der Frequenz idiosynkratischer Nebenwirkungen. In bezug auf die in der Extremitätenangiographie besonders unangenehmen Begleiterscheinungen wie Schmerz und Hitze läßt Ioxaglat allerdings eine tendenziell bessere Verträglichkeit gegenüber Iohexol und möglicherweise auch Iopromid erkennen. Wenn Ioxaglat als erste Substanz injiziert wird, so ist gegenüber Iohexol als Zweitinjektion ein Überhangseffekt nachweisbar ($p < 0{,}01$). Osmolalität und Chemotoxizität werden als ursächliche Parameter der beobachteten Nebenwirkungen ausführlich diskutiert.

## Introduction

The great increase in the fields of application of water-soluble radiographic contrast media (RCM) resulting from technical innovations in the radiological sector (e.g. computerized tomography and digital angiography) calls for the development of new contrast media with optimal tolerance and lowest possible toxicity. Analysis of the side effects of conventional (i.e. high-osmolar) RCM observed after intravascular injections reveals a variety of symptoms which can be divided into idiosyncratic and non-idiosyncratic types (Table 1). While the former type can lead to severe reactions and even to death, the latter lead to frequently harmless, quickly reversible side effects which can, however, be subjectively very unpleasant.

The causes of the side effects observed can be explained by the physicochemical properties of the RCM. While the chemotoxicity and hyperosmolality of the CM can be held responsible for the non-idiosyncratic phenomena, the pathogenesis of idiosyncratic symptoms is the subject of sometimes controversial discussion (4, 7, 21, 24, 28).

However, it has been well documented that the introduction of metrizamide – the first non-ionic contrast medium – in 1972 led to a significant reduction in the side effects rate compared to classical ionic RCM. It is interesting in this respect that not only the dose-dependent symptoms attributable primarily to circulatory effects were reduced (1, 2), but, as recent observations and studies show (31, 46), idiosyncratic phenomena also occur much less frequently.

Table 1 Types and clinical symptoms of adverse reactions to contrast media

| I. *Idiosyncratic reactions* | II. *Non-idiosyncratic reactions* |
|---|---|
| sneezing | vasodilation |
| coughing | hypotension |
| nausea | bradycardia |
| bronchospasm | negatively inotropic effect |
| laryngeal edema | heat sensations |
| angioneurotic edema | pain |
| urticaria | nausea |
| pruritus | neurotoxicity |
| dyspnoea | alteration of renal functions |
| cyanosis | endothelial injury |
| arrhythmia | |
| tachycardia | |
| hypotension | |
| vasomotor collapse | |

In the search for autoclavable, low-osmolar substances which are stable in solution, the non-ionic compound iopamidol[1] and the dimeric, ionic compound ioxaglate[2] were synthesized first of all as successors to metrizamide. As we have shown, both substances are superior to conventional RCM in peripheral angiography by virtue of a drastic reduction of the sensations of pain and heat (13, 15).

Two more substances, namely, iohexol[3] and iopromide[4], are now available for clinical investigation, and we will report in the following on their use in peripheral angiography. Ioxaglate, a substance which has been in routine clinical use since 1979, was used as the reference preparation.

## Contrast Media

The contrast media SHL 412 D (iohexol) and SH 414 E (iopromide) were studied against ioxaglate in a randomized, intra-individual double-blind study. Ioxaglate is the sodium meglumine salt of ioxaglic acid and is present as a monoacid dimer in ionic form. Its iodine content is 320 mg/ml, its osmolality 600 mosmol/kg $H_2O$ and its viscosity 7.5 mpa · s (at 37°C). In the present trial design, iohexol was adjusted by appropriate preparation to an iodine content of 320 mg/ml, at which it displayed osmolality of 770 mosmol/kg $H_2O$* and viscosity of 8.1 mpa · s (at 37°C).

At an iodine content of 320 mg/ml, iopromide displays osmolality of 670 mosmol/kg $H_2O$ and viscosity of 6.2 mpa · s (at 37°C). Like iohexol, it is a non-ionic, monomeric contrast medium.

## Patients, Technique, Methods

98 patients (52 male, 46 female) with an average age of 63 years scheduled for aortofemoral arteriography for chronic arterial occlusive disease were recruited to the study. The extremity with the clinically poorer circulation was investigated first. Since the indication and the tactical procedure for the planned reconstructive operation in the femoro-popliteal segment of the vessel should also be decided on the basis of angiographic criteria, it appeared justifiable here to make two initial injections each of 35 ml investigational substance under standardized conditions. The first injection was given in anteroposterior projection of the leg, the second with the leg rotated inwards to achieve visualization of the femoral bifurcation free from superimposition and for multilateral demonstration of stenoses.

The substance under investigation was administered via a 7 French polyethylene catheter with 8 side holes (Pigtail) by means of a flow-controlled injectomat (10 ml/second). Placing the cathether about 5 cm below the point of departure of the internal iliac artery (anatomical landmark: lower edge of the iliosacral groove) ensured an interindividually identical site of application. At the same time, this selective method of injection provided for optimal visualization of the run-off. The abdominal and pelvic segments and the contralateral side were then visualized by advancing the catheter further into the abdominal aorta.

This trial design had the advantage of eliminating the difficulty in assessing local sensations (such as pain and heat) caused by the often varying severity of the circulatory distrubance in the two extremities on separate right-left administration. On the other hand, hang-over effects must be taken into account with double unilateral injections. To reduce these inevitable effects, the first two injections were given 10 minutes apart. Another 15 minutes were waited before the main injection into the abdominal aorta was made to enable any reactions of an anaphylactoid nature to be assigned to the respective contrast medium.

Furthermore, only reactions of the immediate type were included in the list of identified side effects. The total amount of contrast material administered was between 130 and 150 ml. The somewhat higher iodine concentration of iohexol (350 mg iodine/ml) compared to ioxaglate (320 mg iodine/ml) was balanced out again by appropriate dilution. The "blind" character of the study was ensured by the use of a confidential person.

The double injection therefore resulted in 196 evaluations, 98 injections being made with ioxaglate, 50 with iopromide and 48 with iohexol.

Apart from the idiosyncratic symptoms, particular attention was paid to local reactions, the sensations of pain and heat experienced by the patient being transferred by the investigating physician from a

---

[1] Iopamiro (Bracco Research, Milan; in Germany: Solutrast, Byk Gulden
[2] Hexabrix, Laboratoire Guerbet, S.A., France; in Germany: Byk Gulden
[3] Iohexol, Nyegaard, Oslo/Norway; in Germany: Schering AG
[4] Iopromide, Schering AG
* extrapolated value

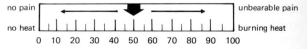

Fig 1 Visual numeric scale for evaluating pain – and heat sensations (scale divided in 20 "dolorimetric" and "calorimetric" units)

visual numerical scale system ("Dolorimeter" and "Kalorimeter", cf. Fig 1) to identical scales in the record form.
These scales contain 20 degrees of intensity between the extreme "0" (absence of any sensation) at the bottom end and the extreme "100" (unbearable pain or burning sensation of heat) at the top. This trial design, which we have described previously (13, 15), has proved its value in clinical studies and is superior to verbal registration of pain (16, 19).
In addition, changes in circulatory parameters were also recorded (blood pressure and pulse checks before and after injection and continuous ECG recording).
No premedication or sedation was employed in view of the use of low-osmolar contrast media, but local anaesthesia was performed with subcutaneous infiltration of 5–10 ml 1% lidocaine-HCL.

## Results

Table 2 shows the number, symptoms and intensity of the anaphylactoid phenomena observed under the different contrast media. Three mild (3%) and four moderate (4%) side effects requiring therapy were observed in 98 injections with ioxaglate. In the 7 cases exhibiting reactions following injection of ioxaglate the ioxaglate had been injected as first substance in 5 cases and as second substance in 2 cases. Consequently, in 2 cases it cannot be assumed unequivocally that the reactions were attributable to the ioxaglate.
Likewise, in the one case (2%) of a moderate reaction observed in 50 iopromide-injections the iopromide had been applied as the second substance. So again an identified association between the contrast medium and the reaction cannot be proven beyond doubt.
No reactions at well were recorded in 48 injections with iohexol.
Cortisone and antihistamine were administered as therapy for the moderate reactions.
The measured values of pain and heat recorded were subjected to multifactorial analysis of variance (12) and analysed by the following model for any sequential effects (hang-over):

$$y_{ijk} = u + r_i + s_{ij} + b_k + (rb)_{1k} + e_{ijk}$$

where
$r_i$ = effect of the i sequence, i=1.2 (hang-over effect) i=1.2 (fixed)
$s_{ij}$ = subject effect j=1, ..... 24, 25, (random)
$b_k$ = effect of the k. treatment, k=1.2 (fixed)

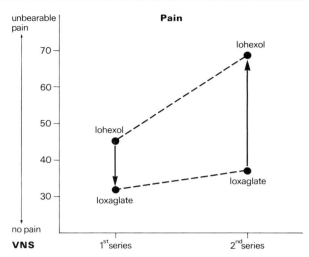

Fig 2 Mean values of pain sensations in the Iohexol/Ioxaglate study

$(rb)_{ik}$ = interaction between sequence and treatment (periodic effect)
$e_{ijk}$ = residual error

A varying sequence effect was established in the *iohexol/ioxaglate* study as an expression of hangover phenomenon (p < 0.01). The mean values for the features "pain" and "heat" and their standard deviations ( )were 45 (28) → 32 (28) for pain and 51 (23) → 48 (21) for heat in the injection sequence iohexol → ioxaglate, and 37 (31) → 69 (30) for pain and 56 (16) → 64 (24) for heat in the sequence ioxaglate → iohexol (Figs 2 and 3).
In opposition to the next study only the data from the first period (first injection) can be evaluated (24 injections per agent) because of the hang-over

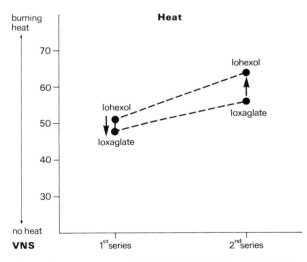

Fig 3 Mean values of heat sensations in the Iohexol/Ioxaglate study

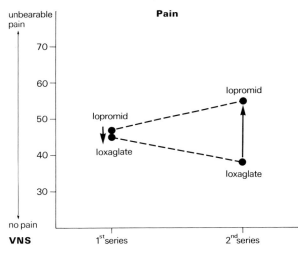

Fig 4  Mean values of pain sensations in the Iopromide/Ioxaglate study

effect. No significant differences are demonstrable between the two preparations (p > 0.05).

There are also no significant differences between the two investigational substances as regards the changes observed in the circulatory parameters.

The sequence effect did not vary in the *iopromide/ioxaglate* study (p > 0.1). The mean values for the features "pain" and "heat" with their standard deviations ( ) were 47 (32) → 45 (29) for pain and 46 (15) → 42 (17) for heat in the injection sequence iopromide → ioxaglate, and 38 (33) → 55 (30) for pain and 50 (23) → 50 (22) for heat in the sequence ioxaglate → iopromide (Figs 4 and 5).

The statistical analysis of these values and the graphic representation show that a periodic effect is present (p < 0.05), i.e. greater pain occurs in the

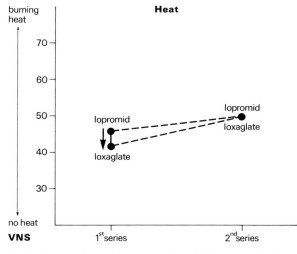

Fig 5  Mean values of heat sensations in the Iopromide/Ioxaglate study

second period (second injection). On top of this, the two preparations differ in that iopromide causes somewhat greater pain than ioxaglate (significance level p < 0.05).

In spite of the fact that the difference between iopromide and ioxaglate is smaller than the difference iohexol – ioxaglate and probably negligable it is statistically significant since all the injections (50 injections per agent) could be included in the calculation. However, the two treatments do not differ as regards the feature "heat".

There are also no demonstrable differences between the two contrast media as regards the circulatory parameters (systolic and diastolic blood pressure and pulse rate), i.e. changes of these parameters were less than 10% of the respective initial values for both RCM.

## Discussion

Since it became evident after the introduction of metrizamide in 1972 that systemic reactions of the anaphylactoid type and local, dose-dependent phenomena such as pain and heat can be significantly reduced by certain physicochemical properties of contrast media, the intensified search for substances with similar favourable properties has led to the synthesis of the contrast media ioxaglate and iopamidol, which are already in use, and to the clinical investigation of iohexol and iopromide.

Ioxaglate, which has been well proved in routine clinical use since 1979, was applied as the reference contrast medium for the clinical investigation (peripheral angiography) of iohexol and iopromide in our intraindividual double-blind study.

Basing on the assignment of the side effects symptoms listed in Table 1, we tried, first of all, to determine the rate of idiosyncratic incidents with clinical relevance.

A frequent difficulty in compiling such a list is that vegetative reactions cannot always be sharply demarcated from anaphylactoid symptoms. Moreover, an exact comparison with the incidents recorded by other investigators can be made difficult by the use of a different method of classifying the type of reaction (27).

Vasovagal incidents are typically accompanied by hypotension and bradycardia. Antihistamines have little or no effect on them, but atropin elicits an immediate response. The differential diagnosis can be complicated by the nausea and bronchospasm (caused by gastric and pulmonary vagus innervation) which is also observed in vagal reactions, and by cholinergic urticaria (10, 17). The presence of bradycardia, which is absent in histamine-induced

Table 2 Anaphylactoid side-effects following injections of ioxaglate (n = 98) iohexol (n = 48) and iopromide (n = 50) in 98 patients

| Pat. | Age | Symptoms | Intensity | Contrast media |
|---|---|---|---|---|
| A. W. | 56 y. | nausea, stridor, conjunctival flush | ++ Th.! | ioxaglate |
| G. D. | 46 y. | local urticaria | + | ioxaglate |
| G. F. | 67 y. | nausea, vomiting tachycardia | + | ioxaglate* |
| R. Sch. | 71 y. | vomiting, respiratory distress | ++ Th.! | ioxaglate* |
| N. N. | 73 y. | generalized urticaria | ++ Th.! | ioxaglate |
| G. J. | 69 y. | nausea, tachycardia, respiratory distress | ++ Th.! | iopromide* |
| J. | 68 y. | nausea, tachycardia, respiratory distress | ++ Th.! | ioxaglate |
| G. B. | 75 y. | nausea, vomiting, tachycardia | + | ioxaglate |

intensity of reactions: slight +, moderate ++, severe +++
Th.! = requiring therapy
* second injection

reactions, serves as a reliable guiding symptom and points the way to adequate therapy (3).
For better comparability, we have recorded only idiosyncratic reactions of the anaphylactoid type in Table 2, and even then only those which could be classified as immediate reactions. A side effects rate of 7% was calculated for ioxaglate, with 4 cases (4%) exhibiting moderate, quickly reversible reactions which required therapy and 3 (3%) displaying milder reactions which did not require therapy. A moderate reaction requiring therapy was found in one case (0.5%) under iopromide, while no reactions at all were observed after the iohexol injections. No serious or fatal incidents were recorded under any of the contrast media.
The unequivocal dominance of ioxaglate in the frequency of anaphylactoid phenomena in comparison to the two other substances shows that even modern developments in the field of contrast media, i.e. low-osmolar substances, apparently do not lead automatically to a reduction of idiosyncratic reactions.
Ioxaglate nevertheless differs considerably from iohexol and iopromide despite virtually isoosmolar conditions: it is an ionic dimeric substance with a meglumine- and a sodium-containing cation component (at a ratio of 2:1). It must therefore be considered whether certain chemotoxic properties of this substance are responsible for the significantly higher rate of side effects.
Briefly, the hypotheses discussed in the literature on the development and causes of idiosyncratic contrast medium incidents can be subdivided into release phenomena, i.e. release of vasoactive substances such as histamine (26, 33), serotonin (32) and kallikrein, activation of the complement cascade (23, 40), the coagulation (45) and fibrinolysin system (37, 38). Finally, antigen-antibody reactions of the IgE (43), IgM (20) and IgG type (8) are described and discussed as another source of adverse reactions to RCM.
However, the tolerance properties of a contrast medium are also determined by interactions with other biological systems, e.g. the protein binding capacity (25), inhibitory effects on enzyme systems (22), and an effect on cell membranes.
It has already been demonstrated that the dimeric molecule ioxaglate with its less hydrophilic structure ring is bound to proteins to a greater extent than iohexol and metrizamide (30). It has also been shown that iohexol and metrizamide exert an inhibitory effect on the enzyme lysozyme only at very much higher concentrations than those of, for example, ioxaglate (30).
The liberation of histamine, which correlates with the magnitude of the protein-binding index, is likewise much more pronounced under ioxaglate than under iohexol and metrizamide (30). Of interest in this connection are the observations by Rockoff et al. (34), which show that histamine release from mast cells of the rat peritoneum is greater under contrast media containing meglumine than under contrast media containing sodium. The cation component of the ioxaglate molecule consists of ⅔ meglumine and ⅓ sodium ions.

It has also been demonstrated that iohexol displays a smaller tendency towards complement activation of human serum than both ioxaglate and metrizamide (30).

In a case collection of 1,200 cerebral angiograms, Aulich recorded objective anaphylactoid symptoms in 6% of cases after intraarterial administration of ioxaglate. Tuengerthal (42) observed urticaria and dyspnoea on i.v. injection of ioxaglate in 7 out of 30 cases (approx. 23%). He also observed that the number of hyperergic reactions was about twice as high under ioxaglate than under the comparative preparation Conray 60, the ionic, hyperosmolar, pure meglumine salt of iothalamic acid.

Together with our own observations, these demonstrate that ioxaglate apparently displays stronger biochemical-pharmacological interactions than the likewise low-osmolar but non-ionic reference preparations metrizamide, iopamidol and iohexol.

The preclinical and preliminary clinical results (13, 39, 44) show that favourable tolerance properties can be expected for iopromide as well.

Apart from observing systemic side effects, we also paid particular attention to local reactions.

Sensations of pain and heat were particularly unpleasant, although harmless, quickly reversible concomitant symptoms of classical ionic contrast media. The causes of these side effects are to be found primarily in the hyperosmolality and, to a lesser extent, also in the chemotoxic properties of the RCM (11, 14, 15, 18, 41).

It has been shown, on the one hand, that even small differences in osmolality can give rise to significant differences in the perception of pain (13); whereas, on the other hand, it has been demonstrated in animal experiments that pure sodium salts of ionic contrast media under iso-osmolar conditions cause greater pseudoaffective reactions than mixed or meglumine salts (36).

Bearing this in mind, it comes as a surprise that iopromide causes significantly greater pain than ioxaglate ($p > 0.05$).

The difference in osmolality between these two agents comes to 70 mosmol/kg $H_2O$ – assuming an iodine concentration of 320 mg/ml. However, in these theoretical calculations of osmolality values the actual osmolality under in vivo conditions (human blood) is not taken into account. It is known that metrizamide as well as dimeric substances (like ioxaglate or iodipamide) develop at high solute concentrations a tendency for molecular association with a consecutive lowering of osmolality below the calculated rate (47, 48).

Moreover, both preparations display a slightly synergistic effect which is reflected in higher pain values after the second injection, regardless of the sequence.

The extremely good pain tolerance of ioxaglate in peripheral angiography has been stressed in earlier studies (18, 29, 41). An indication of this – although not statistically significant – was also seen in a double-blind study against iopamidol (13).

The comparative clinical studies of iopromide and ioxaglate so far available also reveal a possible superiority of ioxaglate in respect of the sensations of both pain and heat (39, 44). However, the injections in these comparative studies were made into the abdominal aorta. Similar to the observations in angiography of the brachial and external carotid arteries, selective injection into the arteries of extremities, the main supply region of which is represented by large masses of striated muscles and extensive areas of skin with minute vascular ramifications, is a more sensitive indicator for the differentiation even of minor differences in the perception of pain and heat than injection into the abdominal aorta or the aortic arch. Selective injection into an artery of the leg therefore appears to be a methodically particularly suitable procedure for the determination of local side effects – especially in a comparison of RCM of equal osmolality but with otherwise different physicochemical properties or in a comparison of RCM of only slightly different osmolality.

As far as the sensations of pain and heat caused by iohexol are concerned, a distinctly different hangover was discovered for the second period (2nd injection) in a direct comparison with ioxaglate. Thus, only the results of the injections of the first treatment period can be used to assess the preparations. In this case, no difference between the two substances was found at the significance level of

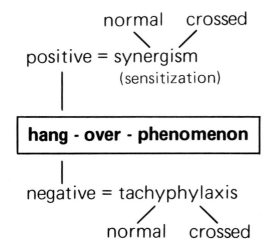

Fig 6 Hang-over phenomena

$p > 0.05$, although the mean values obtained and the graphic representation tend to show that ioxaglate is somewhat better tolerated as regards the sensations of both pain and heat.

However, we must bear in mind here that the osmolality of iohexol (770 mosmol/kg $H_2O$) is distinctly higher than that of ioxaglate (600 mosmol/kg $H_2O$), although the iodine content is identical (320 mg I/ml). Equiosmolar conditions can be achieved only by diluting iohexol to an iodine content of 270 mg/ml. It can be assumed that such a change of concentration would lead to identical values to those of ioxaglate as regards the perception of pain.

As already intimated, hang-over phenomena must be expected in an intraindividual trial design, particularly when double injections are made selectively into the same extremity at relatively short intervals of time.

Hang-over effects can be divided into synergistic and tachyphylactic phenomena (Fig 6). With such subjectively perceived, "extremely complex phenomena" (9) such as pain and heat, it is, under clinical conditions, naturally difficult to separate pharmacological-biological effects from purely psychological phenomena. The close interrelationship between perception and affective reaction (6) with their factors which alter the "sensitivity to pain", e.g. annoyance, fright anxiety, tiredness, distraction and joy, makes it understandable why it is so very difficult to conduct reproducible and conclusive measurements of pain.

Consequently, we have tried to reproduce the above-described hang-over phenomena experimentally in an animal model (14) – an attempt which led to confirmation of the clinical results. In particular, it was shown that ioxaglate (like other ionic substances) displays a distinct hang-over effect when the first injection with ioxaglate is followed at a relatively short interval of time by a second injection with the same or another preparation of equal osmolality. The synergistic effect was found to be most pronounced with iohexol.

## References

1 Almen, I., B. Trägårdh: Effects of non-ionic contrast media on the blood flow through the femoral artery of the dog. Acta radiol. Suppl. 335: 197, 1973

2 Almen, I., P. Aspelin, B. Levin: Effect of ionic and non-ionic contrast medium on aortic pulmonary arterial pressure. An angiocardiographic study in rabbits. Invest. Radiol. 10: 519–525, 1975

3 Andrews, E. J.: The vagus reaction as a possible cause of severe complications of radiological procedures. Radiology 121: 1–4, 1976

4 Arroyave, C. M.: An in vitro assay for radiographic contrast media idiosyncrasy. Invest. Radiol. 15: 21–25, 1980

5 Aulich, A.: Zerebrale Angiographie – Ergebnisse der klinischen Prüfung. Hexabrix – Symposium, Frankfurt 1979. Byk Gulden, Konstanz 1980 (S. 27–33)

6 Beecher, H. K.: The measurement of pain. Pharmacol. Rev. 9: 59–209, 1957

7 Brasch, R. C.: Allergic reactions to contrast media: Accumulated evidence. Amer. J. Roentgenol. 134: 797–801, 1980

8 Brasch, R. C., J. L. Caldwell, H. H. Fudenberg: Antibodies to radiographic contrast agents. Induction and characterisation of rabbit antibody. Invest. Radiol. 11: 1, 1976

9 Chapman. C. L.: The measurement of pain in man. In Kosterlitz, H. W., L. Y. Terenius: Pain and Society. Verlag Chemie, Weinheim 1980 (S. 339–353)

10 Garretts, M.: Cholinergic "urticaria" and miliaria. Brit. J. Derm. 70: 166–170, 1958

11 Grainger, R. G.: Osmolality of intravascular radiological contrast media. Brit. J. Radiol. 53: 739–746, 1980

12 Grizzle, J. E.: The two-period change-over design and its use in clinical trials. Biometrics 21: 467–480, 1965

13 Hagen, B.: Iopamidol, ein neues, nichtionisches Röntgenkontrastmittel. Radiologie, 22: 581–588, 1982

14 Hagen, B.: Contrast media and pain. Hypotheses on the genesis of pain occurring on intra-arterial administration of contrast media. In Taenzer, V., E. Zeitler: Contrast media. Fortschr. Röntgenstr., Erg.-Bd. 118. Thieme, Stuttgart 1983

15 Hagen, B., W. Clauss: Kontrastmittel und Schmerz bei der peripheren Arteriographie: Randomisierter, intraindividueller Doppelblindversuch: Ioglicinat, Ioglicinat-Lidocain, Ioxaglat. Radiologe 22: 470–475, 1982

16 Hardy, J. D., H. G. Wolff, H. Goodell: Pain Sensations and Reactions. Williams & Wilkins, Baltimore 1952

17 Herxheimer, A.: The nervous pathway mediating cholinergic urticaria. Clin. Sci. 15: 195–205, 1956

18 Holm, M., J. Praestholm: Ioxaglate, a new low osmolar contrast medium used in femoral angiography. Invest. Radiol. 52: 169–172, 1979

19 Huskisson, F. C.: Measurement of pain. Lancet II: 1127–1131, 1974

20 Kleinknecht, D., J. Deloux, J. C. Homberg: Acute renal failure after intravenous urography: Detection of antibodies against contrast media. Clin. Nephrol. 2: 116, 1974

21 Lalli, A. F.: Contrast media. Reactions: Data, Analysis and Hypothesis, Radiology 134: 1–12, 1980

22 Lang, J. H., E. C. Lasser: Nonspecific inhibition of enzymes by organic contrast media. J. Med. Chem. 14: 233, 1972

23 Lang, J. H., E. C. Lasser, W. Kolb: Activation of serum complement by contrast media. Invest. Radiol. 11: 303, 1976

24 Lasser, E. C.: Basic mechanisms of contrast media reactions. Theoretical and experimental considerations. Radiology 91: 63–65, 1968

25 Lasser, E. C., J. W. Lang: Contrast-protein interactions. Invest. Radiol. 5: 446, 1970

26 Lasser, E. C., A. J. Walters, J. H. Lang: An experimental basis for Histamine release in contrast material reactions. Diagn. Radiol. 110: 49, 1974
27 Liebermann, P., R. L. Siegle, W. W. Taylor: Anaphylactoid reactions to iodinated contrast material. J. Allergy clin. Immunol. 62: 174–198, 1978
28 Mc Clennan, B. L., P. O. Periman, S. D. Rockoff: Positive immunological responses to contrast media. Invest. Radiol. 11: 240, 1976
29 Moreau, J. F.: Discussion. Supplement: Contrast material symposium. Invest. Radiol. 15/6: 340, 1980
30 Mützel, W., H. M. Siefert, U. Speck: Biochemical – pharmacological properties of Iohexol. Acta radiol. (Stockh.) 362: 111–115, 1980
31 Rapoport, St., J. J. Bookstein, Ch. B. Higgins, P. H. Carey, M. Sovak, E. C. Lasser: Experience with Metrizamide in patients with previous severe anaphylactoid reactions to ionic contrast agents. Radiology 143: 321–325, 1982
32 Ring, J., M. Sovak: Release of serotonin from human platelets in vitro by radiographic contrast media. Invest. Radiol. 16: 254–248, 1981
33 Rockoff, S. D., R. Brasch: Contrast media as histamine liberators. III. Histamine release and some associated hemodynamic effects during pulmonary angiography in the dog. Invest. Radiol. 6: 110, 1971
34 Rockoff, S. D., C. Kuhn, M. Chraplyvy: Contrast media as histamine liberators. V. Comparison of in vitro mast cell histamine release by sodium and methyglucamine salts. Invest. Radiol. 7: 177, 1972
35 Salvesen, S.: Acute intravenous toxicity of Iohexol in the mouse and in the rat. Acta radiol. (Stockh.) Suppl. 362: 73–75, 1980
36 Schmiedel, E.: Präklinische Untersuchungen mit Hexabrix. Symposium, Frankfurt 1979, Byk Gulden, Konstanz 1980 (S. 9–24)
37 Schulze, B., G. Härting, D. Blanke, H. Witte, G. Hauenstein, G. Kotthaus, C. J. Meyen: In-vivo und in vitro-Versuche zur Wirkung trijodierter Röntgenkontrastmittel auf Gerinnung, Fibrinolyse und Komplementsystem. Arzneimittel-Forsch. 28: 755–764, 1978

38 Simon, R. A., M. Schatz, D. D. Stevenson, M. Curry, F. Yamamoto, E. Plow, H. Ring, C. M. Arroyave: Radiographic contrast media infusions. Measurements of mediators and correlation with clinical parameters. J. Allergy clin. Immunol. 61: 145, 1978
39 Skutta, Th.: Erste klinische Erfahrungen mit dem neuen nichtionischen Röntgenkontrastmittel Iopromid. XV. Internationaler Kongreß für Radiologie, Brüssel 1981
40 Till, G.: Röntgenkontrastmittelinduzierte Freisetzung biologischer Aktivitäten aus dem Komplementsystem. In: Neue Aspekte des Kontrastmittelzwischenfalls. Symposium Berlin 1977 (S. 51–56)
41 Tillmann, U., R. Adler, W. A. Fuchs: Pain in peripheral arteriography – a comparison of a low osmolality contrast medium with a conventional compound. Brit. J. Radiol. 52: 102–104, 1979
42 Tuengerthal, S.: Messung des Atemwiderstandes als Parameter einer Röntgenkontrastmittelnebenwirkung (Vergleich zweier Kontrastmittellösungen). Symposium, Frankfurt 1979, Byk Gulden, Konstanz 1980 (S. 73–84)
43 Wakkers-Garritsen, B. G., J. Houwerziji, J. P. Nater, P. J. M. Wakkers: IgE mediated adverse reactivity to a radiographic contrast medium. Ann. Allergy 36: 122, 1976
44 Wolf, H. J.: New Contrast Substances for Angiography. Radiology Today, Salzburg 1982. Springer, Berlin (in press)
45 Zeman, R. K.: Disseminated intravascular coagulation following intravenous pyelography. Invest. Radiol. 12: 203, 1977
46 Nickel, A. R.: Discussion: Contrast Material Symposium. Invest. Radiol., Suppl. 15/6: 341, 1980
47 Violante, M. R., H. W. Fischer, J. A. Mahoney: Particulate Contrast Media. Invest. Radiol., Suppl. 15/6: 329–334, 1980
48 Speck, U., H. M. Siefert, G. Klink: Contrast Media and Pain in Peripheral Arteriography. Invest. Radiol., Suppl. 15/6: 335–339, 1980

# Iohexol and Ioxaglate in Cerebral Angiography

A. Thron, M. Ratzka, K. Voigt and M. Nadjmi

## Summary

Iohexol, a new non-ionic contrast medium similar to metrizamide but in stable solution, was compared with the low-osmolar ionic contrast medium ioxaglate in cerebral angiography. In a double-blind study 60 patients were examined either by transfemorocerebral catheter studies (Group 1) or by direct percutaneous carotid and retrograde brachial arteriography (Group 2).
The incidence of subjective side effects was generally very low and without significant differences in both contrast agents. The image contrast quality was equally good. Less frequent deteriorations of EEG-findings with iohexol suggest lower neurotoxicity of the non-ionic contrast medium.

## Zusammenfassung

Iohexol (Omnipaque) ist ein neues nicht-ionisches Kontrastmittel, das im Gegensatz zu Metrizamid (Amipaque) in stabiler, injektionsfertiger Lösung vorliegt. Seine Kontrastgebung und klinische Verträglichkeit in der zerebralen Angiographie wurde mit der des niederosmolaren ionischen Kontrastmittels Ioxaglat (Hexabrix) verglichen. Die Doppelblindstudie umfaßte 60 Patienten. 30 Patienten wurden selektiv katheterangiographiert (Gruppe 1), die zweite Hälfte mittels Carotisdirektpunktion oder Brachialisgegenstromangiographie untersucht (Gruppe 2). Die Häufigkeit subjektiver Nebenwirkungen war allgemein sehr niedrig und zeigte keine deutlichen Unterschiede für beide Kontrastsubstanzen. Auch die Kontrastqualität war gleichermaßen gut. Seltenere Verschlechterungen des EEG-Befundes unter Iohexol sprechen für eine geringere Neurotoxizität des nicht-ionischen Kontrastmittels.

## Introduction

The good subjective and clinical tolerance of the non-ionic contrast medium metrizamide (Amipaque) (1, 6, 7, 9, 10) made it desirable to develop a corresponding compound as a ready-to-use stable solution for angiography; the monomeric, non-ionic contrast medium iohexol (Omnipaque) appeared to be a suitable substance. Its radiopacity and clinical tolerance at an iodine content of 300 mg/ml was investigated in the present double-blind study. The ionic, dimeric, low-osmolar compound ioxaglate (Hexabrix) with an iodine content of 320 mg/ml, was used as reference substance.

## Material and Methods

The preparations iohexol (n = 30) and ioxaglate (n = 30) were studied in a controlled and double-blind interindividual comparison in 60 patients scheduled for cerebral angiography. The nature and number of subjective complaints, the EEG findings and the neurological status including cardiovascular reactions were recorded.

## Patients

The study was carried out in two groups of 30 patients each who – apart from a few clinically defined exclusion criteria – represented a randomly selected neurological population. There were 36 men and 24 women aged between 20 and 76 years. The indications for cerebral angiography were clinical suspicion of vascular disease in 29 patients, suspected tumor in 26 patients and cerebro-cranial trauma in two cases. In 3 cases the clinical evidence was insufficient to distinguish between a vascular lesion and an intracranial mass.

Table 1  Examination technique (N = 60)

|  | 1st injection | 2nd injection |
|---|---|---|
|  | $x_1/x_2$ | $x_1/x_2$ |
| I. Catheter angiography |  |  |
| common carotid artery | 14 (5/9) | 13 (3/10) |
| internal carotid artery | 11 (8/3) | 7 (5/2) |
| external carotid artery | 3 (1/2) | 8 (5/3) |
| vertebral artery | 2 (1/1) | 2 (2/0) |
| total I | 30 | 30 |
| II. Direct puncture |  |  |
| common carotid artery | 7 (3/4) | 3 (2/1) |
| retrograde brachial angiography | 23 (12/11) | 9 (6/3) |
| total II | 30 | 12 |

$x_1$ = iohexol
$x_2$ = ioxaglate

## Angiographic Technique

In the first group of patients, all 30 cases underwent selective catheter angiography. The second group was examined by means of direct percutaneous puncture of the common carotid artery (7 patients) or by retrograde brachial angiography (23 patients), not all patients receiving a second injection. The name and sequence of the vessels visualized are shown in Table 1. Angiography of the carotid and vertebral arteries was performed by manual injection of 5–10 ml of the respective contrast medium, depending on the selectivity of the investigation. Retrograde brachial angiography was performed with the usual technique with 35 ml contrast medium and a flow rate of 22 ml/sec. The maximum total dose of contrast medium in most cases was 100 ml, but this was exceeded slightly in a few exceptional cases. No premedication was given apart from atropin. There was only local anaesthesia of the puncture site. Neither the examiner nor the patient knew which contrast medium was being injected.

## Tolerance Study

Immediately after the injection, the examiner asked the patient about any side effects and then entered them in the record form. Sensations of heat and pain were quantified subjectively by the patients and recorded in a calorimeter or dolorimeter with values between zero and ten which afterwards were subdivided into 5 main groups (Fig 1). The examiner also noted the mimetic reaction and any movements of the head.

The pulse and blood pressure were measured immediately before and one and ten minutes after the injection, and the EEG was recorded before and immediately after termination of the examination. The neurological status after angiography was also revised. The examiner classified the side effects globally as absent, mild or severe and the opacification as good, adequate or inadequate.

Table 2   Angiographic findings

| Diagnosis | Number of patients |
|---|---|
| no pathological finding | 10 |
| intracranial tumour | 24 |
| arteriosclerotic vascular lesion | 15 |
| inflammatory vascular lesion | 2 |
| orbital tumour | 1 |
| aneurysm | 5 |
| venous thrombosis | 2 |
| haemorrhage | 1 |
| total | 60 |

Table 3   Opacification

|  | Iohexol | Ioxaglate |
|---|---|---|
| good | 26 | 29 |
| adequate | 3 | – |
| inadequate | 1 | 1 |

## Results

In the majority of cases, the angiographic diagnoses were an intracranial tumor or an arteriosclerotic vascular lesion. The findings were normal in only 10 of the 60 patients. The individual angiographic diagnoses are shown in Table 2.

The opacification (Table 3) in the first group with selective injections was classified as good in all patients examined with ioxaglate. Under iohexol, there were two cases after the first injection and three cases after the second injection which were classified as being merely adequate. In the second group, the opacification was adequate in one case and inadequate in two, the latter occurring under both contrast media and in retrograde brachial angiography. It is known that with this examination, depending on the anatomical situation and the circulatory conditions, it is not always possible to obtain a good flow of contrast medium into the carotid artery.

Sensation of heat invariably occurred under both contrast media and in both groups. Other side effects also occurred with equal frequency under both substances – in the first group in 9 out of 15 patients examined with iohexol and in 10 out of 15 examined with ioxaglate; in the second group in 4 out of 15 cases under both substances. By far the most frequent of these other side effects was slight pain. There was one case of nausea and one case of mild and one of severe vomiting under ioxaglate. Temporary dizziness was reported under iohexol in 2 out of 3 selective injections of the vertebral artery. The number of side effects is shown in Table 4.

There were no clear differences between the two preparations in the first group (selective angiography) as regards the subjective sensation of pain classified on a 5-point scale (Fig 1 bottom), although it tended to be somewhat higher after iohexol. 6 patients examined by selective angiography reported mild to moderate pain (grade 3) –

Table 4  Number of side effects

|  | Iohexol | Ioxaglate |
|---|---|---|
| one | 19 | 17 |
| two | 7 | 12 |
| three | 4 | 1 |

mainly after iohexol – while one patient complained of marked pain (grade 4) after angiography of the external carotid artery with ioxaglate. However, no percentages could be evaluated for this parameter, since the number of patients examined by selective angiography was too small and unevenly distributed among the contrast media. In the second group, only two patients examined by retrograde brachial angiography with iohexol reported a dolorimeter value of between 2 and 4 (grade 2).

The findings were similar as regards the subjective sensation of heat, which was recorded as calorimeter values. In the first group, many more patients examined with ioxaglate reported a marked sensation of heat (Fig 1 top), while the second group of patients displayed virtually identical results.

The cardiovascular studies revealed mild tachycardia in only one case examined with ioxaglate. In a few individual cases, the systolic blood pressure 1 minute after injection of the contrast media increased or fell by more than 20 mm Hg with about equal frequency under both preparations. Only one patient displayed a change of this magnitude after the second injection. With two exceptions, the systolic values 10 minutes after injection were constant. Increases of the diastolic blood pressure by more than 10 mm Hg 1 minute after the first injection occurred 5 times under iohexol and two times under ioxaglate, but there were also two decreases under iohexol. Here again, there was only one change downwards under iohexol after the second injection. The diastolic blood pressure values 10 minutes after injection revealed 4 increases under iohexol compared to 2 increases and 1 decrease under ioxaglate.

The EEG studies made immediately after angiography revealed changes in a total of 5 cases after ioxaglate compared to only one case after iohexol with increased beta and theta activity. The changes after ioxaglate consisted of two irregular basic activities, one deceleration, one increase of the focal findings and one inconstant focus.

Therapeutic measures were required in only two cases and were not associated with administration of the contrast media. No unequivocal contrast medium allergy was observed in any of the cases.

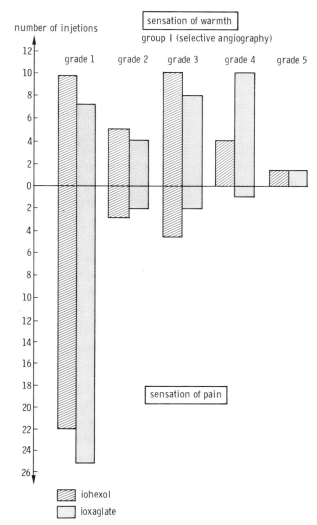

Fig 1  Calorimetry and dolorimetry for injections with iohexol and ioxaglate in 5 grades of severity in selective catheter angiography. Grade 1 = no to mild reaction, Grade 5 = very marked sensation of warmth or pain

Follow-up neurological findings half an hour after termination of the examination revealed no clinical deterioration.

## Discussion

The main result of the present double-blind study of iohexol and ioxaglate in cerebral angiography is the very good subjective tolerance of both preparations compared to previous contrast media. The distinct reduction of sensations of heat and pain under the almost iso-osmolar but ionic substance ioxaglate in peripheral and cerebral angiography is known and has been well-documented (2, 4, 5, 8). Iohexol – a substance similar to metrizamide –, which is present as a stable solution ready for injection and which was tested here in cerebral angiography, displays similar slight subjective side effects and probably also an even lesser sensation of warmth.

In comparison to ioxaglate the somewhat lesser sensation of warmth experienced in selective angiography with non-ionic contrast media is not accompanied by a corresponding reduction in the perception of pain – in fact, the tendency is almost the opposite. The non-ionic character of iohexol does not, therefore, lead to a further reduction of the sensation of pain, a side effect which is attributed primarily to the hyperosmolarity of the "classical" triiodinated ionic contrast media, although the pathomechanism is unknown (3). The osmolality of iohexol is somewhat higher than that of ioxaglate – 0.72 compared to 0.58 Osmol/kg $H_2O$.

The examinations by direct carotid arteriography and retrograde brachial angiography in Group 2 revealed virtually no difference between the two preparations as regards the sensations of warmth and pain. However, the side effects were generally more frequent and severe after bolus injections of large amounts of contrast material.

The comparative evaluation of the above data must take account of the following limitations: small numerical differences must be ignored because of the highly subjective nature of the study parameters. Furthermore, the double-blind technique led to uneven distribution of the two preparations so that, for example, the common carotid artery was investigated more often with ioxaglate, and the internal carotid artery more often with iohexol. However, the distribution of the selective injections was even as regards the external carotid artery, a region which is particularly sensitive to heat and pain. Since selective catheter angiography is the most frequent technique used and the vessels can be studied separately in respect of side effects, we decided to accept these difficulties.

Although the somewhat small number of cases and the use of different angiographic techniques must be borne in mind, the study did not reveal any definite differences in the local tolerance of the two substances either on selective cerebral angiography with small amounts of contrast medium or on use of larger bolus injections such as are required for retrograde brachial angiography.

The radiopacity of the two preparations, which is largely dependent on the iodine content (9), was also virtually identical. Inadequate opacification occurred under both substances only because of the examination technique (brachial angiography). The reason for only adequate opacification in 3 angiograms with iohexol was poor positioning of the tip of the catheter.

Effects on the systolic and diastolic blood pressure values in an upwards and downwards direction were observed in a maximum of 15% of the patients and were almost completely absent after the second injections. In contrast to the results of Dewitz (2), it can be concluded from this that the nervous tension of the patient before the first injection and the slight but, for the patient, unknown sensations on administration of a contrast medium do have an influence on cardiovascular function and overshadow possible direct effects. Any blood pressure changes induced centrally by the contrast medium therefore move over a range of 20 mm Hg systolic and 10 mm Hg diastolic.

Since the EEG studies revealed changes in only one case after angiography with iohexol, but in 5 cases after ioxaglate, the neurotoxicity of the non-ionic contrast medium can be regarded as low.

No serious side effects such as neurological complications, changes of the cardiovascular situation requiring treatment and allergies occurred in the present study population. Because of the only slight subjective side effects, there were no contrast medium-induced movements by the patient which might otherwise have necessitated a repeated injection. Iohexol can, therefore, be recommended for cerebral angiography, displaying about equally good subjective tolerance as ioxaglate and probably less neurotoxicity than ioxaglate.

## References

1 Almén, T., E. Boijsen, S. E. Lindell: Metrizamide in angiography. I. Femoral angiography. Acta radiol. Diagn. 18: 33, 1977

2 von Dewitz, H., M. Langer, W. Th. Glöckler: Verträglichkeit des Kontrastmittels Ioxaglinsäure bei angiographischen Untersuchungen. Eine klinische Studie. Röntgen-Bl. 33: 525–528, 1980

3 Gospos, Ch., N. Freudenberg, K. Mathias: Hyperosmolalität von Röntgen-Kontrastmitteln – ein Faktor für die Endothelschädigung? Fortschr. Röntgenstr. 135, 4: 489–491, 1981

4 Holm, L., J. Praestholm: Ioxaglate, a new isoosmolar contrast medium used in femoral angiography. Brit. J. Radiol. 52: 169, 1979

5 Meves, M., H. Kiefer: Klinische Erfahrungen mit Ioxaglat, einem neuen Kontrastmittel für die Angiographie. Fortschr. Röntgenstr. 113, 6: 657–659, 1980

6 Skalpe, I. O., A. Lundervold, K. Tjørstadt: Cerebral angiography with non-ionic (metrizamide) and ionic (meglumine metrizoate) watersoluble contrast media. A comparative study with double blind technic. Neuroradiology 14: 15, 1977
7 Stoeter, P., M. Schumacher: Direkte und indirekte zerebrale Amipaque-Angiographie. II. Konzentrationsabhängige Untersuchungen der Verträglichkeit und Nebenwirkungen. In: Amipaque Workshop Berlin, 29. Mai 1978, W. Frommhold, H. Hacker, H. E. Schmitt, H. Vogelsang (eds.). Excerpta Medica, Amsterdam 1978
8 Stoeter, P., M. Poremba, M. Schumacher: Zerebrale Angiographie mit Ioxaglat (Hexabrix®): Klinische und densitometrische Ergebnisse bei Verwendung verschiedener Jodkonzentrationen. In: Zukunft der Angiographie – Schmerzfreiheit? Symposium Frankfurt/Main, 7. Juli 1979. Byk Gulden Pharmazeutica, Konstanz 1980
9 Voigt, K., M. Schumacher: Direkte und indirekte zerebrale Amipaque-Angiographien. I. Diagnostische und densitometrische Ergebnisse, Bedeutung und Grenzen in Abhängigkeit von unterschiedlichen Konzentrationen. In: Amipaque Workshop, Berlin, 29. Mai 1978, W. Frommhold, H. Hacker, H. E. Schmitt, H. Vogelsang (eds.). Excerpta Medica, Amsterdam 1978

10 Zachrisson, B.-F., R. Johannson, L. Björk: Two new contrast media in peripheral arteriography. A double blind study in patients with arterial insufficiency in the legs. Fortschr. Röntgenstr. 132, 2: 208–211, 1980

*Addendum:* Since submission of this paper these studies on iohexol have been reported:

Ahlgren, P.: Iohexol compared to Urografin Meglumine in cerebral angiography. A randomized, double blind crossover study. Neuroradiology 23: 195, 1982

Holtås, S., S. Cronqvist, T. Renaa: Cerebral angiography with iohexol. A comparison with metrizamide in man. Neuroradiology 24: 201, 1983

Ingstrup, H. M., P. Hauge: Clinical testing of Iohexol, Conray Meglumine and Amipaque in cerebral angiography. Neuroradiology 23: 75, 1982

Nakstad, P., O. Sortland, O. Aaserud, A. Lundervold: Cerebral angiography with the non-ionic water-soluble contrast medium Iohexol and Meglumine-Ca-Metrizoate. A randomized double blind parallel study in man. Neuroradiology 23: 199, 1982

# Cardiovascular Side Effects of Various Conventional, Low-osmolar and Non-ionic Contrast Media

K. Wink and J. Wissert

## Summary

The cardiovascular side effects of paired, alternating injections of contrast media in selective coronary angiography were studied in 37 patients with coronary heart disease of varying severity. A total of 330 injections was given into right and left coronary arteries.

The decrease in the heart rate and systolic and diastolic aortic pressure and, in the extremity lead I of the ECG, the lifting or lowering of the ST stage on injection into the right or left coronary artery served as the criteria for the cardiovascular side effects – regardless of the coronary artery injected.

As regards the incidence and quantity of these changes based on the behaviour of the heart rate, the systolic and diastolic aortic pressure and, partly, of the ST stage, the least cardiovascular side effects occurred under Hexabrix and Amipaque and the greatest under Urografin, while Rayvist occupied a middle position. A certain parallelism therefore exists between the cardiovascular side effects and the osmolality, while other factors appear to be of secondary importance in our study.

## Zusammenfassung

Bei 37 Patienten unterschiedlichen Schweregrades einer koronaren Herzerkrankung wurden die kardiovaskulären Rückwirkungen von jeweils paarweise bei der selektiven Koronarangiographie alternierend applizierten Kontrastmitteln geprüft. Insgesamt wurden 330 Injektionen in die rechte und linke Koronarie durchgeführt.

Als Kriterien der kardiovaskulären Rückwirkung dienten unabhängig von der injizierten Koronarie die Abnahme der Herzfrequenz und die Senkung des systolischen und diastolischen Aortendrucks sowie im EKG in der Extremitäten-Ableitung I die Hebung bzw. Senkung der ST-Strecke bei Injektion in die rechte bzw. linke Koronararterie.

Nach der Häufigkeit und dem quantitativen Ausmaß dieser Änderungen ergaben sich nach dem Verhalten der Herzfrequenz, dem systolischen und diastolischen Aortendruck sowie zum Teil der ST-Strecke die geringsten kardiovaskulären Rückwirkungen beim Hexabrix und Amipaque, die stärksten Effekte beim Urografin, während Rayvist eine Zwischenstellung einnahm. Es besteht damit eine gewisse Parallelität zwischen den kardiovaskulären Rückwirkungen und der Osmolalität, während andere Faktoren in unserer Studie von untergeordneter Bedeutung zu sein scheinen.

## Introduction

The radiological demonstration of the heart and the vessels in its vicinity with the aid of contrast media has now become an indispensable diagnostic measure for the detection of morphological and functional changes which determines further therapeutic procedure and, in particular, the indication for surgical treatment. Nowadays, however, this method of examination is no longer used for diagnostic purposes only, but has also become a therapeutic measure, e.g. in coronary dilatation with a balloon catheter and in coronary lysis (Figs 1 and 2). This has made contrast radiology of the heart and its vessels a frequently used method even in patients who are seriously ill.

In view of this development, we must be aware of the cardiovascular side effects of contrast media, not only to manage them effectively, but also for choosing the contrast media with the best tolerance.

Today's contrast media can be divided into conventional, low-osmolar and non-ionic preparations, and we have studied representatives from each group. Urografin 76 (meglumine sodium diatrizoate) and Rayvist 350 (meglumine sodium ioglicinate) were studied as conventional contrast media, Hexabrix (meglumine sodium ioxaglate) as a low-

Table 1  Iodine concentration, viscosity and osmolality of the contrast media studied

|  | Iodine concentration (mg/ml) | Viscosity at 37 °C (mPa–sec) | Osmolality at 37 °C (mosm/l) |
|---|---|---|---|
| Meglumine sodium diatrizoate (Urografin 76) | 370 | 8.9 | 2100 |
| Meglumine sodium ioglicinate (Rayvist 350) | 350 | 9.6 | 2240 |
| Meglumine sodium ioxaglate (Hexabrix) | 320 | 7.5 | 600 |
| Metrizamide (Amipaque) | 300 | 6.24 | 485 |

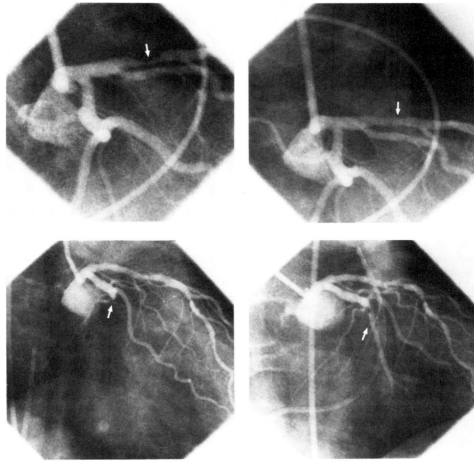

Fig 1 Coronary angiogram before (a) and after (b) dilatation of severe stenosis in the proximal region of the interventricular branch of the left coronary artery

Fig 2 Coronary angiogram before (a) and after (b) re-opening of the circumflex branch of the left coronary artery by intracoronary lysis with streptokinase

osmolar and Amipaque (metrizamide) as a nonionic agent (Table 1).

## Conventional Contrast Media

The diatrizoates replaced the still highly toxic acetrizoates in 1953, and the substances were developed further by changing the substitutes at the $C_3$ atom of the aromatic ring system. In particular, the subsequent years saw the development of preparations which displayed longer hydrophilic side chains.

This gave rise to ioglicinate (meglumine sodium ioglicinate) which, as Rayvist and like Urografin (meglumine sodium diatrizoate), can be regarded as a conventional contrast medium. However, both of these contrast media still produced marked cardiovascular side effects on angiography of the heart and vessels. For example, we observed as adverse effects in personal studies in 37 patients with 330 injections into the right and left coronary arteries, a decrease in heart rate and in systolic and diastolic pressure in the aorta and, in the ECG, lowering of the ST stage on injection into the left coronary artery and lifting of the ST stage on injection into the right coronary artery.

On alternating paired injection of Urografin and Rayvist in two patients (12 injections) into the coronary arteries (Table 2), where only the change in one patient was evaluated further, Urografin led more frequently to a change in heart rate and systolic and diastolic aortic pressure and to lifting of the ST stage on injection into the right coronary artery, than did Rayvist, whereas lowering of the ST stage occurred on every injection of Urografin and Rayvist into the left coronary artery. The magnitude of the change (Table 3) was greater under Urografin than under Rayvist in all parameters.

Therefore, cardiovascular side effects were reduced more by the development of ioglicinate than by that of the diatrizoates. Although the osmolality of Rayvist (2240 mosm/l) is somewhat higher than that of Urografin (2100 mosm/l), its iodine content

Table 2  Incidences of the decrease of heart rate and systolic and diastolic aortic pressure and of lifting and lowering of ST stage on injection into the right and left coronary artery after administration of Urografin (U), Rayvist (R), Hexabrix (H) and Amipaque (A)

| Heart rate | | | | | |
|---|---|---|---|---|---|
| U/R | U/H | U/A | R/H | R/A | H/A |
| 83.0/50.0 | 93.1/34.4 | 100.0/88.8 | 75.8/48.2 | 95.0/72.1 | 23.0/46.1 |
| Systolic aortic pressure | | | | | |
| U/R | U/H | U/A | R/H | R/A | H/A |
| 55.5/44.4 | 80.0/48.0 | 88.8/55.6 | 63.6/4.5 | 84.6/30.7 | 45.0/30.0 |
| Diastolic aortic pressure | | | | | |
| U/R | U/H | U/A | R/H | R/A | H/A |
| 66.6/44.4 | 68.0/16.0 | 66.5/55.5 | 40.9/9.0 | 69.2/19.2 | 10.0/20.0 |
| ST stage Right coronary artery (lifting) | | | | | |
| U/R | U/H | U/A | R/H | R/A | H/A |
| 50.0/25.0 | 40.0/20.0 | 100.0/66.6 | 21.4/14.2 | 73.6/42.1 | 80.0/50.0 |
| Left coronary artery (lowering) | | | | | |
| U/R | U/H | U/A | R/H | R/A | H/A |
| 100.0/100.0 | 75.0/75.0 | 100.0/100.0 | 73.3/73.3 | 95.0/90.0 | 76.9/84.6 |

Table 3  Percental change of the decrease of the heart rate and systolic and diastolic aortic pressure and of lifting and lowering of ST stage on injection into the right and left coronary artery after administration of Urografin (U), Rayvist (R), Hexabrix (H) and Amipaque (A)

| Heart rate | | | | | |
|---|---|---|---|---|---|
| U/R | U/H | U/A | R/H | R/A | H/A |
| 8.7/4.3 | 9.6/2.4 | 16.8/4.2 | 12.2/2.5 | 19.9/3.7 | 1.2/1 |
| Systolic aortic pressure | | | | | |
| U/R | U/H | U/A | R/H | R/A | H/A |
| 8.0/5.4 | 11.2/5.3 | 12.1/7.0 | 7.9/1.7 | 11.1/3.3 | 6.0/3 |
| Diastolic aortic pressure | | | | | |
| U/R | U/H | U/A | R/H | R/A | H/A |
| 7.4/5.4 | 7.8/1.5 | 11.3/7.9 | 579/1.2 | 9.2/1.8 | 3.0/2 |
| ST stage Right coronary artery (lifting) | | | | | |
| U/R | U/H | U/A | R/H | R/A | H/A |
| 27.5/15.0 | 35.0/7.08 | 76.6/66.6 | 14.4/7.8 | 48.7/30.0 | 55.5/36.0 |
| Left coronary artery (lowering) | | | | | |
| U/R | U/H | U/A | R/H | R/A | H/A |
| 98.7/77.2 | 76.5/64.0 | 214.8/116.6 | 100.6/82.6 | 111.5/79.8 | 161.5/107 |

is lower (350 compared to 370 mg/ml) and may be the reason for its more favourable effect.

## Low-osmolar Contrast Media

Ioxaglic acid and, from this, meglumine sodium ioxaglate (Hexabrix) were developed in 1976. This is a low-osmolar contrast medium with an osmolality at 37°C of 600 mosm/l – far lower than that of Urografin (2100 mosm/l) and Rayvist (2240 mosm/l). The most striking thing about Hexabrix was that its injection into the peripheral vessels was virtually painless. Our own studies with paired alternating injection of Urografin and Rayvist in comparison with Hexabrix in 8 patients (116 injections) showed that decreases in heart rate and systolic and diastolic aortic pressure and changes of the ST stage in the ECG were less frequent and pronounced under

Hexabrix than under Urografin and Rayvist (Tables 2 and 3).

The development of ioxaglic acid therefore represents a further improvement of contrast medium tolerance. This was probably brought about primarily by the lower osmolality and viscosity of ioxaglic acid in comparison to the conventional contrast media. In addition, the iodine content of Hexabrix is also lower than that of Urografin and Rayvist (320 compared to 370 and 350 mg/ml, respectively). Despite this, our studies showed that the radiopacity of Hexabrix was at least equal to that of the conventional contrast media.

## Non-ionic Contrast Media

With the development of the non-ionic compound metrizamide (Amipaque) and reduction of the osmolality to 485 mosm/l, the tolerance of contrast media was improved even further.

Our comparative studies (Tables 2 and 3) with Urografin, Rayvist, Hexabrix and Amipaque in 27 patients (192 injections) confirmed this by showing that the incidence and severity of cariovascular side effects are much lower under Amipaque than under Urografin and Rayvist. The differences between Amipaque and Hexabrix were not so great. For example, decreases in heart rate and diastolic aortic pressure and lowering of the ST stage on injection into the left coronary artery were more frequent after Amipaque than after Hexabrix, while decreases in systolic aortic pressure and lifting of the ST stage on injection into the right coronary artery were more frequent after Hexabrix than after Amipaque. However, the magnitude of the changes was greater after Hexabrix than after Amipaque in all parameters.

Summing up, we can say that of all contrast media studied, the best cardiovascular tolerance is displayed by Amipaque, although the differences between the non-ionic preparation Amipaque and the low-osmolar contrast medium Hexabrix are small. This superiority of Amipaque is attributable primarily to its low osmolality, but also to its low viscosity (6.24 mPa·sec) and low iodine content (300 mg/ml). Reducing the iodine content has not, however, reduced the radiopacity of Amipaque compared to the other compounds.

Cardiovascular side effects of contrast media in selective coronary angiography such as a decrease of the heart rate and blood pressure and ECG changes have been known since 1967 (3, 4).

Other contrast medium studies (1, 6, 7, 12, 13, 14, 15, 18, 19) have also shown that these side effects are greater under conventional contrast media than under low-osmolar and non-ionic compounds. The different sodium content of the contrast media has been suggested as the cause (3). It has been shown that complications occur more frequently under both a higher and lower sodium content, meaning that it should equal the physiological milieu as closely as possible (9, 20). However, it is noteworthy that Amipaque, which contains no sodium, also displays the lowest rate of side effects. Thus, the decisive factor is probably the osmolality (2, 5, 16, 17, 21), with the iodine content and the viscosity playing a relatively minor role (8, 21).

An ischaemic explanation for the ECG changes due to displacement of the blood by the contrast medium (10) must be rejected, since balanced physiological solutions have been shown to cause only very small changes (11).

The clinical implications of this are that a low-osmolar or non-ionic contrast medium should be used in patients predisposed to bradycardia or in poor cardiac action with reduced stroke volume and hence, reduced aortic pressures. However, these contrast media should also be used in patients with or liable to cardiac insufficiency. This applies above all to intracoronary lysis of a fresh myocardial infarction. Furthermore, low-osmolar or non-ionic contrast media should be used for investigations in which very large amounts of contrast medium may be required – for example, in coronary artery dilatation with a balloon catheter, where continuous checks of both the coronary stenosis and the position of the balloon catheter may necessitate large amounts of contrast material. On top of this, temporary ischaemia is caused when the balloon is filled and obstructs the coronary artery, and this may impair the action of the heart. The only argument remaining in favour of conventional contrast media is their low price, and even this is now not so important in view of the smaller number of such examinations low conducted.

## References

1 Almen, T.: Effects of metrizamide and other contrast media on the isolated rabbit heart. Acta radiol. (Stockh.) Suppl. 335: 216, 1973
2 Björk, L., P. Eldh, S. Paulin: Non-ionic and dimeric contrast media in coronary angiography. Acta radiol. Diagn. 18: 235, 1977
3 Brown, T. G.: Cardiovascular actions of angiographic media. Angiology 18: 273, 1967
4 Coskey, R. L., O. Magidson: Electrocardiographic response to selective coronary arteriography. Brit. Heart J. 28: 512, 1967
5 Dimsdale, J. E., A. M. Hutter, J. Gelbert, Th. P. Hackett, P. C. Block, D. M. Catanzano: Predicting results of coronary angiography. Amer. Heart J. 98: 281, 1979
6 Erikson, U., I. Cullhed, G. Hemius, G. Ruhn: Erfahrungen mit Amipaque® und Isopaque Coronar® bei der Coronararteriographie. Ein Vergleich. Amipaque Workshop Berlin, 29.5.1978. Excerpta Medica, Amsterdam 1978
7 Hellström, M., B. Jacobson, S.-E. Sörensen, B. O. Erikson: Metrizamide and metrizoate for cardioangiography in infants. Acta radiol. Diagn. 21: 263, 1980
8 Higgins, Ch.: Effects of contrast media in the conducing septum of the heart. Radiology 124: 599, 1977
9 Hildner, F. J., B. Scherlag, Ph. Samet: Evaluation of renografin M-76 as a contrast agent for angiogcardiography. Radiology 100: 329, 1971
10 Maytin, O., C. Castillo, A. Castellanos, jr.: The Genesis of QRS changes produced by selective coronary arteriography. Circulation 41: 247, 1970
11 Ovitt, Th., Gh. Rizk, R. S. Rech, R. Cramer, K. Amplatz: Electrocardiographic changes in selective coronary arteriography: The importance of ions. Radiology 104: 705, 1972
12 Schmitt, H. E., F. Burkart, O. Bertel: Laevokardiographie mit Metrizamid. Amipaque® Workshop Berlin, 29.5.1978. Excerpta Medica, Amsterdam 1978
13 Simon, R.: Interindividuelle randomisierte Studie mit AG 6227 und Conray 60 in der zerebralen Angiographie. Symposium Frankfurt/M., 7. Juli 1979. Byk Gulden Pharmazeutica, Konstanz
14 Stoeter, P., M. Poremba, M. Schuhmacher: Zerebrale Angiographie mit Ioxaglat (Hexabrix®): Klinische und densitometrische Ergebnisse bei Verwendung verschiedener Jodkonzentrationen. Symposium Frankfurt/M., 7. Juli 1979. Byk Gulden Pharmazeutica, Konstanz
15 Stoeter, P., K. Voigt: Ergebnisse zerebraler Angiographien mit Ioglicinat (Rayvist®). Radiologe 19: 494, 1979
16 Trägardh, B., P. R. Lynch, Th. Vinciguerra: Effects of metrizamide, a new nonionic contrast medium on cardiac function during coronary angiography in the dog. Radiology 115: 59, 1975
17 Trägardh, B., P. Lynch, M. Trägardh: Coronary angiography with diatrizoate and metrizamide. Acta radiol. Diagn. 17: 69, 1976
18 Trägardh, B., P. R. Lynch: ECG changes and arrhythmias induced by ionic and non-ionic contrast media during coronary arteriography in dogs. Invest. Radiol. 13: 233, 1978
19 Weikl, A.: Kardiale Nebenwirkungen von Hexabrix bei der Koronarangiographie – ein klinischer Vergleich zu einem Standardmittel. Symposium Frankfurt/M., 7. Juli 1979. Byk Gulden Pharmazeutica, Konstanz
20 Weikl, A., O. E. Durst, E. Lang: Komplikationen der selektiven Koronarangiographie in Abhängigkeit vom verwendeten Kontrastmittel. Fortschr. Röntgenstr. 123: 3, 1975
21 White, C. W., D. L. Eckberg, T. Inasaka, F. M. Abboud: Effects of angiographic contrast media on sino-artrial-nodal function. Cardiovasc. Res. 10: 214, 1976

# Contrast Media in Intravenous Digital Subtraction Angiography (Initial Experience)

W. Seyferth and E. Zeitler

## Summary

The results of use of various ionic and non-ionic contrast agents in over 1300 intravenous digital subtraction angiography patient investigations are reported. In particular, contrast-induced side effects, dependence of subtraction image quality on the total iodine content of the bolus, and the differential employment of ionic and non-ionic agents are discussed.

## Zusammenfassung

Es wird über die Ergebnisse der Anwendung verschiedener ionischer und nicht-ionischer Kontrastmittel nach mehr als 1300 Untersuchungen an Patienten mittels intravenöser digitaler Subtraktions-Angiographie berichtet. Insbesondere werden die kontrastmittelinduzierten Nebenwirkungen, die Abhängigkeit der Qualität des Subtraktionsbildes von dem Gesamtjodgehalt des Bolus und die differenzierte Anwendung ionischer und nicht-ionischer Kontrastmittel besprochen.

## Introduction

In the clinical trials of intravenous digital subtraction angiography (DSA) the primary concerns to date have been the determination of appropriate indications and the estimation of risks in comparison to conventional angiography (2, 3, 11, 13), as well as judging the diagnostic accuracy of the procedure. Meanwhile, technical improvements have been occurring simultaneously (6).

To obtain a favourable signal-to-noise ratio, maximum possible iodine concentration in the arterial filling phase has been sought. This seemed to be guaranteed by using a contrast medium with the highest possible specific iodine concentration.

Another special aspect of intravenous digital subtraction angiography is the mode of application of multiple intravenous boluses of contrast medium, with a resulting high total volume of contrast agent. This may potentially lead to cardiac or renal decompensation. We present here our initial experience with ionic and non-ionic contrast media.

## Materials and Methods

Investigations were carried out with a digital video subtraction angiography device built by Siemens Corporation (Angiotron), the technical specifications of which have been described elsewhere (6, 7, 8).

The factors contributing to image quality, such as decrease in noise through averaging, summation of individual images, coning-down the field of investigation, and maintaining the field and projection of investigation as constant as possible, were all observed during the examinations.

Contrast media were applied through a preatrial (central venous) catheter. The speed of injection was 17 ml per sec. The bolus volume was adjusted to the specific iodine concentration of the employed contrast medium and varied between 20 and 56 ml. The various contrast media (Table 1) were compared according to objectives: time of appearance in the area of investigation (supraaortic neck arteries in the RAO projection), the time of maximum concentration, movement artefacts, and subjective judgement of image quality. The trial proceeded in a controlled cross-over double-blind study (n = 25 as well as n = 50) with evaluation of both initial injections in each patient. The results were considered statistically significant if p was less than 0.05.

Table 1

| Contrast medium | I (mg/ml) |
|---|---|
| Na-meglumine amidotrizoate (Urografin 45) | 218 |
| Meglumine amidotrizoate (Angiografin) | 306 |
| Na-meglumine amidotrizoate (Urografin 76) | 370 |
| Iohexol | 350 |

## Results

There was essentially no difference in the time of the first appearance of contrast medium in the field. The timing of contrast maximum could be optically differentiated in those instances only where considerably different contrast volumes were employed, that is in the iodine-equivalent doses of Urografin 76 and Urografin 45 (33 and 56 ml respectively).

## Movement and Swallowing Artefacts

With respect to examinations of the arteries of the neck, certain unfortunate responses are elicited by the use of contrast media, that is, swallowing motions of the larynx, contraction of cervical muscles, and resulting misregistration through movement of the cervical spine. These movements appear to be primarily related to the sensation of heat induced by the contrast agent, a sensation which may be perceived by some as a choking sensation.

In each case, we conduct the investigation after adequately informing the patient of the sensations to be expected and emphasizing the necessity for complete co-operation (refraining from swallowing and remaining relaxed). Under these conditions, we could not establish any significant differences between the ionic contrast media and also between ionic and nonionic contrast media, as far as the frequency of movement artefacts was concerned.

Certainly, after the application of iohexol, the sensation of heat was clearly graded lower than after ionic contrast media. This subjective difference was confirmed statistically in the course of the double-blind study, but was not reflected in a statistically significant decrease in motion artefacts.

Nonetheless, there were individual patients in whom movement artefacts, incorrigible by postprocessing, arose with the use of ionic contrast media, but who could still be successfully studied, free of artefact, by employing iohexol.

## Subjective Image Quality (Table 2)

The impressions of image quality and detail recognition were made by two different observers, both on the basis of television picture and hard-copy.

Our results seem to indicate that when using a digital subtraction system capable of maintaining a constant summation image, the total amount of iodine applied is the deciding factor. In this regard, an iodine dose of between 12 and 15 grams appears sufficient, while 8 grams of iodine in the objection bolus lead to a considerable subjective deterioration in the image quality. This impression was constant whether Urografin 45 or Urografin 76 were employed.

Table 2

| Iod. (g) | Δ image quality | |
|---|---|---|
| 8 | Na-Megl'amidotrizoate | 218 |
|   | Na-Megl'amidotrizoate | 370 |
| 12 | Na-Megl'amidotrizoate | 218 |
|    | Megl'amidotrizoate | 306 |
|    | Na-Megl'amidotrizoate | 370 |
| 14 | Iohexol | 350 |
|    | Na-Megl'amidotrizoate | 370 |
| 15 | Na-Megl'amidotrizoate | 370 |

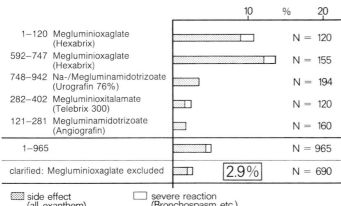

Fig 1   Contrast medium complications (N = 965)

## Contrast Agent Side Effects

Also evaluated were mild contrast reactions, such as allergic urticaria, as well as the more severe reactions of bronchospasm, pulmonary oedema, etc. (Fig 1).

Sodium meglumine amidotrizoate, meglumine ioxithalamate, and meglumine amidotrizoate were subjected to evaluation. The resulting 2.9% rate of contrast media reactions after multiple intravenous injections of the individual contrast media proved to be no greater than that observed in single contrast injections, such as used in i. v. pyelography. The number of patients thus far examined with iohexol is as yet insufficient for us to draw a conclusion.

## Medical Complications (Table 3)

Independent of the type of ionic contrast medium given, symptoms of angina pectoris occurred in 2.8% of the patients. This does not appear to be influenced by the central venous application, since similar symptoms were reported after multiple injections in the cubital region (6, 10). Symptoms of angina pectoris were also observed with the use of iohexol, occurring in 1.8% (n = 50).

Table 3  Medical complications (n = 1000)

| | | | | |
|---|---|---|---|---|
| Acute renal failure | | | 1 | |
| Angina pectoris | | | | |
| 1–120 | Meglumine ioxaglate (Hexabrix) | L<br>S | 2<br>1 | 2.5% |
| 121–281 | Meglumine amidotrizoate (Angiografin) | L<br>S | 3<br>– | 1.9% |
| 282–402 | Meglumine ioxithalamate (Telebrix) | L<br>S | –<br>1 | 0.8% |
| 592–747 | Meglumine ioxaglate (Hexabrix) | L<br>S | 4<br>1 | 3.2% |
| 748–942 | Na-meglumine amidotrizoate (Urografin) | L<br>S | 4<br>– | 2.1% |
| 1–965 | | L<br>S | 21<br>6 | 2.8% |

## Discussion

A high-contrast visualisation of the vascular system and an image free from artefacts are two of the most important goals of digital subtraction angiography. Our investigations indicate that the specific iodine content of the contrast agent employed is not the deciding factor, but rather it is the total amount of iodine injected in the bolus. This result provides a point of departure for future investigations to determine the minimum amount of contrast dose necessary. The production of an artefact-free image depends considerably upon the cooperation of the patient, and is decidedly influenced by the use of ionic or non-ionic contrast agents in very few cases. In this regard, we cannot confirm the results of previous investigations (5).

The use of non-ionic materials may still be influenced by purely cardiologic features, such as the decreased haemodynamic effects induced by non-ionic contrast media, as well as their decreased detrimental influence on myocardial contractility (1, 5). The frequency of skin reactions related to the use of ionic contrast media, sodium meglumine amidotrizoate, meglumine ioxithalamate, and meglumine amidotrizoate remains, at 2.9%, within the range to be expected from intravenous injection in other studies, such as i. v. pyelography. A possible explanation for the special effects of meglumine ioxaglate may be the observed increased release of histamine resulting from the intravenous bolus application of this medium, as opposed to the other contrast media (12). Cells containing histamine are concentrated particularly in the lung. That the release of histamine may be a function of repeated, shortterm high concentrations of meglumine ioxaglate, can be presumed on the basis of our experiences in spermatic phlebography. We used small quantities of meglumine ioxaglate in spermatic phlebography, with repeated manually applied boluses in the renal vein, without observing an increased number of contrast reactions (9).

At present, we cannot confirm whether the amount of contrast agent used in intravenous digital subtraction angiography will have any effect on the possible number of reactions induced by later repeated examinations. It also remains an open question whether the employment of non-ionic contrast media in digital subtraction angiography will lead to a decrease in risk, as proved in conventional arteriography (4). Larger patient numbers are required for this purpose.

Angina pectoris provides a typical complication for DSA. The appearance of angina shows no dependence on the kind of contrast medium employed, or on a central versus peripheral site of application. It would be good to determine if the patients' repeated breath-holding plays a causal role through the cardiac loading induced, this in combination with the contrast injection. Here, too, the use of non-ionic contrast media does not seem to provide a beneficial effect.

Thus, one may advance the following, last but by no means least from the economic viewpoint:

The use of non-ionic contrast media is possible on the basis of the quality of the resulting studies, and the complication rates. Non-ionic contrast agents may be of special advantage in patients with known risk factors for contrast studies, as well as in quantitative cardiac studies.

## References

1 Gerber, K. H., C. B. Higgins, Y. S. Yuh, J. A. Keziol: Regional myocardial hemodynamic and metabolic effects of ionic and nonionic contrast media in the normal and ischemic state. Circulation (in press)
2 Mistretta, Ch. A., A. B. Crummy, Ch. M. Strother, J. F. Sackett: Digital Subtraction Arteriography: An Application of Computerized Fluoroscopy. Year Book Med. Publ., Chicago 1982
3 Pond, G. D., J. R. L. Smith, B. J. Hillmann, Th. W. Ovitt, M. P. Capp: Current clinical applications of clinical subtraction angiography. Applied Radiology 71, Nov/Dec. 1981
4 Rapoport, S. et al: Experience with Metrizamide in patients with previous severe anaphylactoid reactions to ionic contrast agents. Radiology 143: 321, 1982
5 Sackett, J. F., F. A. Mann: Contrast media for digital subtraction arteriography of cerebral arteries. In Mistretta, Ch. A., A. B. Crummy, Ch. M. Strother, J. F. Sackett: Digital Subtraction Arteriography. An Application of Computerized Fluoroscopy. Year Book Med. Publ., Chicago 1982 (p. 23)
6 Seyferth, W., G. Dilbat, R. Herde et al.: Digitale Subtraktionsangiographie (DSA) an einem konventionellen Röntgen-Durchleuchtungsgerät. Electromedica 4: 120, 1982
7 Seyferth, W., P. Marhoff, E. Zeitler: Transvenöse und arterielle digitale Videosubtraktionsangiographie (DVSA). Fortschr. Röntgenstr. 136: 301–309, 1982
8 Seyferth, W., P. Marhoff, E. Zeitler: Digitale Subtraktionsangiographie: Diagnostischer Stellenwert und Risiko. Electromedica 2: 60–68, 1982
9 Seyferth, W., E.-I. Richter, R. Grosse-Vorholt: Phlebographie der Vena spermatic interna. Radiologe 20: 440–444, 1980
10 Stark, E., P. Harth, J. Kollath et al.: Klinische Erfahrungen mit der digitalen Subtraktionsangiographie. (in press)
11 Stieghorst, M. F., Ch. Strother, Ch. A. Mistretta, A. B. Crummy et al.: Digital subtraction angiography – a clinical overview. Applied Radiology 43, Nov./Dec. 1981
12 Tuengerthal, S.: Physiologie und Nebenwirkungen der Kontrastmittelapplication in Bolustechnik bei der CT. In J. Lissner, J. L. Doppmann: Internationales CT-Symposium, Seefeld 1982. Schnetztor-Verlag, Konstanz 1982 (p. 296–304)
13 Weinstein, M. A., M. T. Modic, E. Buonocore, Th. F. Meaney: Digital subtraction angiography. Clinical experience of the Cleveland Clinic Foundation. Applied Radiology 53, Nov./Dec. 1981

# Urography

## The Risk Liability of Nephrotropic Contrast Media: Clinical and Experimental Results

T. Kröpelin, Ch. Gospos, X. Papacaralampous and N. Freudenberg

### Summary

The pharmokinetics of renal contrast media (= CM) are first of all explained as a base for understanding the risks of CM. It is stressed that the risks – general reactions and local, nephrogenic damage and disorders of the blood-clotting system – are dependent not only on the nature, dose and mode of administration of the CM, but also on various endogenous and exogenous factors. The time factor, incidence and forms of general reactions are compared after intravenous and intraarterial administration of different CM in nephrological and heterogeneous study populations. Local damage is discussed and experimental results regarding the injurious effect of different CM on the endothelium of the aorta and vena cava of rats are described. As regards organ damage, nephrogenic CM damage is dealt with in greatest detail; attention is drawn to the fact that dilute CM drip infusions are tolerated better than undiluted bolus injections by patients with chronic renal disease with and without impaired renal function. CM-induced deterioration of renal function can be avoided in this way. Transient disorders of renal function were observed in patients without renal disease as a result of a shock syndrome. The histology of direct nephrotoxic CM damage cannot always be clearly delineated from the changes occurring in shock kidneys without CM administration.

### Zusammenfassung

Zum Verständnis der KM-Risiken wird zunächst auf die Pharmakokinetik der renalen Kontrastmittel (= KM) eingegangen. Es wird betont, daß die Risiken: Allgemeinreaktionen sowie lokale, organ-nephrogene Schäden und Blut-Gerinnungssystemstörungen nicht nur von der KM-Art, -Dosis und dem -Applikationsmodus abhängig sind, sondern auch von verschiedenen endogenen und exogenen Faktoren. Von Allgemeinreaktionen werden Zeitfaktor, Häufigkeit und Formen verglichen nach intravenösen und intraarteriellen Gaben unterschiedlicher KM beim nephrologisch und heterogen zusammengesetzten Krankengut. Die lokalen Schäden werden erwähnt und die experimentellen Ergebnisse über die endothelschädigende Wirkung verschiedener KM an der Aorta und Vena cava von Ratten dargestellt. Bei den Organschäden wird vorwiegend auf die nephrogenen KM-Schäden eingegangen und darauf hingewiesen, daß bei chronischen Nierenkranken mit und ohne eingeschränkter Nierenfunktion verdünnte KM-Tropfinfusionen besser toleriert werden, als unverdünnte Bolusinjektionen. So läßt sich eine KM-induzierte Nierenfunktionsverschlechterung vermeiden. Bei nicht nierenkranken Patienten sahen wir vorübergehende Nierenfunktionsstörungen als Folge einer Schocksymptomatik. Die Histologie der direkten nephrotoxischen KM-Schäden läßt sich gegenüber den Veränderungen von Schocknieren ohne KM-Gabe nicht immer sicher abgrenzen.

### Introduction

The use of nephrotropic contrast media is no longer restricted to conventional urographic and angiographic examinations, but is increasing steadily with the introduction of new methods (Table 1). Large amounts of contrast media are administered intravenously in new non-invasive methods, e. g. in various computerized tomographic examinations with different modes of administration and in computerized digital transvenous video subtraction angiography (4, 36). Smaller amounts of renal contrast media are also being used for localization in new therapeutic catheter techniques. Thanks to improved, modern contrast media, however, the rate of side effects and incidents does not appear to be increasing to any significant extent despite this increased use, although there are no up-to-date statistical surveys on this.

The various tri-iodobenzoic acid derivatives now on the market are distinguished by their different side chains and halogens. The latter are sodium or methyl glucamine salts, although they are often present as mixtures. Some contrast media (= CM), however, are used as pure methyl glucamine salts.

# Urography

Table 1a  Non-invasive methods

| Conventional | New |
|---|---|
| – excretory urography | – computerized tomography vascular-parenchymal phase |
| – phlebography | – i.v. arteriography: digital vascular imaging = DVI |

Table 1b  Invasive methods

| Conventional | New |
|---|---|
| – aorto-, arteriography<br>– cardiac, pulmonary angiography<br>– selective phlebography<br>– retrograde pyelogram | – catheter dilatation<br>– catheter embolisation<br>– catheter embolectomy – thrombolysis<br>– percutaneous nephropyelostomy<br>– percutaneous renocystography |

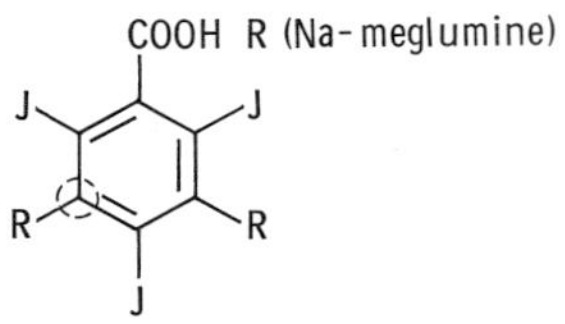

COOH R (Na-meglumine)

Nephrotropic (parenteral)

Diatrizoate (e.g. Urografin)
Metrizoate (e.g. Isopaque)
Iothalamate (e.g. Conray)
Ioxitalamate (e.g. Telebrix)
Ioxaglate (e.g. Hexabrix)

Fig 1  Water-soluble contrast media (2-4-6-triiodobenzoic acid)

## Pharmacokinetics

Understanding the mode of action of CM requires a knowledge of their pharmacokinetics. Most of the nephrotropic CM injected into the bloodstream is eliminated via the kidneys – at the usual dosage (30–60 ml), about 10–20% after 10 minutes, about 50% after 1 hour and more than 90% after 24 hours. The renal elimination of modern CM is effected by glomerular filtration. Extrarenal elimination via the liver, small bowel, rectum and salivary glands is negligibly small when renal function is normal, but increases in impaired renal function in relation to the degree of renal insufficiency. Nephrotropic CM flow via the preglomerular bloodstream and the vasa afferentia to the glomeruli, where they undergo glomerular filtration and are excreted into the renal pelvis via the renal tubule system. When an excess of contrast material is present (e.g. in high-dose urography and angiography) or where the glomerular filtration rate is reduced, the unfiltered portion of the contrast medium passes through the vasa efferentia, becomes dispersed throughout the peritubular capillary networks and leaves the kidney via the venous route. Later on, this portion – minus the extrarenal and renal elimination rates – returns to the kidney via the arteries in a more dilute form until it is finally eliminated via the renal tubules. Because it must first pass through the lung, intravenously administered nephrotropic CM is usually diluted to a greater extent on reaching the kidney than is CM injected directly into an artery under high-pressure conditions. When the contrast material is diluted in this way, the unfiltered portion leaving the kidney via the vasa efferentia shifts in favour of the portion undergoing glomerular filtration.

In impaired renal function, the amount of CM eliminated per time unit is reduced in relation to the reduced filtration rate. The amount of contrast medium in the primary urine is therefore dependent on (22):

1. the blood concentration of contrast material,
2. the glomerular filtration rate,
3. the extrarenal elimination rate (minimal).

## Risks

Even modern nephrotropic CM are drugs with potential risks, the occurrence of which greatly depends on the points in Table 2.

Contrast medium risks can be divided into the following groups:

1. General reactions
2. Local damage
3. Organ damage
4. Systemic damage

All reactions of these four groups can vary in severity; however, symptoms from the different

Table 2

Nature of the contrast media
Mode of administration and dose
Endogenous factors – patient situation
    allergic diathesis
    underlying disease (nephro-hepatogenic, cardiac, CNS)
    paraproteinaemias
    hyperuricaemias
    electrolyte disorders, state of hydration
    general condition
Exogenous factors – examination situation
    technical equipment – apprehension
    nature of explanation
    reassuring attitude: doctor + staff
    fluctuating weather

groups can also interact and provoke a chain reaction, e.g. an intravascular or paravascular injection of contrast medium (local damage) leads, via an attack of severe pain and a vascular lesion, to hypotension and shock (general reaction), and the prolonged shock symptoms lead to acute renal failure (organ damage).

Table 3

| Form of reactions | CM effect | | |
|---|---|---|---|
| | dose | nature | mode of administration |
| general | ? | + | + |
| local | ? | + | + |
| organic, systemic damage | + | + | + |

according to Kröpelin et al. 1982 (4)

The general reactions and local CM damage do not usually display a dose-effect relationship, but the nature of the contrast media and their mode of administration can have a provocative effect. In contrast, special organ and systemic damage frequently shows a dose-effect relationship, but even here the nature of the CM and their mode of administration can increase or reduce the risk liability of contrast media.

## General Reactions

The general reactions shown in Table 4 are of most clinical importance:
The mild and severe reaction-specific symptoms may occur in isolation or combined. In severe respiratory distress it is important to establish whether bronchial asthma or pulmonary oedema is present. The latter may be of cardiac origin, but can also be caused by capillary permeability resulting from shock or renal insufficiency. Status anginosus with threatening cardiac infarct can occur above all during coronarography (7). The commonest symptoms on the part of the autonomic nervous system are nausea and vomiting. We observed an increase of these symptoms particulary during fluctuating weather and in apprehensive patients. Severe CNS symptoms with eclamptic convulsions are usually a sign that the contrast medium has broken through the blood-brain barrier, a situation which can easily arise in cerebral damage, infants or after cerebral angiography.

## Time Factor and Incidence of Reactions

It is true for all general reactions that they occur within the first 0–5 minutes in 50 to 80% of cases (10).

Moreover, there are relevant differences in the incidence not only between nephrotropic and biliary contrast media, but also apparently between intravenous and arteriographic administration of renal contrast media, as shown by the following graph (Fig 2) based on the numerical data of Shehadi (38).

Immediate, severe reactions usually occur as shock symptoms, and the implementation of therapy within the first few minutes may be life-saving. Elke and Ferstl (10) have described the importance of the time factor for successful resuscitation in graphic form (Fig 3).

Shock, a dramatic development, usually occurs without any particular subjective or objective prodromes after the administration of a few ml of contrast medium. The cause lies not so much in the nature, dose and mode of administration of the

Table 4

| Mild | Severe | Mild | Severe |
|---|---|---|---|
| *Skin – Mucosa* | | *Respiratory* | |
| – flush | – urticaria, generalised | – tachypnoea | – dyspnoea – cyanosis |
| – itching | – Quincke's oedema of the glottis | – hyperpnoea | – bronchospasm – asthma |
| – urticaria | | – coughing | – pulmonary oedema |
| – hydroblepharon | | | – respiratory arrest |
| *Cardiovascular* | | *CNS Autonomic* | |
| – hypertension | – hypertensive crises | – salivation – dryness | – profuse sweating |
| – hypotension | – shock | – nausea – vomitting | – severe excitation |
| – bradycardia | – arrhythmias | – nervousness – restlessness | – unconsciousness – coma |
| – tachycardia | – status anginosus | – sensation of heat | – tonic-clonic convulsions |
| – anginose complaints | – heart failure | – yawning and sneezing reflex | – paralyses |
| | | – dizziness | |
| | | – tinnitus | |

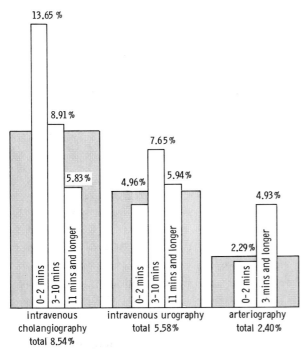

Fig 2  Time factor and incidence of reactions
Comparison of different examination methods. (Modified [graphic presentation] from numerical data of Shehadi 1978)

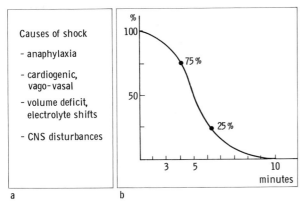

Fig 3
a) Causes of shock
b) Importance of the time factor for successful resuscitation after Elke and Ferstl (1978)

contrast medium as in a poor endogenous or exogenous initial situation. The individual causes of shock listed in Fig 3 are not immediately recognizable, but this is of little importance as regards the immediate countermeasures. The ready availability of full resuscitative facilities including all necessary drugs is essential, and an emergency treatment plan should always be displayed in a prominent position.

*Late reactions* are less frequent. We have experienced a few after ambulatory high-dose urography when the patient had a long journey home in a fasting state. Since then we have always observed the rule that the patient should eat something and drink copiously immediately after the examination. We have also observed allergic, cutaneous reactions with itching a few hours after contrast medium administration in patients with chronic renal disease with severely impaired function and, usually, oliguria who had undergone infusion urography. We attribute these symptoms to the greatly retarded contrast medium elimination and the resultant prolonged circulatory CM persistence with potentially increased histamine liberation. However, late reactions in these patients can be managed easily by providing prophylactic cover with cortisone and antihistamine (23).

## Reported Incidence and Personal Results

There are great differences in literature regarding the incidence and intensity of general reactions (3, 17). The reasons for this are the different examination techniques used, the use of different modes of administration and types of contrast media, and the heterogeneous study population of the different clinics. The data on the incidence of reactions based on the results of inquiries at different centres can, therefore, only provide an approximate, unreliable indication. It is better to compare recent study series conducted with modern contrast media in certain clinics.

A comparison between intravenous and intra-arterial administration of renal contrast media reveals different reaction rates which, according to Shehadi's data (38) and our own results, are of almost

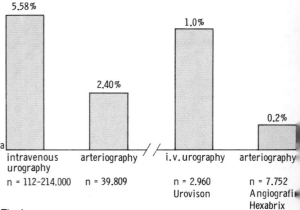

Fig 4
a) Incidence of reactions (%). Modified (graphic presentation) from numerical data of Shehadi (7)
b) Incidence of reactions (%). University of Freiburg 1977–1982

Table 5a  i.v. urography, n = 2,960. Urovison®

| Reactions | n | % |
|---|---|---|
| mild | | |
| – nausea, vomiting, blood pressure | 17 | } 0.98 |
| – generalized urticaria | 12 | |
| severe | | |
| – shock, persistent nephrogram | 2 | |
| – shock, tachycardia, paraesthesias, persistent, nephrogram | 1 | } 0.17 |
| – bronchospasm, cyanosis | 1 | |
| – hypertensive crises, convulsions (cerebral tumour) | 1 | |
| total | 34 | 1.15 |

Table 5b  Arteriography, n = 7,757. Organs = Angiografin®, peripheral = Hexabrix®

| Reactions | n | % |
|---|---|---|
| mild | | |
| – nausea, vomiting, blood pressure | 6 | } 0.18 |
| – generalised urticaria | 8 | |
| severe | | |
| – shock, unconscious (carotid angiography) | 1 | |
| – loss of vision and consciousness vertebral angiography) | 1 | } 0.04 |
| – shock, resuscitated* 10 mins. after aortic arch angiography, transaxillary | 1 | |
| total (1977 – May 1982) | 17 | 0.22 |

* Resuscitation successful

Table 6a  Complications in angiographic examinations (results of inquiries at 519 hospitals in the USA) (*Hessel* et al. 1976 [10])

| | Femoral catheter | Axillary catheter | Translumbar aortography |
|---|---|---|---|
| number of cases | 83,068 | 4,590 | 4,418 |
| cardiovascular | 0.29% | 0.26% | 0.36% |
| neurological | 0.23% | 0.61% | 0.02% |
| death | 0.03% | 0.09% | 0.05% |

Table 6b  Severe complications in 4,348 patients with 8417 arteriograms (*Zeitler* 1978 [9])

| | | |
|---|---|---|
| 1. CNS disorders | | 15 (0.34%) |
| 2. circulatory disorders | | 12 (0.28%) |
| 3. pulmonary disorders | | 2 (0.05) |

4049 under local anaesthesia
299 under general anaesthesia

Aggertal clinic 1969–1973)

equal proportions in urographic and arteriographic examinations despite a greatly differing number of examinations, as Fig 4 shows.
The reason for the differences in the reaction rates may be that intravenously administered contrast material reaches the lung more quickly and in a less diluted form – thereby provoking the liberation of histamine in the large intrapulmonary mast cell and basophil depot – than intra-arterially administered contrast medium, which reaches the lungs in more diluted form only after dispersion throughout the periphery of the body. Milder allergic and anaphylactoid reactions in particular may therefore occur more frequently after urography than after arteriography.
As regards our own results, this comparison reveals a predominance of mild autonomic and allergic reactions under urography compared to arteriography (only reactions requiring therapy were evaluated). Severe CNS symptoms (loss of visual acuity, coma, unconsciousness) were caused by selective demonstration in the case of arteriography, and consisted in the case of urography of a shock syndrome with persisting nephrogram in 3 cases, severe bronchospasm in one case and hypertonic crises with convulsions in another case with a cerebral tumour. The severe incidents reported in the literature following urographic investigations also consist for the greater part of shock symptoms, while neurological and cardiac complications predominate in arteriography. They are associated less frequently with the catheter technique than with demonstration of the organ, as the surveys by Zeitler 1978 (44) and Hessel et al. 1976 (17) show (Table 6).
In this respect, the pre-existence of relevant organ damage may be a particularly predisposing factor. For example, cardiac arrest occurring in one of our patients 10 minutes after the end of transaxillary angiography of the aortic arch appeared to be induced more as a result of pre-existing severe impairment of the cardiac circulation and less by the contrast medium, since the catheter had already been removed and the compression concluded a few minutes beforehand.
The incidence of urographic CM complications also varies according to the mode of administration employed. According to Ansell (3) and Shehadi (38) it is higher with drip infusion than with bolus injection.
In contrast, Da Silva et al. (8) and Brutschin et al. (6) have reported a greater incidence of cardiovas-

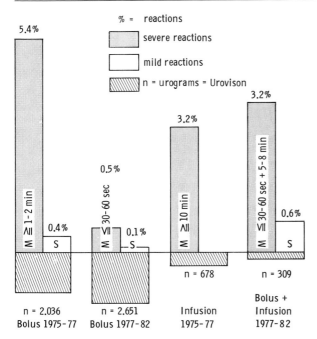

Fig 5 Own results: mild (M) and severe (S) reactions requiring therapy in urographic examinations with Urovison and different modes of administration in a nephrological study population

cular reactions in particular after bolus injections than after infusion. These discrepancies are due not only to the mode and duration of administration, but also to the nature, dose and dilution of the contrast medium. Using our own study model, we investigated the risks associated with different durations and modes of administration of a urographic contrast medium in two commercial concentrations in a special nephrological case collection. The results are presented in Fig 5.

Only the urographic examinations in which Urovison with the bigger proportion of sodium salt was used were evaluated. The bolus injection always consisted of two ampoules, while the drip infusion consisted of a dilute, commercial ready-to-use solution of Urovison in which 100 ml CM are diluted in 150 ml aqueous solution. From 1975 to 1977 we practised slower bolus injection within 1–2 minutes, but since 1977 we inject 2 ampoules in quick succession – usually within 30–60 seconds, but in even less than 10–15 seconds in the clarification of hypertension in order to obtain an angiogram as well as a vascular nephrogram (22).

Milder reactions requiring therapy were found to occur more frequently with the slower than with the quicker bolus injection. From 1975 go 1977 we practised infusion of a ready-to-use solution of Urovison within 10 minutes, mainly in patients with incipient renal insufficiency. In 1977 we switched to a biphasic examination procedure consisting of a rapid bolus injection followed by a drip infusion of Urovison, the drip speed being also reduced from previously 10 minutes to about 5 minutes. The indication for infusion urography (including the combined technique) in our clinic is nephropathy (usually chronic) of various origin. Incipient impairment of renal function is already present in many cases. We observed no severe incidents during our earlier practice of infusion alone. The percentage of mild reactions requiring therapy was less than with the previous slower bolus injection (23). In contrast, the combined technique which we now use displays a moderate increase of mild reactions compared to infusion alone, but still fewer such reactions compared to slower bolus injection alone. Our severe incidents, which occurred only with the bolus injection and combined technique, were as follows:

Severe reactions
1. slow bolus technique 1975–1977, n = 9 (= 0.45%)
   1 × hypertonic crises, convulsions (cerebral tumour)
   2 × attack of bronchial asthma
   3 × vomiting, tremor, hypotension, cold sweat, paleness, bradycardia
   2 × vomiting, flush, hypertension, paroxysmal tachycardia
   1 × generalized urticaria, Quincke's oedema
2. rapid bolus technique 1977–1982, n = 3 (= 0.1%)
   2 × shock syndrome, persistent nephrogram
   1 × bronchospasm – cyanosis
   1 × shock syndrome, persistent nephrogram (abuse of analgesics)
   1 × shock syndrome, tachycardia, paraesthesias, persistent nephrogram
3. combined technique 1977–1980, n = 2 (= 0.6%)
   1 × shock syndrome, persistent nephrogram (hypokalaemia)
   1 × hypertonic crises, convulsions (cerebral tumour)

There was no impairment of renal function prior to urography in the total of 16 cases with severe reactions.

The dilute contrast medium infusion solutions are well tolerated by our patients with chronic renal disease – and even by those with more severe renal insufficiency. We observed no serious incidents in any of these – not even in the few cases in which we had to perform infusion urography in the stage of oliguria. The urographic contrast effect is also good despite impaired renal function as long as the urea level is less than 100 mg/ml. Our results agree with those by Taenzer et al. (40) in that the radiopacity of contrast media with a higher proportion of sodium salt (e.g. Urovison) is better precisely in the diagnosis of patients with chronic renal disease, while the side effects rates are relatively low. The indication from our results that the risk liability of a contrast medium can change when it is administered in different ways and different concentration appears to be important for two reasons:

1. Biphasic contrast medium applications with various modifications (bolus injections with drip infusions and perfusions) have recently been published in association with computerized tomographic investigations (20, 28, 30). An increase of the CM risk therefore appears possible, but a lower CM concentration (dilution) should be tolerated better while still guaranteeing adequate opacification in the computed tomogram.
2. A rapid bolus injection is called for in i. v. arteriography with both conventional and modern techniques (4, 19, 36). This does not appear to increase the side effects rates to any particular extent compared to the slow bolus injection.

We consider it important to mention in this connection that a renal contrast medium of lower concentration usually provides adequate opacification in computerized tomographic and intravenous computerized angiography while possibly reducing the side effects rate. This is borne out by our results as shown in Table 7.

Over the period of time stated, we observed no side effects requiring treatment on intravenous administration of Telebrix 30 for computerized tomography either as a bolus injection (which, however, was usually given more slowly than in urography) or as a drip infusion. Despite the intravenous route of administration, the side effects rate was lower than in the arteriographic examinations, which were likewise performed with well-tolerated contrast media. The heterogeneity of the study populations was about equal. The highest side effects rate was found in urographic examinations of nephrological patients. However, it should be added that milder side effects such as nausea, vomiting and isolated urticaria were not recorded in the computerized tomographic studies with Telebrix 30. These side effects, which were not severe enough to require treatment, occurred somewhat more frequently with bolus injection of Telebrix 30 than with the infusion. Their incidence was not, however, increased on urography with Urovison.

Table 7a  i.v. urography in a nephrological study population

| Urovision | Examinations n | Reactions n | % |
|---|---|---|---|
| bolus | 2,651 | 17 | 0.3 |
| infusion | 309 | 12 | 2.0 |
| 1977 – V/82 | 2,960 | 29 | 1.0 |

Table 7b  i.v. CM computerized tomography in a heterogeneous study population

| Telebrix 30 | n | n | % |
|---|---|---|---|
| bolus | 112 | – | – |
| infusion | 667 | – | – |
| 18/12/80 – 3/5/82 | 779 | | |

Table 7c  Arteriography in a heterogeneous study population

| Hexabrix Angiografin | n | n | % |
|---|---|---|---|
| 1977 – V/82 | 7,757 | 17 | 0.2 |

*The risk of general reactions at repeat examinations and in a history of allergy.*

According to a prospective study by Rothenberger and Ring (34), there appears to be no statistical significance for the risk at repeat contrast examinations. Although they observed mild repeat reactions, there were no definite, verifiable complaints during repeat examinations – a finding which is in agreement with our own experience. The "anxiety" factor appears to be very important here: if the patient is convinced that he is going to feel "sick", we frequently observe nausea and vomiting even at puncture before administration of the contrast medium. A reassuring approach by the doctor and his assistants is vital in such cases (25).

In contrast, it is a well-documented fact that the incidence of allergic general reactions is increased in patients with a history of allergy. According to Elke and Brune (9), CM side effects occurred in 1–2% of cases without a history of allergy and in 2–6% of cases with a pertinent history following intravenous injection of nephrotropic CM. It has also been our experience that mainly allergic cutaneous and bronchospastic reactions are likely to occur.

## Special CM Side Effects

Before the side effects of contrast media can be placed in their correct relationship to local and certain organic and systemic damage, it is necessary to distinguish between direct and indirect effects and also to consider disturbances which are not a result of the CM. The factors can be additive and provoke a chain reaction.

Table 8   CM side effects: local, organic, systemic

| direct | indirect |
|---|---|
| – endothelium | – result of general reactions |
| – blood clotting system | – result of underlying disease |
| – organs | – result of vaso-vagal reflex |
| | Addition |
| | No |
| | – puncture trauma |
| | – catheter trauma |
| | – neuro-vegetative disturbances |

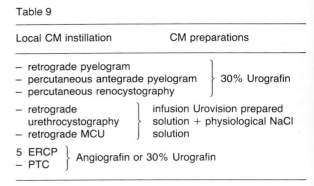

Table 9

| Local CM instillation | CM preparations |
|---|---|
| – retrograde pyelogram<br>– percutaneous antegrade pyelogram<br>– percutaneous renocystography | 30% Urografin |
| – retrograde urethrocystography<br>– retrograde MCU | infusion Urovison prepared solution + physiological NaCl solution |
| 5 ERCP<br>– PTC | Angiografin or 30% Urografin |

Mention of the interaction between different functional mechanisms appears important for correct categorization and interpretation of the reactions. Direct damage occurs more frequently on arteriographic perfusion of CM than on intravenous administration, but it can also be caused by CM potentiation due to excretory disturbances of the liver and kidneys or by shifts in the electrolyte and water balance. The main contributory factors in the development of direct CM side effects are:

1. The protein binding of the CM (negligible in nephrotopic CM)
2. The hyperosmosis of the entire molecule
3. The viscosity of the salts: methyl glucamines are more viscous than sodium salts
4. The pharmacodynamic activities of the salts: Histamine liberation is said to occur more readily under methylglucamine salts (3, 26), whereas cardiovascular effects are more prominent under sodium salts (11).
5. Adjuvants: sodium citrate, sodium or calcium EDTA (42)
6. Impurities: free iodide, toxins etc. (42).

## Local Damage

Renal contrast media are used for local, diagnostic instillation in preformed cavitis and duct systems, and we prefer the following (Table 9).
The intact mucosa of the urinary tract tolerates the stress well despite the frequently long period of contact; we have very rarely observed local irritation, and this was caused mainly by insertion of the catheter. The absorption rate of the instilled CM is so low that allergic reactions are unlikely – in contrast to intravascular administration. We ourselves have never observed an allergic reaction. Highly concentrated CM solutions can, however, damage the delicate duct structures of parenchymal organs and, hence, lead to a disturbance of organ function (42). Examples are pancreatitis and even pancreatic apoplexy, which have been described as complications of ERCP. This damage occurs mainly when highly concentrated CM solutions enter the delicate pancreatic duct system under high pressure and, because of obstructed drainage and previous damage to the wall of the pancreas, act as a persisting local injurious noxa. The CM instillation potentiates the pre-existing damage in the cavities or parenchyma.

A similar situation can arise with percutaneous transhepatic cholangiography (PTC) if the biliary tract is damaged by inflammation and drainage is also obstructed. Warmed-up low-osmolar CM of low concentration should always be used for local instillation, particularly in ERCP and PTC. With intravascular administration, the vascular pain, thrombosis and phlebitis are attributed to endothelial irritation and damage. According to studies by Penry et al. (31), such local intravascular damage occurs more frequently after injection of mainly sodium salt-containing CM than after methylglucamine salts, although clinical studies by Taenzer et al. (40) suggest that this is not so for urography. Our own observations that, despite rapid intravenous injection, venous irritation is negligible after administration of the mainly sodium salt-containing CM Urovison for urography support this latter finding. On the other hand, severe vascular irritation is known to occur in arteriography, particularly in the periphery. Because of this, recent years have seen the development of mainly methylglucamine-containing, low-osmolar CM for arteriography. The local pain syndrome has consequently been considerably reduced or eliminated by the following CM: Hexabrix, Amipaque and Solutrast. A Freiburg study group under Gospos et al. (13, 14, 15, 16) compared the injurious effect of different CM – diatrizoate (Angiografin), metrizamide (Amipaque), ioxaglate (Hexabrix) and a 20% sorbit solution – on the endothelia of the rat aorta and vena cava. 1 ml of the 22% sorbit solution (with the same osmotic pressure as diatrizoate) and 1 ml of each of the contrast media with an iodine content of 300 mg/ml were injected via the intraaortic and intravenous route. The parameter for the degree of endothelial damage was the increase in DNA synthesis by the vascular endothelium (repair process after damage) compared to the DNA synthesis of controls, which was determined autoradiographically in the "membrane preparation" (12) by calculation of the proliferation quotient (PQ).

Figs 6 and 7 show the kinetics of DNA synthesis by the endothelium of the aorta and vena cava of control animals and of rats treated with contrast media and with the hyperosmolar sorbit solution. The observed increase of DNA synthesis, which displays some significant differences from the controls after injection of contrast media, permits conclusions about the degree of damage to the endothelium. The endothelium of the aorta and vena cava is damaged after intra-aortic and intravenous injection of the hyperosmolar contrast media diatrizoate and ioxithalamate and of the low-osmolar substance metrizamide, the degree of damage being far greater in the case of the venous endothelium (PQ 10) than in the aortic endothelium (PQ

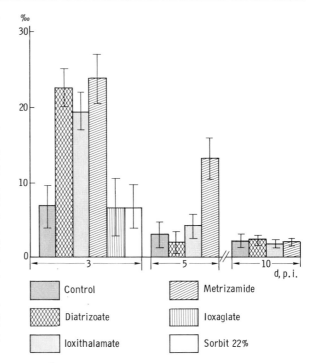

Fig 6 ³H-thymidine indices (as ‰) of endothelial cells of the aorta at various times (d = days, p. i. = post injection) in controls and after injektion of diatrizoate (Angiografin), ioxithalamate (Telebrix 300), metrizamide (Amipaque), ioxaglate (Hexabrix) and a 22% sorbitol solution

3). The repair process of the endothelium of both vessels takes longer under metrizamide (DNA synthesis does not return to normal until the 10th day after the injection).

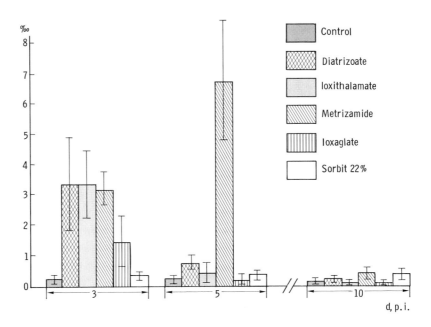

Fig 7 ³H-thymidine indices (as ‰) of endothelial cells of the vena cava at different times (d = days, p.i. = post injection) in controls and after injections of diatrizoate (Angiografin), ioxithalamate (Telebrix 300), metrizamide (Amipaque), ioxaglate (Hexabrix) and a 22% sorbitol solution

These differences between the two vessels as regards the degree of damage suggest that venous endothelium is more sensitive to contrast media – a finding which is supported by our studies with the lowosmolar contrast medium ioxaglate, which causes damage to the endothelium of the vena cava – albeit less than with other contrast media –, but no damage to the aortic endothelium. The following factors have been suggested as the cause of the endothelium-damaging effect of contrast media (35):

1. The chemical structure of the contrast media
2. The cation used to form the salt of the solution
3. Physico-chemical properties of the solutions such as the pH value, osmotic properties, protein binding capacity and lipophilia
4. The mode of administration of the contrast media, e. g. its temperature on injection and the rate of injection.

According to the literature, the most important factors leading to endothelial damage are, apart from the chemical structure and cation, the physico-chemical properties of the CM such as their hyperosmolarity and protein binding capacity. However, the present results show that a hyperosmolar sorbitol solution with an osmotic pressure comparable to that of diatrizoate does not cause any damage to the endothelium of the aorta and vena cava. In our opinion, therefore, the hyperosmolarity known for most contrast media is not a major injurious factor. This conclusion is supported by the finding that the two virtually isotonic contrast media metrizamide and ioxaglate cause different degrees of endothelial damage.

## Sytemic Damage

For the greater part, changes caused by different CM in the blood-clotting system have been studied in vitro and are not discussed here. Recent in vivo studies by Albert et al. (1) have revealed statistically significant clotting disorders in patients following arteriographic and urographic examinations and also in patients after stressful examinations without contrast medium administration (e. g. after gastroscopy). They therefore consider clotting disorders after CM examinations to be biologically and clinically irrelevant and suggest that thrombotic complications are rather a consequence of trauma to the vascular wall and of the release of clotting factors.

The cellular elements of the blood also undergo changes when they come into contact with CM solutions. For example, osmotic dehydration of erythrocytes, which can greatly increase the viscosity of blood, has been reported. Furthermore, changes of the thrombocyte surface can lead to agglutination of the cellular components of the blood; however, the phenomenon of bogging-down of erythrocytes in the peripheral bloodstream, which is known as sludging and results in tissue hypoxia, is also observed in states of shock (42). We have observed neither a tendency to haemorrhage nor thrombosis following contrast examinations.

## Organ Damage

As has already been shown, the nervous and cardiovascular systems react particularly sensitively to direct CM perfusion during arteriography. An increased incidence is likely above all where organ damage already exists. Patients with cerebral damage react quite frequently to the administration of CM. Shifts in the cell membrane potential are apparently the reason why the CM can overcome the blood-brain barrier. This is probably also the reason for the central convulsions which occur in infants without cerebral damage when excessively high doses of CM are given.

The cardiovascular damage occurring after coronarography in particular has been studied in depth by a Freiburg group under Wink, whose results are published in this volume. Beyond these results, it should also be mentioned as regards cardiac damage that an increase in the intrapulmonary vascular resistance following CM administration (particularly for pulmonary angiography) in existing right heart insufficiency can induce severe cardiac CM side effects (42).

## Nephrogenic CM Damage: Reported Incidents and Own Results

Because of the special excretory mechanism of nephrotropic CM, organ-specific renal CM damage is of particular interest. Several authors have recently reported on reversible and even irreversible impairment of renal function following administration of nephrotropic CM (29, 32, 37, 43). Patients with renal insufficiency and serum creatinine values of more than 2–3 mg% are regarded as being at particular risk (9).

Although more than 60% of the urographic examinations at our clinic are performed in patients with chronic nephropathy and, frequently, impaired renal function of varying severity, we have not observed any transient or permanent deterioration of renal function either during the first or during repeat examinations. This applies not only to present examinations, but also to all examinations over the last 11 years, and we perform urography up to a serum creatinine value of 6 mg% and, in special indications, even higher if the serum urea is less than 100 mg% and the patient is not dehydrated. On the other hand, over the last few years we have observed 3 cases of transient acute impairment of renal function as part of a general reaction in patients without renal disease. We apply a rule that undiluted high-dose urography should never be performed in patients with chronic renal disease with a serum creatinine value of more than 2 mg% – we always perform infusion urography (biphasic – cf. Fig 5). Most reports of the recent past have concerned high-dosed, undiluted bolus injections, which are certainly not adequately tolerated by a kidney with already reduced function. Although a rapid, high-dosed bolus injection can provide information about the vascular situation, excretion of the contrast medium via the tubular and urinary system is retarded and this diagnostic effect in such patients is, in any case, recognizable only on late films. The slow, plasma-borne contrast enhancement provided by a drip infusion is adequate for this. The sudden arrival of a high CM plasma level resulting from a high-dosed bolus injection could, in fact, have a direct nephrotoxic effect, but it could also cause deteriorating renal function indirectly via general reactions in kidney patients in particular, who frequently have pre-existing cardiovascular and pulmonary damage. In this connection we consider it important to point out that a clear distinction must be made between direct and indirect CM effects in functional disorders of the kidney following CM administration:

Table 10a  Indirect CM effect: renal function

- persistent nephrogram
- shock – acute renal failure
- change of renal size

Table 10b  Direct CM effect: renal function

1. Nature, dose, mode of administration of the CM
2. Dehydration
   - renal insufficiency
   - hyperuricaemia
   - paraproteinaemia
   - diabetes mellitus
3. Electrolyte disturbances in patients
   - with renal disease
   - without renal disease
4. Renal *and* hepatogenic insufficiency

We believe that not every acute impairment of renal function with and without pre-existing nephropathy should be regarded as a direct nephrotoxic effect of the contrast medium. It may also be an indirect consequence of hypotension or a shock syndrome, in which a persistent nephrogram occurs and an ischaemic disturbance of circulation can progress into acute renal failure with oligoanuria leading to distinct renal enlargement from the second or third day (21). An acute impairment of renal function can, nevertheless, also occur as a direct result of the contrast medium – on the one hand due to the nature, dose and mode of injection of the CM (intravenous, intraarterial – selective) and, on the other hand, due to CM potentiation caused by dehydration and electrolyte disturbances. Intracellular and extracellular shifts in the electrolyte balance apparently also induce a different distribution of hyperosmotic CM substances. This applies not only to patients with renal insufficiency, in whom shifts in the water and electrolyte balance readily occur, but also to non-kidney patients given effective diuretic therapy before the CM examination. Because of the considerable CM potentiation, severe renal and hepatogenic disorders of excretion constitute an absolute contraindication for contrast medium administration.

The following are possible causes of a persistent nephrogram:

1. Hypotension, shock after CM administration (vascular CM stasis)
2. Acute stone occlusion (tubular CM stasis)
3. Acute renal insufficiency before CM administration (the CM enters the kidneys via the arteries, but cannot be eliminated via the venous or tubular routes because of intrarenal circulatory or excretory disorders)
4. Direct nephrotoxic CM effect (a persistent nephrogram is not always present!), e. g. CM accumulation in dehydration and electrolyte disturbances and in pre-existing renal damage etc.

A persisting nephrogram is a sign of a transient or permanent acute impairment of renal function, but it does not always correlate with a direct nephrotoxic CM effect. It is the phenomenon which results when the CM remains in the parenchyma until circulation and excretion are restored. Once circulation is restored, e. g. by elimination of the shock syndrome and electrolyte compensation, the persistent nephrogram decreases to the same extent as the cavity demonstration increases (Fig 8). However, protracted shock – without or after CM administration – can progress into acute renal

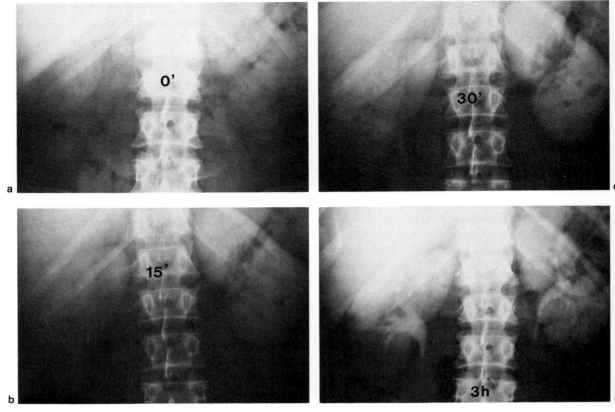

Fig 8 a–d  A. Sch., female, born 1952, persistent nephrogram:
i. v. bolus injection of Urovision within 30 seconds. 2 minutes later: hypotension, cerebral confusion, cold sweat. Films 15 and 30 minutes p. i. (b + c): persistent nephrogram, poor opacification of cavities. 3 hours p. i. (d) persistent nephrogram, better opacification of cavities – increase of diuresis after mannitol 20%. Hypokalaemia of 2.0 mval/l before urography (retrospective finding)

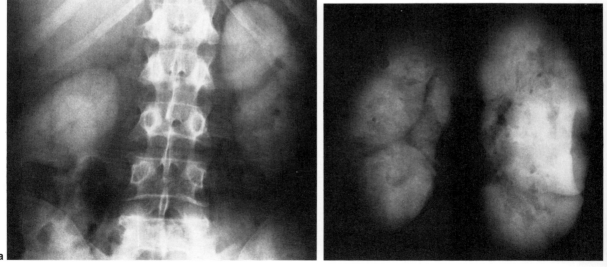

Fig 9  L. W., female, born 1939. Persistent nephrogram, no contrast medium incident
a) Urographic clarification – acute postoperative renal insufficiency (probably prerenal): persistent nephrogram, no cavity demonstration after infusion urography
b) Postmortem film (death 6 days after surgery = 3rd day after urography): persistent nephrogram, no contrast medium elimination into hollow regions
Pathological diagnosis: shock kidneys

failure, in which case the persistent nephrogram remains and the kidney enlarges considerably over the following few days (Fig 9). This situation calls for dialysis treatment until normal conditions are fully restored. Control films are therefore important to permit evaluation of the persistent nephrogram as a critical sign of a transient or permanent disorder of function. Some emergency treatment plans recommend i. v. administration of Lasix as treatment for contrast medium-induced oliguria. We consider this wrong for the following reasons:

1. It has a further adverse effect on hypotension,
2. The diuretic has no effect at all on the nephrogenic functional situation in existing oliguria.

We practise the following technique as a test for the return of normal micturition following acute oliguria: 80–100 ml 20% mannitol are given as a rapid i. v. bolus injection and diuresis via an in-dwelling bladder catheter awaited. Mannitol improves the renal blood circulation, which results in renewed stimulation of diuresis. If diuresis fails to occur, acute renal failure must be treated by means of dialysis.

The fact that the CM remains in the renal parenchyma can, of course, lead secondarily to a nephrotoxic effect in the above-mentioned causes of the persistent nephrogram. It is possible for disorders of renal function which are primarily not – or only indirectly – due to a CM effect to progress to direct contrast medium-induced damage. If at all possible, therefore, a CM examination to clarify acute renal insufficiency of various etiology should be avoided.

Histological evaluation of nephrotoxic CM damage is difficult because the nephrogenic cellular damage in the proximal and distal tubular epithelium and in the interstitium resulting from direct and indirect CM effects also occurs in shock kidneys without CM administration and can also be simulated by intra- and postmortem cellular changes; the histological results after exsanguination and histamine shock without CM administration resemble those after direct perfusion (after selective renal arteriography) of various CM. This has been demonstrated in animal studies and also in human shock kidneys (2, 5, 18, 41, 33).

## Prophylaxis of CM Risks

To conclude, a reminder about the guidelines for the prophylaxis and, hence, reduction of CM risks and serious CM incidents (24).

1. Good clinical data are absolutely essential for a CM examination. One should also have the courage to refuse a CM examination because of a lack of data. This applies especially to patients with preexisting kidney disease and liver damage, paraproteinaemia, pre-existing disturbances of the electrolyte and water balance and to patients with hyperuricaemia and diabetes mellitus.
2. All patients must be questioned about any history of allergy before the CM is administered; where applicable, the provision of prophylactic antihistamine or cortisone cover is indicated before the examination takes place (27).
3. The emergency resuscitation facilities must be checked carefully and all the staff involved given regular training.
4. In high-risk patients requiring arteriography, access to a vein must be created before the investigation.
5. In intravenous CM examinations, the puncture should always be made with an indwelling needle.

So that the impression is not created that all side effects of nephrotropic CM are adverse, mention should finally be made of a positive side effect observed in a clinical study by Strohm (39): Urografin injections considerably improved the hearing of patients with labyrinthine deafness.

## References

1 Albert, J. P., R. Bernsmeier, H. D. Bruhn: Einfluß von Röntgenkontrastmitteln auf das Blutgerinnungs- und Fibrinolysesystem. Med. Klin. 74, 48: 1811–1817, 1979
2 Ansar, A., D. S. Baldwin: Acute renal failure due to radiocontrast agents. Nephron 17: 28–40, 1976
3 Ansell, G.: Adverse reactions to contrast agents. Scope of problem. Invest. Radiol. 5: 374–391, 1970
4 Baert, A. L., G. Wilms, G. Marchal et al.: Intravenous digital subtraction angiography. Europ. J. Radiol. 1: 97–103, 1891
5 Bohle, A.: Pathologische Anatomie des akuten Nierenversagens. Verh. dtsch. Ges. Path. 49: 53, 1965
6 Brutschin, P., P. Vock, W. A. Fuchs: Die klinische Prüfung kardiovasculärer Reaktionen auf nephrotope Kontrastmittel unter Anwendung der Impedanz-Methode. Fortschr. Röntgenstr. 125, 4: 365–371, 1976
7 Bussmann, W. D.: Drohender Herzinfarkt. Dtsch. Ärztebl. 47: 2793–2800, 1980
8 Da Silva, O., R. C. Stadalnik, R. Davies, Z. Vera: Elektrocardiographie effects of two types of contrast agents

during intravenous urography using the bolus and infusion. Clin. Res. 23, 3: 178, 1975
9 Elke, M., K. Brune: Prophylaktische Maßnahmen vor Kontrastmittelinjektion. Dtsch. med. Wschr. 105: 250–252, 1980
10 Elke, M., A. Ferstl: Zur Behandlung des akuten Kontrastmittelzwischenfalls. In Zeitler, E.: Neue Aspekte des Kontrastmittelzwischenfalls. Symposion, Berlin 1977. Schering AG, Berlin 1978 (S. 129–137)
11 Fischer, H. W.: Hemodynamic reactions to angiographic media a survey and commentary. Radiology 91: 66–73, 1968
12 Freudenberg, N., U. Häublein: The effect of endotoxin shock on the aortic endothelium of young rats. Beitr. Path. 156: 1–15, 1975
13 Gospos, Ch., N. Freudenberg: Hyperosmolalität von Röntgenkontrastmitteln – ein Faktor für die Endothelschädigung? Fortschr. Röntgenstr. 135: 489–491, 1981
14 Gospos, Ch., N. Freudenberg, J. Staubesand: Wirkung von Röntgenkontrastmitteln auf das Endothel der Aorta. Pathologe 2: 247, 1981
15 Gospos, Ch., N. Freudenberg, A. Stephan: Wirkung von Diatricoat (Angiografin®) auf das Aortenendothel der Ratte. Fortschr. Röntgenstr. 133: 654–656, 1980
16 Gospos, Ch., N. Freudenberg, J. Staubesand, K. Mathias: The effect of x-ray contrast media on the aortic endothelium in rats. Radiology (in press)
17 Hessel, S. J., D. F. Adams, H. L. Abrams: Complications of angiography – a nationwide survey. RSNA 1976, 172
18 Huth, F.: Morphologische Befunde bei Schockniere. Ärztl. Forsch. 1: 3, 1969
19 Ingrisch, H., H. Holzgreve, B. Sommer, K. W. Westerburg, K. W. Frey: Technik der Nierenarteriendarstellung im Rahmen des Ausscheidungsurogramms. Bolustechnik––Zeitbestimmung–Simultantomographie. Fortschr. Röntgenstr. 132, 4: 422–427, 1980
20 Kirschner, H., A. Kremp, H. Poppe: Vergleich der Häufigkeit von Nebenwirkungen zwischen zweiphasigen Bolusperfusor- und der einphasigen Bolusinjektion eines Röntgenkontrastmittels in der kranialen Computertomographie. Fortschr. Röntgenstr. 133, 2: 119–124, 1980
21 Kröpelin, T.: Radiologische Methoden und Befunde: Nierenbefunde im Verlauf des akuten Nierenversagens. In Sarre, H.: Nierenkrankheiten. Thieme, Stuttgart 1976 (S. 139–158)
22 Kröpelin, T.: Functional urography. In Donner, M. W., F. H. W. Heuck: Radiology Today 1. Springer, Berlin 1981 (S. 217–228)
23 Kröpelin, T., Y. Heuser, Ch. Gospos: Kontrastmittelrisiko bei der Ausscheidungsurographie. In Zeitler, E.: Neue Aspekte des Kontrastmittelzwischenfalls. Symposion, Berlin 1977. Schering AG, Berlin 1978 (S. 103–115)
24 Kröpelin, T., W. Wenz, W. R. Seemann, Ch. Gospos: Nebenwirkungen und Zwischenfälle gallen- und nierengängiger Kontrastmittel. In: IV. Radiologische Woche, München 1980. Referate, hrsg. von J. Lissner, Schnetztor-Verlag, Konstanz 1982 (S. 213–232)
25 Lalli, A. F.: Urographic contrast media reactions and anxiety. Radiology 112: 267–271, 1974
26 Lasser, E. C., A. J. Walters, J. H. Lang: An experimental basis for histamine release in contrast material reactions. Radiology, 110: 49–59, 1974
27 Lasser, B. C., J. H. Lang, M. Sovak, W. P. Kolb, S. G. Lyon, A. E. Hamblin: Steroids: Theoretical and experimental basis for utilization in prevention of contrast media reactions. Radiology 125: 1–9, 1977
28 Norton, G. A., P. R. S. Kishore, J. Lin: CT contrast enhancement in cerebral infarction. Amer. J. Roentgenol. 131: 881–885, 1978
29 Older, R. A., M. Korobkin, D. M. Cleeve, R. Schaaf, W. Thompson: Contrast-induced acute renal failure: Persistend nephrogram as clue and early detection. Amer. J. Roentgenol. 134: 339–342, 1980
30 Paling, M. R.: Contrast dose for enhancement of computed tomograms of the brain. Brit. J. Radiol. 52: 620–623, 1979
31 Penry, J. B., Livingston: A comparison of diagnostic effectiveness and vascular side-effects of various diatrizoate salts used for intravenous pyelography. Clin. Radiol. 23: 362–369, 1972
32 Pierach, C. A.: Transitorische Urämie durch Kontrastmittel – ein Risikofaktor bei niereninsuffizienten Diabetikern. Dtsch. med. Wschr. 104: 148–149, 1979
33 Rohrbach, R., D. Weingard: Zur Nephrotoxizität wasserlöslicher Kontrastmittel bei der Nierenangiographie. Referat 14, Symposion Ges. f. Nephrologie 1980. Abstract: Nieren-Hochdruckkrankh. 9, 5: 219, 1980
34 Rothenberger K., J. Ring: Das Wiederholungsrisiko von Kontrastmittel-Reaktionen bei der Urographie. Fortschr. Med. 97, 33: 1429–1432, 1979
35 Schmid, H. W.: Untersuchungen der Toxizität der physikalisch-chemischen Eigenschaften und der hämolytischen Aktivität von trijodierten Röntgenkontrastmittelsalzen in wässrigen Lösungen. Pharm. Acta Helv. 46: 134–313, 1971
36 Seyferth, W., P. Marhoff, E. Zeitler: Transvenöse und arterielle digitale Videosubtraktionsangiographie (DVSA). Fortschr. Röntgenstr. 136, 3: 301–309, 1982
37 Shafi, T., S. Y. Chou, J. G. Porush: Infusion intravenous pyelography and renal function. Effects in patients with chronic renal insufficiency. Arch. intern. Med. 138: 1218–1221, 1978
38 Shehadi, H.: The risks involved in the use of contrast media in cholecystocholangiography. In Zeitler, E.: Neue Aspekte des Kontrastmittelzwischenfalls. Symposion, Berlin 1977. Schering AG, Berlin 1978 (S. 91–102)
39 Strohm, M.: Erfahrungen mit der Gabe von Urografin® bei Innenohrschwerhörigkeit. Larying. Rhinol. 59: 159–162, 1980
40 Taenzer, V., W. Clauss, J. Simon: Natrium- oder Methylglukaminsalze der Kontrastmittel für die Urographie? Fortschr. Röntgenstr. 133, 1: 78–83, 1980
41 Thoenes, W., K. H. Langer: Beitrag zur Pathomorphologie des Tubulussystems beim akuten Nierenversagen (nach Modellversuchen an der Rattenniere). Symposion, Nürnberg 1971
42 Tuengerthal, S.: Röntgenkontrastmittel – Pathophysiologische Ursachen. In: IV. Radiologische Woche, München 1980. Referate, hrsg. von J. Lissner, Schnetztor-Verlag, Konstanz 1982 (S. 200–212)
43 Warren, S. E., J. C. Bott, C. Thornfeldt, A. H. Swerdlin, S. M. Steinberg: Hazards of computerized tomography: Renal failure following contrast injection. Surg. Neurol. 10: 335–336, 1978
44 Zeitler, E.: Kontrastmittelrisiko arterieller Angiographie. In Zeitler, E.: Neue Aspekte des Kontrastmittelzwischenfalls. Symposion, Berlin 1977. Schering AG, Berlin 1978 (S. 117–121)

# Double Blind Comparison of Ioglicate and Iothalamate in Intravenous Urography

T. Baitsch, D. Beduhn and G. Klink

## Summary

Ioglicate was compared with iothalamate in three controlled, randomized multicentre studies on 995 patients. The studies differed in dose and application technique: Ioglicate was administered in a 40-ml (14.8 g iodine) rapid injection, in 100-ml (30 g iodine) and 250-ml (44 g iodine) infusions; adequate amounts of iothalamate were administered. Sodium-meglumine mixed salts were used for rapid injection and meglumine salts for the other two investigations.

For demonstration of renal parenchyma, pelvi-calyceal system and ureters ioglicate proved equivalent to iothalamate in all three studies, but with some qualifications. The proportion of patients with side effects was between 6% (high dose) and 22% (rapid injection), where this increase was caused by a more significant occurrence of vascular pain and heat sensation. In all three comparisons ioglicate was tolerated somewhat better than iothalamate.

## Zusammenfassung

In 3 kontrollierten multizentrischen Prüfungen an 995 nicht ausgewählten Patienten wurde Ioglicinat mit Iothalamat verglichen.

Die 3 Prüfungen unterschieden sich durch die Dosis und Applikationstechnik: vom Ioglicinat wurden verabreicht 14,8 gJ in 40 ml als Schnellinjektion, 30 gJ in einer 100 ml-Infusion und 44 gJ in einer 250 ml-Infusion, vom Iothalamat adäquate Mengen. Für die Schnellinjektion wurden Natrium-Meglumin-Mischsalze, für die anderen beiden Prüfungen Megluminsalze verwendet.

Für die Darstellungen von Parenchym, Becken-Kelch-System und Ureter erwies sich Ioglicinat als gut geeignet und in allen 3 Prüfungen dem Iothalamat gleichwertig. Die Anzahl der Patienten mit Nebenwirkungen lag zwischen 6% (hohe Dosis) und 22% (Schnellinjektion), wobei diese Zunahme durch ein verstärktes Auftreten von Venenschmerz und Hitzegefühl bedingt war. Ioglicinat war bei allen 3 Vergleichen etwas besser verträglich als Iothalamat.

## Introduction

Nowadays urologic contrast media are expected to satisfy many requirements. Optimal nephrograms and urograms and also utilization of the contrast agent in new roentgenologic techniques necessitate high dosages and rapid injection. In the synthesis of new compounds consideration should therefore be given to the demand for improved tolerance. This is especially true for ionic urographics, which also in future will be of great significance because of low toxicity and low production costs.

Ioglicate acid* is an ionic agent derived from iothalamic acid. It contains the amino acid glycine within one side chain of the molecule. As a derivative of iothalamic acid, ioglicate combines excellent neural tolerance with decreased cardiovascular, vascular and general toxicity due to its increased hydrophilicity. Some features of ioglicate such as weak protein binding and a short half-life in the blood make the compound particularly suitable for excretory urography (3, 6). The preparation has already proved its worth in several minor clinical studies and also as an angiographic (2, 3, 7, 9).

The cations sodium and meglumine also have an effect on the properties of an urographic agent: the favourable influence which a high proportion of sodium in mixed salts has on contrast (especially in the efferent urinary passages) (1, 8) and on viscosity is somewhat offset by the disadvantage of a rather reduced tolerance (9). These considerations formed the background to three comparative studies with three different formulations and application techniques using iothalamic acid as a reference substance.

## Method

The controlled, randomized multicentre examinations of a total of 995 patients consisted of three double-blind studies in the indication excretory urography, which were carried out separately. They differed in total iodine dose, rate of injection and concentration of contrast media. Pure meglumine salts were used in two studies (A and B) and mixed salts in the third.

A: A high total dose was infused in a low concentration in 8–10 minutes.

B: A medium dose was infused in a higher concentration in 4–5 minutes.

C: A highly concentrated preparation was to be injected in as short a time as possible (1–2

---

* Rayvist

Table 1  Formulation, dosages, application techniques and number of patients

| study number | preparation | injection/infusion | concentration mg I/ml | dose g I | no. of patients |
|---|---|---|---|---|---|
| A 1 | ioglicate meglumine | 250 ml 8–10 min | 176 | 44 | 150 |
| A 2 | iothalamate meglumine | | 170 | 42,5 | 150 |
| B 1 | ioglicate meglumine | 100 ml 4–5 min | 300 | 30 | 150 |
| B 2 | iothalamate meglumine | | 282 | 28,2 | 149 |
| C 1 | ioglicate sodium: meglumine = 2 : 1 | 40 ml 1–2 min (except for 39 patients: 5–10 min) | 370 | 14,8 | 198 |
| C 2 | iothalamate sodium: meglumine = 9 : 1 | 40 ml 1–2 min (except for 46 patients: 5–10 min) | 410 | 16,4 | 198 |

minutes). In this case the less viscous mixed salts were selected because of their better injectability. For practical reasons, the ratio of sodium salt to meglumine salt was kept at 2 : 1 or 9 : 1. The total dose was at its lowest in this study.

For formulations, dosages and patient numbers see Table 1. The ioglicate and iothalamate preparations were distributed at random among the patients, whose ages ranged mostly between 10 and 85 years. Only 5 patients were less than 10 years of age. Criteria for exclusion were the already known contra-indications for application of x-ray contrast media.

Recording of indications for examination, history-taking, preparation of patients according to type an extent was left to the examiners. These and the results of diagnoses, contrast evaluation and side effects were recorded on a special report form. The analyses on conclusion of the tests revealed an approximately symmetrical distribution of patients by age and sex, history of allergy, indications for diagnosis, preparation of patients and technical execution. The quality of the films was evaluated by visual observation. The examiners estimated the films at equal periods of time without previous knowledge of the preparation to be tested. Abdominal compression was not applied.

In study C it was not possible to keep to the injection rate of 1–2 minutes (as specified in the trial protocol) in 85 cases, it being extended to 5–10 minutes. X-rays were mostly taken 5, 10 an 20 minutes after administration had been completed.

## Results

*Diagnosis:* Normal x-ray findings were obtained in 46%–63% of the cases examined.

*Quality of x-rays:* A glance at the overall results reveals that in 93–99% of the cases in all three studies the parenchymal pattern, pelvi-calyceal system and urethers were visualized well or satisfactorily (Tables 2 and 4). The highest proportion of unsatisfactory radiographic quality occurred in one group with 8.1% (evaluation "poor", B 1, in Table 4). In some cases the unsatisfactory radiographs were a result of restricted kidney function and, therefore, could only be partially blamed on the contrast media. In view of these figures the differences in contrast (insignificant, anyway) between the individual groups allow no distinction to be drawn between the two contrast media.

Comparing the influence of doses on quality of radiographic films, it can be concluded that the best opacification and lowest rates of unsatisfactory radiographs were achieved with the highest doses of iodine. Thus, the proportion of nephrograms and urograms rated "good" in study A was over 84%, while unsatisfactory roentgenograms reached a maximum of only 2.7% (Table 2).

*Side effects:* Between 6 and 22% of the patients suffered one or more side effects, which occurred most frequently in study C with the most highly concentrated formulations and quickest injections. Vascular pain and heat sensation were noticeably increased in this study.

Table 2  Evaluation of opacification. Percentages 1 : ioglicate, 2 : iothalamate

| study | opacification | parenchyma | | pelvi-calyceal system | | ureters | |
|---|---|---|---|---|---|---|---|
| | | 1 | 2 | 1 | 2 | 1 | 2 |
| A | good | 85.3 | 85.3 | 87.3 | 84.7 | 94.0 | 92.7 |
| | satisfactory | 13.3 | 14.0 | 12.0 | 12.7 | 5.3 | 5.3 |
| | poor | 1.3 | 0.7 | 0.7 | 2.7 | 0.7 | 1.3 |
| | none | 0 | 0 | 0 | 0 | 0 | 0.7 |
| B | good | 77.3 | 73.8 | 79.3 | 76.5 | 81.3 | 79.9 |
| | satisfactory | 17.3 | 23.5 | 17.3 | 21.5 | 12.7 | 13.4 |
| | poor | 4.7 | 2.7 | 2.7 | 2.0 | 4.7 | 6.0 |
| | none | 0.7 | 0 | 0.7 | 0 | 1.3 | 0.7 |
| C | good | 79.8 | 76.3 | 78.8 | 82.3 | 77.3 | 74.8 |
| | satisfactory | 17.2 | 19.7 | 16.2 | 14.7 | 15.2 | 20.7 |
| | poor | 3.0 | 4.0 | 5.1 | 3.0 | 5.6 | 3.5 |
| | none | 0 | 0 | 0 | 0 | 2.0 | 1.0 |

In all three studies ioglicate was tolerated better than the control substance. The greatest difference occurred in study A with the highest dosage (statistically significant; Tables 3 and 4). In this study treatment with corticoids or anti-histamines was required in the case of five urograms with ioglicate and 13 with the reference substance. The examination had to be discontinued in one case with ioglicate and in three cases with the reference substance. In studies B and C medical treatment or premature termination of the injection were required 1 and 7 times after ioglicate and 3 and 16 times after iothalamate.

## Discussion

For the purpose of these studies, the suitability of ioglicate for intravenous urography was to be compared with that of a preparation used clinically on a regular basis. This suitability was to be expected in

Table 3  Frequency of side effects and number of patients with one or more side effects in the studies A, B, and C. 1 : ioglicate, 2 : iothalamate

| | A 1 | A 2 | B 1 | B 2 | C 1 | C 2 |
|---|---|---|---|---|---|---|
| vascular pain and phlebitis | 0 | 0 | 1 | 5 | 9 | 16 |
| heat sensation | 0 | 8 | 2 | 4 | 12 | 15 |
| tachycardia | 1 | 7 | 0 | 1 | 0 | 1 |
| intra-ocular pressure | 0 | 0 | 0 | 0 | 1 | 0 |
| nausea | 3 | 12 | 6 | 9 | 10 | 15 |
| vomiting | 0 | 4 | 1 | 6 | 2 | 4 |
| dizziness | 0 | 0 | 0 | 1 | 3 | 0 |
| colic | 1 | 0 | 0 | 0 | 0 | 0 |
| breathing difficulties | 0 | 4 | 0 | 1 | 2 | 1 |
| skin reactions | 3 | 7 | 3 | 1 | 1 | 6 |
| coughing, sneezing | 1 | 0 | 1 | 1 | 2 | 0 |
| angioneurotic edema | 0 | 1 | 0 | 0 | 0 | 0 |
| collapse | 0 | 1 | 0 | 1 | 0 | 0 |
| sensation of coldness | 1 | 0 | 0 | 0 | 0 | 0 |
| sensation of taste | 0 | 0 | 0 | 0 | 1 | 0 |
| total number of side effects | 10 | 44 | 14 | 30 | 43 | 58 |
| patients with side effects | 9 | 23 | 9 | 16 | 35 | 44 |
| in pecent | 6.0 | 15.3* | 6.0 | 10.7 | 17.7 | 22.2 |
| total number of patients | 150 | 150 | 150 | 149 | 198 | 198 |

* $p < 0.05$ (A1/A2; Fisher's exact test)

Table 4 Overall evaluation of opacification and tolerance of ioglicate (1 A–C) and iothalamate (2 A–C) in percent

| evaluation | A 1 | A 2 | B 1 | B 2 | C 1 | C 2 |
|---|---|---|---|---|---|---|
| | opafication | | | | | |
| good | 82.7 | 84.7 | 64.4 | 66.2 | 69.0 | 67.0 |
| satisfactory | 14.7 | 11.3 | 27.5 | 31.1 | 23.9 | 27.9 |
| poor | 2.7 | 2.7 | 8.1 | 2.7 | 6.6 | 5.1 |
| none | 0 | 1.3 | 0 | 0 | 0.5 | 0 |
| | tolerance* | | | | | |
| good | 95.3 | 89.3 | 96.6 | 93.9 | 88.8 | 85.6 |
| moderate | 3.3 | 7.3 | 3.4 | 6.1 | 9.1 | 10.8 |
| poor | 1.3 | 3.3 | 0 | 0 | 2.0 | 3.6 |

* In study A the tolerance is significantly better for ioglicate ($p < 0.05$; Fisher's exact test)

view of the preclinical and pharmacokinetic data available. Ioglicate was obtained chemically by introducing the highly hydrophilic amino acid glycine into iothalamate molecules. Pharmacological differences between this and iothalamate were weaker lipophilic properties, reduced protein binding and fewer membrane-damaging characteristics, though neural tolerance was roughly equal (3, 5, 6). Therefore, iothalamate was selected as a reference substance for the clinical trials because of this chemical relationship.

With various dosages and application techniques normally used in practice, advantages and disadvantages were to be brought to light and thereby the optimum relationship between contrast and tolerance traced. For example, in study A a high dose (over 40 g of iodine) was administered in the form of a low-concentration, high-volume solution (infusion), whereas in study C highly concentrated solutions were injected as quickly as possible in the usual dose of about 15 g iodine. As was to be expected, the greatest number of radiographs rated "good" and also the smallest proportion of unsatisfactory radiographs occurred in study A. However, it must be emphasized that a comparison between the three studies is only partially possible because of the subjective component in evaluation (different examiners!). On the other hand, consideration of the examiners' expectations on application of a higher dose lends more weight to allocation of the rating "good" in study A.

However, thanks to the double-blind nature of the study the evidence yielded by a comparison of the contrast media is clear. There are no differences in radiographic quality between them. If such differences were even vaguely expected in studies A and B (since solutions with almost equal iodine content were used), then differences in study C caused by a higher proportion of sodium in one of the two preparations would have been more likely. However, even in this case they could not be determined (apart from slight insignificant differences).

Side effects were slight to moderate in nature. In study C the high concentration of contrast medium and probably even the sodium salt content in the formulations (4) were marked by an increase in vascular pain and heat sensation. The results of study A bear out the well-known advantages of infusion urography: – high doses are conducive to optimum contrast without putting a greater strain on the patient. Ioglicate proves especially suitable for this purpose. Optimal opacification was combined with a low occurrence of side effects. A comparison of tolerance in all three studies brings a further trend to light in that side effects always occur less frequently under the influence of ioglicate than of iothalamate: the higher the dose, the better the difference between ioglicate and iothalamate was shown. An objective view of the occurrence of vomiting (by way of comparison) makes the difference particularly clear: – only three cases of vomiting were recorded among a total of 498 patients when ioglicate was administered (iothalamate 14 cases).

In conclusion, it may be stated that ioglicate met the demands placed on a modern contrast medium for excretion urography: – demands such as good contrast quality and good tolerance when dosages are high and injection of highly concentrated solutions is rapid.

# References

1 Dacie, J. E., I. K. Fry: Comparison of sodium and methylglucamine diatrizoate in high dose urography. Brit. J. Radiol. 45: 385–387, 1972
2 Hayek, H. W., G. Fleischhauer, R. Fehr: The use of a new renotropic contrast medium in infants with special reference to magnesium metabolism. Radiologe 19: 94–98, 1979
3 Nagel, R., W. Leistenschneider, U. Speck, W. Clauss: Pharmacokinetics and clinical studies of ioglicate, a new contrast medium for intravenous urography. Int. J. clin. Pharmacol. Biopharm. 16: 49–53, 1978
4 Penry, J. B., A. Livingston: A comparison of diagnostic effectiveness and vascular side-effects of various diatrizoate salts used for intravenous pyelography. Clin. Radiol. 23: 362–369, 1972
5 Speck, U., H.-M. Siefert: Unpublished data.
6 Speck, U., R. Nagel, W. Leistenschneider, W. Mützel: Pharmakokinetik und Biotransformation neuer Röntgenkontrastmittel für die Uro- und Angiographie beim Patienten. Fortschr. Röntgenstr. 127: 270–274, 1977
7 Stoeter, P., K. Voigt: Cerebral angiography with Ioglicinate (Rayvist®). A double blind study of image quality and clinical side effects. Radiologe 19: 494–498, 1979
8 Taenzer, V., W. Clauss, I. Simon: Sodium or methylglucamine salts as contrast media for urography? Fortschr. Röntgenstr. 133: 78–83, 1980
9 Taenzer, V., A. Albrecht, W. Clauss, I. Held: Sodium salts or methylglucamine salts in contrast media for infusion pyelography? Radiologe 21: 288–290, 1981

# Urography with Non-ionic Contrast Media:

## I. Diagnostic Quality and Tolerance of Iohexol in Comparison with Meglumine Amidotrizoate

V. Taenzer, H. Heep and W. Clauss

## Summary

The double-blind study described in this paper shows that the non-ionic substance iohexol is superior to meglumine amidotrizoate in intravenous urography. Visualization of the urinary system and the general tolerance are better.

## Zusammenfassung

Bei der intravenösen Urographie ist im Doppelblindversuch das nicht-ionische Iohexol dem Meglumin-Amidotrizoat überlegen. Die Darstellungsqualität der ableitenden Harnwege und die allgemeine Verträglichkeit sind besser.

## Introduction

In animal experiments, the excretory kinetics of non-ionic contrast media are superior to those of ionic agents (2, 4, 6, 7, 9, 12, 16). Urographic studies in patients, particulary in children, are available which show the same results (1, 8, 10, 11). The following report describes the clinical experience gained in a double-blind comparative study between iohexol (Omnipaque, Schering AG) and meglumine amidotrizoate (Urovist, Schering AG).

## Material and Methods

The randomized, double-blind comparative study was conducted in two independent radiological departments in Frankfurt/M (F) and Berlin (B) in a mixed sample of patients. Each centre studied two groups of 15 patients each (60 patients) aged from 18–75 years. The sex distribution was almost the same with 29 men and 31 women. Patients with serum creatinine values of more than 1.5 mg%, known hypersensitivity to contrast media and severely impaired general condition of various etiology were excluded from the study. Specific preparation was achieved in almost all the patients, i.e. withdrawal of fluids and food to achieve a comparable state of hydration: 95% of the patients adhered to the instruction not to drink, laxatives were administered in 56%, and 20% also received an antiflatulent.

30 patients received iohexol and 30 meglumine amidotrizoate at a dosage of 1 ml/kg body weight with almost the same iodine content of 300 and 306 mg/ml, as an intravenous injection given in 1 to 2 minutes. Neither the examining doctor nor the patient knew which contrast medium was being administered.

Standardized, large-format x-ray films for complete coverage of kidneys and urinary tract were made by examiner (B) at 10 and 20 minutes after the injection, and by examiner (F) at 1, 5 and 10 minutes after the injection. .Additional films and radiological methods such as tomography and others required for the diagnosis were not included in the comparative assessment.

## Evaluation Criteria

The x-ray films were analysed by the respective examiner for the quality of visualization of the renal parenchyma, pelvicalyceal system and ureters, and separately by one examiner (B) for contrast quality and state of filling of the urinary tract. As in previous studies (14, 15), the qualitative assessment was made in the categories good, adequate, poor and no demonstration. The contrast quality was classified as "good" if it permitted perfect diagnostic evaluation with a contrast density in the urinary tract higher than the x-ray absorption of the bones of an approximately 30-year old healthy person. "Adequate" meant contrast density less than this but still permitting reliable diagnostic evaluation. The contrast was classified as "poor" if visualization of the urinary tract was inadequate and diagnosing was difficult, uncertain or impossible.

The evaluation criteria for filling of the urinary tract irrespective of the opacification were similar. Complete filling of the calyces, renal pelvis and ureters was classified as "good", filling of these sections of the urinary tract to about two thirds which still permitted diagnosis was classified as "adequate", while only partial opacification of the calyces or filling of the ureters to only about one third was classified as "poor".

Contrast medium tolerance:
a) Clinical: The results of the tolerance study were evaluated and classified as good, moderate or poor. The tolerance was classified as "good" if no or only transient, slight side effects (slight sensation of warmth or heat) occurred. Depending of their extent and duration, respiratory complaints, nausea, vomiting or skin eruptions were classified as either "moderate" or "poor" tolerance.
b) Haemodynamic: The blood pressure and pulse rate were recorded immediately before the contrast medium administration, and immediately, five and twenty minutes after the end of the injection.
c) Laboratory: Blood samples were taken immediately before and six and twenty four hours (Trialist F) or 48 hours (Trialist B) after administration of the contrast media and the following parameters determined:
Creatinine, urea-nitrogen, alkaline phosphatase, sodium, calcium and potassium, SGOT, SGPT, Gamma GT, LDH, Hb, hematocrit, differential blood picture with erythrocyte and leukocyte counts.
The early morning urine was analysed before the examination and 24 hours later for:
Total protein, urea, erythrocytes, creatinine, potassium, sodium and calcium.

The numerous data determined in the study were evaluated by computer.

## Results

### Radiodiagnosis

An overall comparative assessment of the quality of the contrast films is shown in Table 1. Good and adequate films were obtained in all 30 patients, i.e. in 100%, examined with iohexol, but in only 25 (= 83%) of the patients examined with meglumine amidotrizoate ($p < 0.05$). The quality of the individual sections of the kidney, i.e. the parenchyma, renal pelvicalyceal system and the ureters, is shown individually in Table 2 for the films taken 5, 10 and 20 minutes after the injection.

If the renal elimination of the two substances is judged by the best assessment of the contrast achieved at the respective time point (= good), the films taken 5, 10 and 20 minutes after the injection

Table 1  Overall assessment of the quality of opacification

| classification | iohexol | meglumine amidotrizoate |
| --- | --- | --- |
| good | 15 (50.0%) | 12 (40.0%) |
| adequate | 15 (50.0%) | 13 (43.3%) |
| poor | 0 (0%) | 5 (16.7%) |
| not demonstrable | 0 (0%) | 0 (0%) |
| n | 30 (100%) | 30 (100%) |

show that the nephrographic effect, which was equally good under both preparations 1 minute after injection, decreased more quickly after iohexol than after meglumine amidotrizoate. Iohexol leads to good opacification of the pelvicalyceal system and the ureters more frequently at an earlier time and also for a longer period. The tabular comparison of the filling states (Table 3) shows that, at the dose of 1 ml contrast medium per kg body weight studied here, there are no differences between the filling of the urinary tract at the times 10 and 20 minutes after the injection ($p > 0.05$, Fischer's exact method for the qualities good and adequate on the one hand, poor and no demonstration on the other).

Pathological x-ray findings were made in six patients and normal findings in 24 after injection of iohexol, and in 11 and 19 patients, respectively, after administration of meglumine amidotrizoate.

### Side Effects

The overall assessment of the tolerance shows a significant difference between the two preparations in favour of iohexol. Side effects, most of them clinically insignificant, were observed in 12 (40%) of the patients examined with iohexol and in 19 (63%) of those examined with meglumine amidotrizoate. The incidence of the different side effects is shown in Table 4. Whereas only one side effect – classified as mild – was reported per patient after iohexol, multiple side effects which were also more serious as regards their nature and intensity were a quite frequent occurrence after meglumine amidotrizoate.

Apart from the clinically relevant blood pressure changes shown in Table 4, the routine blood pressure checks revealed no deviation of the mean systolic values by more than 20 mm Hg, of the mean diastolic values by more than 10 mm Hg and of the pulse by more than 10 signals per minute. Beyond these limits, meglumine amidotrizoate has a somewhat greater effect on the blood pressure

Table 2  Assessment of the opacification at 5, 10 and 20 minutes (%)

| classification | parenchyma | | pelvicalyceal system | | ureters | |
|---|---|---|---|---|---|---|
| | iohexol | meglumine amidotrizoate | iohexol | meglumine amidotrizoate | iohexol | meglumine amidotrizoate |
| *5 minutes* | | | | | | |
| good | 16.7 | 43.3 | 33.3 | 16.7 | 20.0 | 10.0 |
| adequate | 53.3 | 13.4 | 56.7 | 40.0 | 23.3 | 33.3 |
| poor | 30.0 | 43.3 | 10.0 | 43.3 | 43.3 | 50.0 |
| not demonstrable | 0 | 0 | 0 | 0 | 13.4 | 6.7 |
| examinations evaluated (n) | 15 | 15 | 15 | 15 | 15 | 15 |
| *10 minutes* | | | | | | |
| good | 21.7 | 37.3 | 50.0 | 47.5 | 38.3 | 45.8 |
| adequate | 40.0 | 32.2 | 40.0 | 35.6 | 33.3 | 30.5 |
| poor | 38.3 | 30.5 | 8.3 | 16.9 | 20.0 | 16.9 |
| not demonstrable | 0 | 0 | 1.7 | 0 | 8.4 | 6.8 |
| examinations evaluated (n) | 30 | 29 | 30 | 29 | 30 | 29 |
| *20 minutes* | | | | | | |
| good | 3.3 | 24.1 | 73.4 | 41.4 | 63.4 | 24.1 |
| adequate | 63.4 | 48.3 | 23.3 | 55.2 | 20.0 | 51.7 |
| poor | 33.3 | 27.6 | 3.3 | 3.4 | 6.6 | 17.3 |
| not demonstrable | 0 | 0 | 0 | 0 | 10.0 | 6.9 |
| examinations evaluated (n) | 15 | 14 | 15 | 14 | 15 | 14 |

The percentages are calculated from the mean values of the assessment of the right and left kidney

Table 3  Assessment of the filling state at 10 and 20 minutes (%)

| classification | pelvicalyceal system | | ureters | |
|---|---|---|---|---|
| | iohexol | meglumine amidotrizoate | iohexol | meglumine amidotrizoate |
| *10 minutes* | | | | |
| good | 75.9 | 79.3 | 27.6 | 41.4 |
| adequate | 20.7 | 20.7 | 34.5 | 34.5 |
| poor | 3.4 | 0 | 37.9 | 13.8 |
| not demonstrable | 0 | 0 | 0 | 10.3 |
| n | 29 | 29 | 29 | 29 |
| *20 minutes* | | | | |
| good | 60 | 62.1 | 20.7 | 20.7 |
| adequate | 33.3 | 27.6 | 37.9 | 51.7 |
| poor | 6.7 | 10.3 | 34.5 | 20.7 |
| not demonstrable | 0 | 0 | 6.9 | 6.9 |
| n | 30 | 29 | 29 | 29 |

The percentage are calculated from the mean values of the assessment of the right and left kidney

Table 4  Number, nature and severity of the side effects

| side effects | iohexol (n = 30) mild | severe | meglumine amidotrizoate (n = 30) mild | severe |
|---|---|---|---|---|
| venous pain | 0 ( 0%) | 0 | 1 ( 3.3%) | 0 |
| nausea | 1 ( 3.3%) | 0 | 1 ( 3.3%) | 3 (10.0%) |
| vomiting | 0 ( 0%) | 0 | 1 ( 3.3%) | 0 |
| sensation of warmth/heat | 11 (36.7%) | 0 | 12 (40.0%) | 6 (20.0%) |
| tachycardia | 0 | 0 | 2 ( 6.7%) | 1 ( 3.3%) |
| blood pressure change | 0 | 0 | 5 (16.7%) | 0 |
| respiratory complaints | 0 | 0 | 1 ( 3.3%) | 0 |
| urticaria | 0 | 0 | 2 ( 6.7%) | 0 |
| other side effects | 0 | 0 | 4 (13.3%) | 1 ( 3.3%) |

and pulse rate than iohexol in the form of a slight increase. The blood pressure values return to the initial level at the latest after 20 minutes.

Clinico-chemical analyses of the blood and urine revealed only slight changes within the normal values without any indication of statistically significant differences. This applies in particular to the serum creatinine and urea-nitrogen values, which are used to assess renal function. It must be borne in mind here, however, that patients with distinctly pathological creatinine values were excluded from this study.

## Discussion

### Urographic Quality

With conventional ionic contrast media, the urographic contrast – the concentration of contrast material in the urine – is greatly influenced by the nature of the radiolucent cations (14, 15). Compared to meglumine-containing salts, sodium salts of the contrast media cause less osmotic diuresis – probably because of reabsorption of the sodium$^+$. In practical use, better results can be achieved after administration of Urovison-Natrium or Urovison (mixed salt with a preponderance of $Na^+$) than after the meglumine salts of amidotrizoate (Urovist).

The double-blind study between the meglumine salt of amidotrizoate and the non-ionic substance iohexol confirms earlier observations (5, 10) of a reduced nephrographic effect after administration of non-ionic uro-angiographic agents. The renal pelvicalyceal system and the urinary tract are enhanced to a relatively greater extent after iohexol, confirming experimental studies reporting on higher urinary iodine concentrations resulting from a reduced osmodiuretic effect of non-ionic contrast media. Generally speaking, however, the inadequate filling of the urinary system which one would expect as a consequence of this was not confirmed at the times 10 and 20 minutes after the injection at the dose of 1 ml/kg body weight used in our study. Although a tendency towards more frequent good filling of the ureters after meglumine amidotrizoate is recognizable temporarily 10 minutes after the injection, this has disappeared after 20 minutes.

In children, the superior contrast density of the bladder filling offers the advantage to perform voiding cystograms without any additional methods (12). According to Aakhus et al., iohexol is completely eliminated with the urine in unchanged form. Bianchi et al. have shown that the reduced osmodiuretic effect of non-ionic contrast media in comparison to traditional ionic contrast media is also of great diagnostic value in patients with severe renal insufficiency.

For the reasons mentioned at the start of the discussion, the findings of better contrast quality for iohexol in comparison to the pure meglumine salt of amidotrizoate cannot so easily be extrapolated to preparations with sodium salts which are often used because of their high urographic contrast.

### Tolerance

In theory and according to the results of animal experiments, the reduction of osmotic activity under non-ionic contrast media should lead to better tolerance on intravenous injection as well (13), the reasons being:

reduced cardiovascular stress due to lower hypervolaemia, less impairment of the flow properties of the blood, extremely low binding to plasma proteins and no more electrical charging.

Despite the relatively small number of patients, the double-blind study reveals a clear-cut reduction in the side effects rate after intravenous use of the non-ionic substance iohexol for urography.

A slight sensation of warmth is almost the only side effect observed after iohexol. The greater cardiovascular stress caused by Urovist manifests itself not only in the development of tachycardia and respiratory complaints, but also in a greater effect on the blood pressure and pulse rate ($p > 0.05$).

Non-ionic substances have been used in babies and infants because of their better tolerance and improved opacification (3, 8). The use of these substances is advantageous not only in babies, but also in patients with severe cardiovascular diseases who are particularly sensitive to osmotic hypervolaemia.

At the present time, the high price prohibits the general use of non-ionic urographic agents.

The reduced osmotic diuresis means that higher renal concentrations can be achieved than after ionic contrast media. There are no indications in the literature that this might result in poorer renal tolerance (9, 16), and our laboratory analyses also failed to reveal any evidence for a negative effect on renal function.

## References

1. Aakhus, T., S. Ch. Sommerfelt, H. Stormorken, K. Dahlström: Tolerance and excretion of iohexol after intravenous injection in healthy volunteers. Acta radiol. (Stockh.) Suppl. 362: 131, 1980
2. Bianchi, S. D., A. Granone, G. Gatti, B. Meozzi: La nefroangiotomografia con Iopamidolo nelle insufficienze renali. Minerva med. 72: 1531, 1981
3. Brun, B., M. Egeblad: Metrizamide in pediatric urography. Ann. Radiol. 22: 198, 1979
4. Evill, C. A., G. T. Benness: Urographic excretion studies with metrizamide and "dimer". A high dose comparison in dogs. Invest. Radiol. 13: 325, 1978
5. Fischer, K., C. Javot: Die intravenöse Urographie mit Aortogramm unter Verwendung eines Kontrastmittels mit geringer Osmolalität. Röntgen-Bl. 33: 496, 1980
6. Golman, K., T. Almén: Metrizamide in experimental urography: I. Iodine concentration and flow of urine following intravenous injection of an ionic and a nonionic contrast medium in rabbits. Acta radiol. (Stockh.) Suppl. 335: 312, 1973
7. Golman, K., J. Wilk: Renal excretion of a non-ionic contrast agent. Invest. Radiol. 14: 224, 1979
8. Hayek, H. W., G. Fleischhauer: Metrizamid (Amipaque) in der Ausscheidungsurographie von Neugeborenen und Säuglingen. Amipaque Workshop, Berlin 1978, Excerpta Medica, Amsterdam 1978
9. Holtås, S., K. Golman, C. Törnquist: Proteinuria following nephroangiography. VIII. Comparison between diatrizoate and iohexol in the rat. Acta radiol. (Stockh.) Suppl. 362: 53, 1980
10. Kolbenstvedt, A., E. Andrew, B. Christophersen, K. Golman, B. Kvarstein, H. H. Lien: Metrizamide in high-dose urography. Acta radiol. Diagn. 20: 39, 1979
11. Oppermann, H. C., M. Klett, E. Willich: Metrizamid in der kinderurologischen Röntgendiagnostik. Amipaque Workshop, Berlin 1978, Excerpta Medica, Amsterdam 1978
12. Sjöberg, S., T. Almén, K. Golman: Excretion of urographic contrast media. I. Iohexol and other media during free urine flow in the rabbit. Acta radiol. (Stockh.) Suppl. 362: 93, 1980
13. Speck, U.: Neue intravenöse Kontrastmittel für die Cholegraphie, Urographie und Computertomographie. Röntgenpraxis 35: 47, 1982
14. Taenzer, V., W. Clauß, I. Simon: Natrium- oder Methylglucaminsalze der Kontrastmittel für die Urographie? Fortschr. Röntgenstr. 133: 78, 1980
15. Taenzer, V., A. Albrecht, W. Clauß, I. Held: Natrium- oder Methylglucaminsalze der Kontrastmittel für die Infusionsurographie? Radiologie 21: 288, 1981
16. Törnquist, C., T. Almén, K. Golman, S. Holtås: Proteinuria following nephroangiography. VII. Comparison between ionic monomeric, monoacidic dimer and non-ionic contrast media in the dog. Acta radiol. (Stockh.) Suppl. 362: 49, 1980

# Urography with Non-ionic Contrast Media:
## II. Diagnostic Quality and Tolerance of Iopromide in Comparison with Ioxaglate

V. Taenzer, P. Meiisel and P. Hartwig

## Summary

The intravenous administration of the contrast agents iopromide and ioxaglate at a dose of 1 ml/kg body weight leads to good urographic results. Iopromide is suitable for urography in particular because of its excellent tolerance.

## Zusammenfassung

Iopromid und Ioxaglat führen nach intravenöser Kontrastmittel-Applikation bei einer Dosis von 1 ml/kg Körpergewicht zu guten urographischen Ergebnissen. Iopromid ist besonders wegen der ausgezeichneten Verträglichkeit zur Urographie geeignet.

## Introduction

Iopromide is a new non-ionic radiographic contrast medium displaying physico-chemical, pharmacological and toxicological properties similar to those of metrizamide. In contrast to the latter, however, it can be produced as a stable solution ready for injection.
In animal experiments, 94 ± 6% of the intravenously administered dose of iopromide is eliminated with the urine (2 ±1 % with the faeces) in the dog, and 90% with the urine (10% with the faeces) in the rat. In man, the pharmacokinetics are analogous to those of amidotrizoate and metrizamide, 94% of the substance administered being eliminated with the urine. The results suggest that iopromide is highly suitable as a contrast agent for urography and angiography. A pilot study (information of Schering AG) in excretory urography with 14 volunteer subjects demonstrated that the best radiographic quality is obtained after injection of a dose of 100 ml, which is well tolerated. The following report on clinical experience from a double-blind comparative study between the ionic, low-osmolar contrast medium ioxaglate (Hexabrix, Guerbet) and the non-ionic contrast medium iopromide, Schering AG, complements the urographic comparison between the non-ionic substance amidotrizoate and the ionic contrast medium iohexol conducted in part I.

## Material and Methods

The double-blind comparative study was conducted in the radiological departments of the Wenckebach Hospital, Berlin-Tempelhof, and the Hospital Moabit, Berlin-Tiergarten, in a mixed group of patients.
A randomization plan was drawn up according to which 30 patients aged from 18 to 75 years received ioxaglate and 30 patients of the same age range received iopromide at a dosage of 1 ml/kg body weight given within 2 mins. as an intravenous injection. The iodine dose was almost the same at 300 and 320 mg/ml, respectively. 98% of the patients had undergone preparation (dehydration in 69%, laxatives in 68%, antiflatulents in 48%). The study design was otherwise the same as the guidelines described in Part I in respect of the exclusion criteria for the inspection of the radiological documentation, the recording of laboratory parameters and the evaluation for urographic quality and contrast medium tolerance.

## Results
### Radiodiagnosis

It can be seen from Table 1, which shows the overall assessment of the contrast quality, that the number of evaluations classified as good tends to be larger after iopromide (59%) than after ioxaglate (47%). Analysis of the quality of the contrast in individual sections of the organ (Table 2) shows that good parenchymal enhancement was obtained more frequently after iopromide (50%) than after ioxaglate (33%) in the film taken 10 minutes after the injection. However, these differences are no

Table 1 Overall assessment of the contrast quality

| assessment | iopromide | ioxaglate |
| --- | --- | --- |
| good | 17 (58.6%) | 14 (46.7%) |
| adequate | 10 (34.5%) | 15 (50.0%) |
| poor | 2 ( 6.9%) | 1 ( 3.3%) |
| not demonstrable | 0 | 0 |
| n | 29 (100%) | 30 (100%) |

longer present 20 minutes after the injection. There are no differences between the two filming times as regards opacification of the renal pelvicalyceal system and the ureters. Assessment of the filling states (Table 3) 10 minutes after the injection shows that good filling of the ureters is achieved more frequently after ioxaglate (33%) than after iopromide, whereas there are no differences as regards filling of the pelvicalyceal system. There is no difference between the two contrast media in respect of filling of the renal cavity system and the ureters 20 minutes after the injection.

Table 2 Assessment of the contrast quality at 10 minutes and 20 minutes (%)

| assessment | parenchyma | | pelvicalyceal system | | ureters | |
| --- | --- | --- | --- | --- | --- | --- |
| | iohexol | ioxaglate | iopromide | ioxaglate | iopromide | ioxaglate |
| *10 minutes* | | | | | | |
| good | 50.0 | 33.3 | 81.1 | 80.0 | 55.2 | 65.5 |
| adequate | 27.5 | 30.0 | 13.8 | 15.0 | 20.7 | 13.8 |
| poor | 22.5 | 36.7 | 5.1 | 5.0 | 13.8 | 5.2 |
| no demonstration | 0 | 0 | 0 | 0 | 10.3 | 15.5 |
| number of examinations evaluated (n) | 29 | 30 | 29 | 30 | 29 | 30 |
| *20 minutes* | | | | | | |
| good | 29.3 | 20.0 | 77.6 | 80.0 | 48.2 | 50.0 |
| adequate | 51.7 | 41.8 | 15.5 | 18.3 | 22.5 | 32.8 |
| poor | 19.0 | 37.2 | 6.9 | 1.7 | 15.5 | 10.3 |
| no demonstration | 0 | 0 | 0 | 0 | 13.8 | 6.9 |
| number of examinations evaluated (n) | 29 | 30 | 29 | 30 | 29 | 30 |

Table 3 Assessment of the filling state at 10 minutes and 20 minutes (%)

| assessment | pelvicalyceal system | | ureters | |
| --- | --- | --- | --- | --- |
| | iopromide | ioxaglate | iopromide | ioxaglate |
| *10 minutes* | | | | |
| good | 69.0 | 71.7 | 13.8 | 32.8 |
| adequate | 27.6 | 25.0 | 41.8 | 17.2 |
| poor | 3.4 | 3.3 | 34.5 | 34.5 |
| no demonstration | 0 | 0 | 10.3 | 15.5 |
| n | 29 | 30 | 29 | 30 |
| *20 minutes* | | | | |
| good | 60.5 | 58.4 | 20.7 | 29.3 |
| adequate | 32.8 | 38.3 | 36.2 | 27.6 |
| poor | 6.9 | 3.3 | 29.3 | 36.2 |
| no demonstration | 0 | 0 | 13.8 | 6.9 |
| n | 29 | 30 | 29 | 30 |

## Side Effects

The overall tolerance was classified as good after all injections of iopromide (=100%), whereas after ioxaglate it was assessed as good in only 77% and as moderate in 23% (venous pain in 10%, nausea in 20%, urticaria in 3%). Evaluation of the blood pressure and laboratory values revealed no significant differences.

## Discussion and Conclusions

Overall, there are no recognizable differences between iopromide and ioxaglate as regards the urographic quality. The two contrast media are equally suitable for urography. Despite the relatively small sample, however, impressive differences exist as regards the tolerance. Side effects such as venous pain and nausea – mainly harmless – were observed in almost a quarter of the patients after ioxaglate, while no side effects at all were observed after injection of iopromide in our sample of 30 patients. Ioxaglate is an ionic dimer which, like the dimers used for intravenous cholegraphy, displays comparatively different liophilia and high protein binding of almost 8% (2).

The general association between the side effects rate and protein binding is well-known (1). Comparative studies between iohexol, metrizamide and ioxaglate conducted by Mützel et al. demonstrated that histamine release and complement activation are greatest after administration of ioxaglate. Our clinical results are supported or explained by these experimental studies.

## References

1 Lasser, E. C., J. W. Lang: Contrast-protein interactions. Invest. Radiol. 5: 446, 1970
2 Mützel, W., H.-M. Siefert, U. Speck: Biochemical-pharmacologic properties of iohexol. Acta radiol. (Stockh.) Suppl. 362: 111, 1980
3 Speck, U., G. Mannesmann, W. Mützel, G. Schröder: Preliminary evaluation of new non-ionic contrast media. Radiology Today, Salzburg 1980. Springer, Berlin 1981

# Computerized Tomography

## Contrast Medium Tolerance in Computed Tomography

H. Tschakert

### Summary

In 6 randomized double-blind studies in 1000 patients the tolerance of various x-ray contrast media with comparable iodine contents was studied.
Apart from the different injection speeds all other conditions of the investigation were kept constant. With a low speed of injection (½ ml/sec) the pure meglumine salt of amidotrizoic acid showed better tolerance than the pure sodium salt or the mixed salt. When the injection speed was first incresed (1 ml/sec) meglumine ioglicate was judged to be superior to meglumine amidotrizoate. Its tolerance is finally (2–5 ml/sec) clearly exceeded by that of the two non-ionic preparations Iohexol and Iopromide.

### Zusammenfassung

In 6 randomisierten Doppelblindstudien wurde bei 1000 Patienten die Verträglichkeit verschiedener Röntgenkontrastmittel mit vergleichbarem Jodgehalt untersucht.
Abgesehen von der unterschiedlichen Injektionsgeschwindigkeit wurden sämtliche sonstige Untersuchungsbedingungen gleichgehalten. Bei niedriger Injektionsgeschwindigkeit (½ ml/sec) zeigt das reine Megluminsalz der Amidotrizoesäure gegenüber dem reinen Natriumsalz und dem Mischsalz die bessere Verträglichkeit. Bei Erhöhung der Injektionsgeschwindigkeit wird zunächst (1 ml/sec) das Megluminioglicinat als dem Megluminamidotrizoat überlegen beurteilt. Dessen Verträglichkeit wird schließlich (2–5 ml/sec) deutlich von den beiden nicht-ionischen Präparaten Johexol und Jopromid übertroffen.

### Introduction

Computed tomography has undergone rapid technological development in the last 5 years. The reduction in the scanning times to below 2 sec. per single slice and the possibility of rapid succession of slices has made it possible to perform dynamic contrast medium examinations of single organs or of the large blood vessels. It was possible to increase the diagnostic value with bolus injections of contrast medium (6, 9, 10, 17, 18, 24, 30, 39). This means that new demands are made on the contrast media. On the one hand, in order to permit broad application of these specific computed tomographic examinations the risk of intolerance reactions when the injection speed is raised must be kept low. On the other hand, subjective feelings of discomfort frequently make the patient restless or unable to hold his breath during the examination. This then leads to artefacts or makes it necessary to break off the examination.
The aim of the contrast medium studies performed was to examine the frequency and severity of the side-effects of various contrast media at different injection rates.

### Methods

Between 1979 and 1982 six double-blind studies were performed with two of the contrast media to be compared respectively. Before the contrast medium injection all the patients were informed about possible side-effects.
After the examination the subjective feelings of discomfort reported in response to unspecific questioning and the objectively verifiable side-effects were recorded. Dysphasic or confused patients were excluded from the study and only patients aged between 18 and 70 years were included.
In all cases the administration of contrast medium was in the context of a cranial computed tomographic examination. The respective contrast media, which were at a room temperature of 21 °C, were injected into the right cubital vein via a 19-Butterfly in a dose of 300 mg iodine per kg body weight; the injection time was measured with a stop-watch.
All the studies took the form of randomized double-blind investigations in which neither the patient nor the examining doctor knew which type of contrast medium was being used.

Table 1  Physicochemical properties of the examined contrast media

| Generic name | 1 ml CM contains | | osmolality osm/kg H$_2$O 37 °C | molecular weight | viscosity 20 °C mPa · s | 37 °C |
|---|---|---|---|---|---|---|
| | mg CM | mg iodine/ml | | | | |
| Na-amidotrizoate | 80 | 292 | 1.50 | 786.04 | 7.2 | 4.0 |
| Meglumine amidotrizoate | 520 | | | | | |
| Na-amidotrizoate | 300 | 500 | 1.57 | 635.90 | 4.1 | 2.4 |
| Meglumine amidotrizoate | 650 | 306 | 1.53 | 809.13 | 9.3 | 5.0 |
| Meglumine ioglicate | 683 | 300 | 1.79 | 866.18 | 11.5 | 6.0 |
| Iohexol | 647 | 300 | 0.72 | 821.17 | 11.0 | 5.7 |
| Iopromide | 623 | 300 | 0.62 | 791.14 | 9.7 | 5.0 |

Table 1 shows the different contrast media with their physical and chemical properties. All the side-effects were entered on uniform questionnaires after each contrast medium administration. At the end of each study the individual contrast medium reactions were classed in side-effect groups (Table 2) by an independent evaluator.

## Results

In the first part of our study we examined the type and frequency of side-effects of the various salts of amidotrizoate, a conventional monomeric ionic contrast medium, at a uniform injection speed of ½ ml/sec.

While in the case of the pure sodium salts of amidotrizoate nausea was reported most often and mild side-effects were recorded, in the case of the sodium-meglumine salt mixture more patients complained of a feeling of warmth. The overall rate of side-effects and of reactions requiring treatment after injection of pure sodium salts does not differ from that of the sodium-meglumine salt mixtures. The pure meglumine salts, however, show the lowest rate of side-effects in all groups (Table 3).

In the second phase of our comparative studies the pure meglumine salt of ioglicic acid was compared with the monomeric ionic meglumine amidotrizoate and with the monomeric non-ionic iohexol and iopromide at various injection speeds.

At the injection speed of 1 ml/sec the ioglicate is found to have better tolerance in all side-effect groups while at the higher injection speeds the monomeric non-ionic contrast media (iohexol, iopromide) are significantly superior to it; in all side-effect groups the frequency of contrast medium reactions is significantly lower.

When the injection speed is increased the patients complain more often of a feeling of warmth after injection of meglumine ioglicate, likewise the overall rate of side-effects increases to about double. The side-effects requiring treatment surprisingly show a reverse pattern; at higher injection speeds the therapeutic measures are less often necessary (Table 3).

In 591 patients the contrast medium reactions were also studied as a function of age and sex (Table 4). Young patients complain more often of a sensation of heat and of non-anaphylactoid side-effects than older patients; comparison of the two sexes shows this tendency to be more marked in female patients.

Table 2  Classification of the subjective and objective side effects after contrast medium administration

1. Sensation of warmth or heat
2. Nausea, queasiness
3. Mild side effects
   - vomiting
   - pain
   - dizziness
   - headaches
   - urticaria
   - tachycardia (mild)
   - bradycardia (mild)
   - respiratory complaints (mild)
   - desire to sneeze
   - taste sensations
   - paresthesia
   - psychic or vegetative disturbances (mild)
4. Severe side effects
   - collapse
   - respiratory complaints (severe)
   - tachycardia (severe)
   - bradycardia (severe)
   - cardiac arrest
   - Quincke's oedema
   - arrhythmia (severe)
5. Side-effects requiring treatment

Table 3  Frequency of the side effects after administration of the examined contrast media

|  | Sodium megl.-amido-trizoate | Sodium amido-trizoate | Meglumine amido-trizoate | Meglumine amido-trizoate | Meglumine ioglicinate | Meglumine ioglicinate | Iohexol | Megl. ioglicinate | Iopromide |
|---|---|---|---|---|---|---|---|---|---|
| No. of cases | 100 | 100 | 200 | 100 | 200 | 100 | 100 | 50 | 50 |
| sensation of heat | 38% | 34% | 31% | 50% | 33% | 40% | 19% | 71% | 31% |
| nausea | 11% | 15% | 9% | 12% | 9% | 7% | 0% | 37% | 2% |
| mild side-effects | 18% | 24% | 14% | 21% | 15% | 9% | 4% | 33% | 8% |
| severe side-effects | – | – | – | – | 0.5% | – | – | – | – |
| total side-effects | 42% | 43% | 35% | 55% | 37% | 56% | 23% | 76% | 33% |
| side-effects requiring treatment | 5% | 6% | 3% | 5% | 6% | 3% | 1% | – | – |
| injection speed | ½ ml/sec | | | 1 ml/sec | | 2 ml/sec | | 5 ml/sec | |

Table 4  Sex and age distribution of adverse reactions after contrast medium administration

| age distribution | severe side effects | mild side effects | sensation of heath | no side effects | total |
|---|---|---|---|---|---|
| | | *male* | | | |
| 18–40 | – | 24 (23%) | 24 (23%) | 55 (54%) | 103 (100%) |
| 41–60 | 1 | 23 (14%) | 37 (23%) | 102 (63%) | 163 (100%) |
| 61–70 | – | 8 (15%) | 10 (20%) | 33 (65%) | 51 (100%) |
| total | 1 | 55 (17%) | 71 (23%) | 190 (60%) | 317 (100%) |
| | | *female* | | | |
| 18–40 | – | 18 (17%) | 33 (32%) | 52 (51%) | 103 (100%) |
| 41–60 | – | 25 (20%) | 27 (22%) | 70 (57%) | 122 (100%) |
| 61–70 | – | 7 (14%) | 7 (14%) | 35 (72%) | 48 (100%) |
| total | – | 50 (18%) | 67 (24%) | 157 (58%) | 274 (100%) |
| | | *total* | | | |
| 18–40 | – | 42 (20%) | 57 (28%) | 107 (52%) | 206 (100%) |
| 41–60 | 1 | 48 (17%) | 64 (23%) | 172 (60%) | 285 (100%) |
| 61–70 | – | 15 (15%) | 17 (17%) | 68 (68%) | 100 (100%) |
| total | 1 | 105 (18%) | 138 (23%) | 347 (59%) | 591 (100%) |

## Discussion

On the basis of a large patient sample W. H. Shehadi found a side-effect rate after intravascular contrast medium administration of about 5% and a mortality rate of 0.006%. It was mostly anaphylactoid reactions which were concerned here (37). Depending on the value attached to the side-effects, the type of examination procedure and the use of contrast medium and depending on the type of contrast medium, the site and speed of injection the figures given vary considerably (2, 11, 13, 20). The present investigations make it clear how great the differences in the side-effect rates are when only the speed of injection and the type of contrast medium are changed even though the iodine concentrations and the other conditions of the study were practically the same.

In accordance with the usual experience with contrast media the comparison of different salt components showed the pure meglumine salts to have the best tolerance, in particular less nausea and sensation of heat. Meglumine salts cause less endothelial irritation (28), in large doses they are found to be less toxic to the brain and myocardium (8).

The age and sex distribution shows no significant sex dominance for the individual side-effect groups. Younger patients, especially female ones, complain relatively more often of a sensation of heat and other subjective complaints such as dizziness, headaches and taste sensations. There are undoubtedly many reasons for this fact; greater fear of the contrast medium administration and possibly a lower tolerance limit may be factors which play an important part here (19). The objectively verifiable side-effects were distributed evenly between both sexes and the age groups as expected (37).

On consideration of the different injection speeds of one and the same contrast medium, e.g. of meglumine ioglicinate, two contrary tendencies were observed. On the one hand, as expected the overall side-effect rate increased with an increased injection speed, in particular there were more and intenser complaints of sensations of heat. On the other hand, the number of side-effects requiring treatment decreased when the injection speed was increased.

Studies on contrast medium tolerance in urography produce similar results: with an increase in injection speed there are increased complaints of a sensation of heat but the rate of contrast medium incidents requiring treatment remains at least the same or is lower (5, 13, 16, 36). Systemic contrast medium incidents of low or moderate severity are also rarer in angiography than in urography (36) although such a comparison must be regarded with caution as the conditions of the investigation were not the same.

A possible explanation for the higher rate of systemic side-effects at lower injection speeds could be that the longer contact time on the first heart and lung passage before dilution in the systemic circulation leads to more interaction between the contrast medium and the mast cell and basophil depot of the lung and is thus more likely to cause an anaphylactoid reaction.

A number of more recent studies and papers have shown that, with practically the same qualities of contrast (14, 15, 40), the new, non-ionic, monomeric contrast media have significantly better tolerance (here we only mention some general papers – 8, 32). Comparative studies emphasize particularly the better tolerance compared with the conventional ionic compounds at high injection speeds, in arteriographic examinations for example (7, 23, 38).

A number of studies confirm that most non-anaphylactoid contrast medium side-effects can be attributed to the high osmolality and the molecular toxicity of the individual contrast media (8, 32, 34). The non-ionic contrast media with their considerably reduced osmolality and lower molecular toxicity show less effects on haemodynamics – such as vasodilatation, changes in heartbeat sequence and flush symptoms, for example – reduced neurotoxicity and injury to the vascular endothelium, less influence on renal and myocardial function and less deformation and tendency towards aggregation of erythrocytes (3, 4, 12, 26, 27, 31, 32, 33, 34).

A study conducted in 1980 points out that the rate of anaphylactoid reactions is also lower with non-ionic contrast media (1). The reason discussed for this is, apart from the lower osmolality, the lower protein-binding capacity (25, 35) which appears to be responsible for the serum complement activation (22, 25). Further reasons for the low rate of anaphylactoid side-effects of the non-ionic contrast media could be on the one hand the reduced histamine release (25), on the other hand the reduced endothelial damage (26, 29). This, furthermore, is held responsible for the activation of coagulation factor XII as a consequence of which, via several intermediate steps, the elicitation of an anaphylactoid reaction is possible (21, 22).

In agreement with previous results the new, non-ionic contrast media are characterized by better tolerance, as was demonstrated in the double-blind studies performed. At higher injection speeds the side-effect rate of non-anaphylactoid reactions is distinctly lower, at an injection rate of 5 ml/sec into the V. cubitalis the incidence of side-effects is less than half of that with the ionic monomeric ioglicate.

On account of the only limited numbers of cases conclusive statements of the incidence of anaphylactoid reactions, in particular severe reactions, are not possible.

In all six studies only one severe contrast medium incident with bronchospasm and asystole was observed; thanks to immediate intervention this severe reaction was brought under control without detrimental consequences.

In spite of the present relatively high cost of the non-ionic preparations and the increasing price-consciousness in medicine their use in computed tomography in the so-called "angio-computed tomographic examinations„ is meaningful; with their help the most frequent subjective complaints such as feeling of heat, nausea with vomiting, dizziness, visual disturbances and severe taste sensations can be alleviated or even eliminated. This contributes to more distrubance-free examination and this could lead to a saving in repeat or additional examinations.

As there are indications that there is also a reduction in anaphylactoid reactions with metrizamide, a non-ionic contrast medium which has been on the market for about 10 years, further long-term studies should determine exact figures on the inci-

dence of moderate and severe contrast medium reactions.
If the lower incidence of reactions found for metrizamide is confirmed for the other non-ionic preparations, depending on future cost relations, the use of the non-ionic contrast media should be discussed in general, in particular for patients with an allergoid contrast media history.

## References

1 Almen, T., A. Nickel: In: Discussion, new contrast media. Symposion on contrast media toxicity. Invest. Radiol. Suppl. 340–344, 1980
2 Ansell, G.: Adverse reactions to contrast agents. Scope of problems. Invest. Radiol. 5: 374–394, 1970
3 Aspelin, P. et al: Effect of iohexol on human erythrocytes. Changes of red cell morphology in vitro. Acta radiol. (Stockh.) Suppl. 362: 117–122, 1980
4 Aspelin, P. et. al: Effect of iohexol on human erythrocyts. Red cell aggregation in vitro. Acta radiol. (Stockh.) Suppl. 362: 123–126, 1980
5 Davies, P., M. B. Roberts, J. Roylance: Acute reactions to urographic contrast media. Brit. J. Radiol. 434–437, 1975
6 Emde, H., N. Braun-Feldweg, U. Piepgras: Die quantitative Bildanalyse im Rahmen der kranialen Computertomographie. Fortschr. Röntgenstr. 131: 356, 1979
7 Fletcher, E. W. L.: A comparison of iopamidol and diatrizoate in peripheral angiography. Brit. J. Radiol. 55: 36–38, 1982
8 Grainger, R. G.: Osmolality of intravascular radiologic contrast media. Brit. J. Radiol. 53: 739–746, 1980
9 Hacker, H., H. Becker: Time controlled computed tomographic angiography. J. Comput. Ass. Tomogr. 1: 405, 1977
10 Harris, R. D., J. A. Usselman, V. D. Vint, M. A. Warmath: Computerized tomographic diagnosis of aneurysms of the thoracic aorta. Comput. Tomogr. 3: 81–91, 1979
11 Hessel, S. J., D. F. Adams, H. L. Abrams: Complications of Angiography – a nationwide Survey. RSNA 172, 1976 (Radiology 138: 273–281 [1981])
12 Higgins, C. B. et al.: Evaluation of the hemodynamic effects of intravenous administration of ionic and non-ionic contrast materials. Implications for deriving physiologic measurement from computed tomography and digital cardiovascular imaging. Radiology 142: 681–686, 1982
13 Jensen, N., S. Dorph: Adverse reactions to urographic contrast medium. Rapid versus slow injection rate. Brit. J. Radiol. 53: 659–661, 1980
14 Kormano, M. J.: Kinetics of Contrast Media after Bolus Injection and Infusion. Vortrag: Contrast Media in Computed Tomography. Int. Workshop, Berlin 1981. Excerpta Medica Int. Congr. Series 561. Excerpta Medica, Amsterdam
15 Kormano, M. J.: Basics on contrast enhancement in computed tomography. Vortrag: Radiology Today, Salzburg 1982. In: Donner/Heuck: Radiology Today, Vol. II., Springer, Berlin 1983
16 Kröpelin, T., Y. Heuser, Ch. Gospos: Kontrastmittelrisiko bei der Ausscheidungsurographie. In Zeitler, E.: Neue Aspekte des Kontrastmittelzwischenfalls. Symposion, Berlin 1977. Schering AG, Berlin 1978 (S. 103–115)
17 Lackner, K., H. Simon, P. Thurn: Kardio-Computertomographie – Neue Möglichkeiten in der radiologischen nichtinvasiven Herzdiagnostik. Z. Kardiol. 68: 667–675, 1979
18 Lackner, M., R. Felix, H. Oeser, O. H. Wegener, E. Buecheler, R. Buurmann, L. Hauser, U. Moedder: Erweiterung der Röntgendiagnostik im Thoraxbereich durch die Computer-Tomographie. Radiologe 19: 79, 1979

19 Lalli, A. F.: Urographic contrast media reactions and anxiety. Radiology 112: 267–271, 1974
20 Lalli, A. F., R. Greenstreet: Reactions to contrast media. Radiology 138: 47–49, 1981
21 Lasser, E. C.: New aspects of contrast reactions: considerations, ideology, and prophylaxis. Vortrag: Contrast Media in Computed Tomography. Int. Workshop, Berlin 1981 In: Excerpta Medica, Int. Congress Series 561. Excerpta Medica, Amsterdam 1981
22 Lasser, E. C.: Adverse systemic reaction to contrast media. In Sovak, M.: Handbook of Experimental Pharmacology, Contrast Media Colume. Springer, Heidelberg 1982
23 Molyneux, A. J., P. W. E. Sheldon: A randomized blind trial of Iopamidol and meglumine calcium metrizoate (Triosil 280, Isopaque Cerebral) in cerebral angiography. Brit. J. Radiol. 55: 117–119, 1982
24 Moss, A. A., J. Schrumpf, P. Schnyder, et al.: Computed tomography of focal hepatic lesions – a blind clinical evaluation of the effect of contrast enhancement. Radiology 131: 427–430, 1979
25 Mützel, W. et al.: Biochemical-pharmacological properties of iohexol. Acta radiol. (Stockh.) Suppl. 362: 111–115, 1980
26 Nyman, U., T. Almén: Effects of contrast media on aortic endothelium. Experiments in the rat with non-ionic and ionic monomeric and monoacidic dimeric contrast media. Acta radiol. (Stockh.) Suppl. 362: 65–71, 1980
27 Nyman, U. et al.: Effect of contrast media on femoral blood flow. Comparison between non-ionic and ionic monomeric and monoacid dimeric contrast media in the dog. Acta radiol. (Stockh.) Suppl. 362: 43–48, 1980
28 Penry, J. B., A. Livingston: A comparison of diagnostic effectiveness and vascular side-effects of various diatrizoate salts used for intravenous pyelography. Clin. Radiol. 23: 362–369, 1972
29 Raininko, R.: Role of hypertonicity in the endothelial injury caused by angiographic contrast media. Acta radiol. (Stockh.) 20: 410–416, 1979
30 Raininko, R., M.-L. Majurin, P. Virtama, P. Kangasniemi: Value of high contrast medium dose in brain CT. J. Comput. Ass. Tomogr. 6: 54–57, 1982
31 Rapoport, S. L., H. J. Thomson, J. M. Bidinger: Equiosmolol opening of the blood-brain barrier in the rabbit by different contrast media. Acta radiol. Diagn. 15: 21–32, 1974
32 Rapoport, S., J. J. Bookstein, C. E. Higgins, P. H. Carey, M. Sovak, E. C. Lasser: Experience with metrizamide in patients with previous severe anyphylactoid reactions to ionic contrast agents. Radiology 143: 321–325, 1982
33 Romano, J. J., D. D. Shaw: Hemodynamic and Cardiovascular Effects during Canine Carotid Arteriography. A comparison of iohexol (Win 39, 424), Renografin 60, Conray 60 and Isopaque. Report of 19. Sept. 1980 in the files of Sterling-Winthrop Research Institute
34 Salvensen, S.: Acute intravenous toxicity of iohexol in the mouse and in the rat. Acta radiol. (Stockh.) Suppl. 335: 5–13, 1973

35 Salvesen, S., K. Frey: Protein binding of metrizamide and the effect on various enzymes. Acta radiol. (Stockh.) Suppl. 355: 247–252, 1977
36 Shehadi, H.: The risks involved in the use of contrast media in cholecystocholaniography. In Zeitler, E.: Neue Aspekte des Kontrastmittelzwischenfalls. Symposion, Berlin 1977. Schering AG, Berlin 1978 (S. 91–102)
37 Shehadi, W. H., G. Toniolo: Adverse reactions to contrast media. Radiology 137: 299–302, 1980
38 Tillmann, U., R. Adler, W. A. Fuchs: Pain in peripheral arteriography – a comparison of a low osmolality contrast medium with a conventional compound. Brit. J. Radiol. 52: 102–104, 1979
39 Tschakert, H.: Zeitlicher Ablauf des Dichteverhaltens von Lebermetastasen nach Kontrastmittelgabe. Fortschr. Röntgenstr. 133: 171, 1980
40 Tschakert, H.: New contrast substances for angiography. Vortrag, Radiology Today, Salzburg 1982. In: Donner/Heuck: Radiology Today Vol. II. Springer, Berlin 1983

# Experiences with Rayvist and Iopromid in Head and Body CT

E. Zeitler, K. Böhnlein, H. Gailer, R. Lindner and E.-I. Richter

## Summary

The results of application of Rayvist 300 as an infusion for computed tomography are reported, including the small number of contrast reactions observed. Furthermore, a randomised comparison between Iopromid and Rayvist as bolus injection, demonstrated that reactions occurred only after Rayvist administration. The behaviour of both contrast media as a function of time is virtually identical. Small degrees of difference were perceived in the enhancement of tumors and in the timing of contrast enhancement of the renal medulla. The latter could have practical importance in evaluating diseases affecting primarily the renal cortex, or medulla, as well as in the detection of rejection reactions in renal transplant patients.

## Zusammenfassung

Ergebnisse von Rayvist-300-Infusion bei der Computer-Tomographie werden einschließlich der geringen Anzahl beobachteter Nebenwirkung berichtet. Darüber hinaus zeigt ein randomisierter Vergleich zwischen Iopromid und Rayvist als Bolusinjektion, daß Nebenwirkungen nur nach Rayvist-Applikation auftreten. Das Verhalten beider Kontrastmittel als eine Funktion der Zeit ist nahezu identisch. Geringe Unterschiede werden beim "enhancement" von Tumoren und beim "timing" des Enhancement des Nierenmarks beobachtet. Letzteres hat praktische Bedeutung bei der Erkennung von Nierenerkrankungen, die primär die Nierenrinde oder das Mark betreffen, aber auch bei der Entdeckung von Abstoßungsreaktionen von Transplantatnieren.

## Choice of Contrast Agent

The means of administration and amount of contrast medium used in diagnostic CT of the brain and body have special importance in the evaluation of parenchymal organs and vessels (1–9).

The following modes of administration are possible:

1. Infusion of 100–250 cc of contrast agent within 6 to 10 minutes
2. Single bolus injection of 30–100 cc by hand or power injector
3. Injection of multiple 30–40 cc contrast agent boluses.

Administration of a large amount of contrast medium as a prolonged i.v. drip is designed primarily to provide uniform enhancement of parenchymal organs, with the intensity of enhancement comparable from one slice to the next. Bolus injection is used primarily to provide transient high-grade enhancement (particularly in vascular structures) (1, 2, 9). One can further differentiate dynamic contrast enhancement (4) into angio CT, which concerns the demonstration of vessels primarily, and sequential CT, with the objective of determining time-dependent density changes throughout a given level.

Angio CT serves not only to substantiate pathologic arterial or venous structures, but also to separate vascular structures from parenchymal changes. In the context of head CT this is of particular importance in documenting aneurysms and angiomas. In the upper abdomen, angio CT allows better evaluation of pathologic changes in the region of the pancreas and porta hepatis, in the retroperitoneum, one may impressively document the atypical course of renal vessels with respect to the vena cava, as well as tumour extension into the vena cava from hypernephromas.

Sequential CT allows the clear evaluation of the ebb and flow of contrast medium within a CT slice, as well as its distribution. This is most clearly substantiated in the region of the aorta and surrounding vessels, and also permits differentiation of renal cortex from medulla. Sequential CT also can document the passage of contrast medium through tumours, making the formulation of differential diagnoses possible from the resulting pattern.

The increasing importance of contrast medium application in the context of CT examinations sets particular prerequisites for the applied contrast agent. In the following, we report our experience with Rayvist 300 and Iopromid 300 in diagnostic CT. The structural forms, as well as characteristics of both contrast agents are portrayed in Table 1 and Figs 1 and 2. While Rayvist 300 is a ionic contrast medium with osmolality of 1.79 Osm/kg $H_2O$, the newly developed contrast medium Iopromid has an osmolality of only 0.58 Osm/kg $H_2O$. The iodine concentration in both solutions is 300 mg per ml.

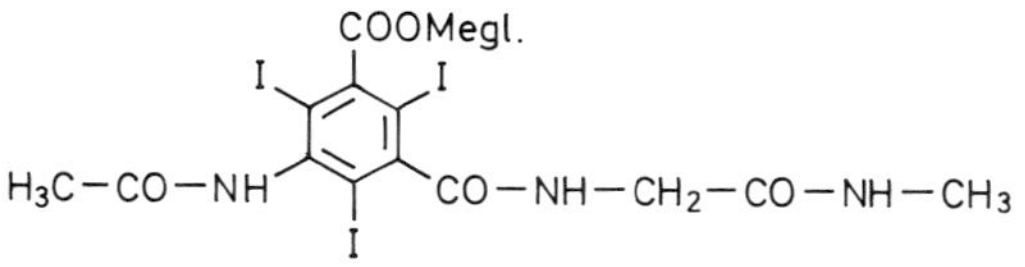

5-Acetamido-2,4,6-triiod-[CN-methyl=carbamoyl)methyl]-isophthalamic acid N-Methylglucaminsalt
Molecular weight: 866.18
Iodine content: 43.95%

Fig 1  Rayvist 300 (Megluminioglicinate)

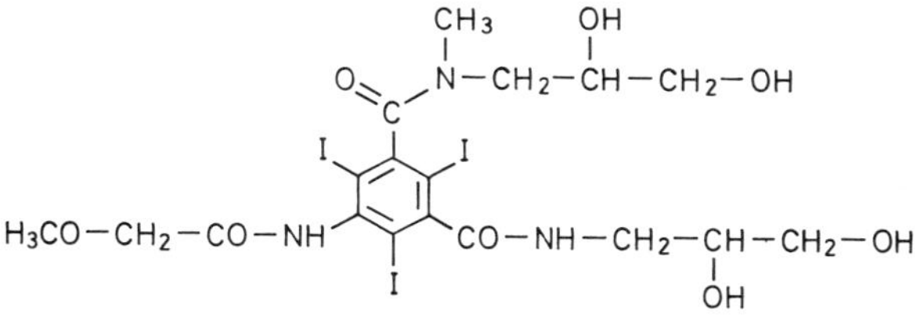

5-Methoxyacetylamino-2,4,6-triiodisophthalsäure- (2,3-dihydroxy-N-methylpropyl)-((R,S)-2,3-dihydroxypropyl) diamid (lupac)
Molecular weight  791.144
Iodine content:  48.1%

Fig 2  Iopromid (ZK 35 760)

Table 1  Characteristics of Rayvist 300 and Iopromid 300

|  | Rayvist 300 | (Iopromid 300) |
|---|---|---|
| Generic name | ioglicinic acid N-methylgluc.-salt | Iopromid SHL 414 C |
| Molecular weight | 866.18 | 791.14 |
| Iodine content of the substance (% of weight) | 43.95 | 48.10 |
| Contrast media content of the solution (g/100 ml) | 68.3 | 62.3 |
| Iodine content of the solution (mg/ml) | 300 | 300 |
| Osmotic pressure at 37° C (Mpa) | 4.61 | 1.50 |
| Osmolality at 37° C (Osm/kg H$_2$O) | 1.79 | 0.58 |
| Viscosity at 37° C (mpa.s) | 6.0 | 4.9 |

Table 2  Head – CT. 1. 1. 81 – 22. 12. 81

| 3285 | with Rayvist 300 (Ioglicinate) 1576 (48%) | | |
|---|---|---|---|
|  | contrast reactions |  | 1.14% |
|  | mild | 10 | 0.63% |
|  | moderate | 7 | 0.44% |
|  | severe | 1 | 0.06% |

Table 3  Body – CT. 1. 1. 81 – 22. 12. 81

| 3020 | with Rayvist 300 (Ioglicinate) 1319 (44%) | | |
|---|---|---|---|
|  | contrast reactions |  | 0.83% |
|  | mild | 4 | 0.3 % |
|  | moderate | 7 | 0.53% |

The following questions were investigated:

1. How is ioglicinate tolerated as a 100 ml infusion in adults in the context of head and whole body CT?
2. A double-blind study was performed comparing the side effects of Ioglicinate and Iopromid when applied as a bolus by power injector in a dose of 1.5 cc/kg body weight.
3. Time-density curves were prepared for aorta, celiac artery, vena cava, pancreas, liver, spleen, kidneys, and renal veins after bolus injections and checked for any significant differences.

## Side Effects and Their Frequency with the Infusion Method of Contrast Agent Application

In 1981, computer tomographic studies of the body and head were almost equally divided in number in the diagnostic radiology section of the Klinikum Nürnberg. The number of examinations, frequency of contrast administration as Ioglicinate infusion, and the frequency of side effects are set forth in tables 2 and 3.

100 cc of Rayvist 300 were given as a rapid infusion within 5 to 10 minutes. Of the 3285 CT examinations of the head and brain, contrast medium was administered in this matter in 1576 cases (48%). Systemic contrast medium reactions were observed in 1.14%, among which there was one severe reaction.

44% of body CT studies were carried through with contrast agent infusions. Systemic reactions were encountered in 0.83%. No severe reactions occurred. Patients often spontaneously remarked about a sensation of heat caused by the contrast medium, but without additional symptoms, this was rarely perceived as objectionable.

## Double-blind Study Comparing Ioglicinate and Iopromid

To compare the patient tolerance of ionic contrast medium Ioglicinate with the non-ionic Iopromid, a bolus injection of 1.5 ml contrast medium per kilogram body weight was employed. The injection was performed through a plastic catheter or butterfly needle in an arm vein, and was driven by an automatic injector at a standard rate of 8 ml/sec.

Patients under 40 years of age or over 70 were not included in the study. Such exclusions were due to the frequency of cardiac insufficiency in the older patients, and the intent to minimize radiation exposure in those patients requiring a sequential CT study. Under these conditions, 50 patients were studied with either Rayvist or Iopromid. Contrast reactions appeared in 3 patients who received Rayvist. Of these, 2 involved an objectionable sensation of heat in conjunction with mild tachycardia, and 1 patient experienced an intense sensation of heat with hypotension, urticaria, and angio-oedema. Among those patients who had received Iopromid, no side effects were observed beyond a mild sensation of heat. In any case, patients spontaneously remarked about sensations of heat more frequently after Rayvist administration than after Iopromid. Thus, the patient tolerance of the latter contrast medium is quite satisfactory in this mode of administration.

## Contrast Enhancement in Various Vessels and Parenchymal Organs

Contrast changes in CT exams after administration of Rayvist or Iopromid were measured by obtaining average density values, expressed in Hounsfield units, in various regions of interest. Among the 50 patients receiving Rayvist, 49 cases could be evaluated. Of the group receiving Iopromid, 2 of the 50 patients could not be evaluated, since the examinations were interrupted.

Sequential CT examination consisted of 10 consecutive scans, with the first performed at the start of contrast injection and serving as a standard for later contrast enhancement. Subsequent scans were obtained in 10 sec. intervals (after 12, 22, 32, 52 and 62 sec.) using the quick scan mode of a SOMATOM-SD with the cardiac angio series option. Scanning was performed in the region of the pancreas, where the aorta, vena cava inferior, liver, spleen and pancreas could be evaluated in the majority of examined patients (Fig 3).

To complete the procedure, the examination table would be quickly moved 8 to 12 cm to a preselected level, containing not only aorta, vena cava and portions of liver and spleen, but also kidneys and renal veins. In 10 patients we were able to see kidneys, liver and spleen in the initial sequential CT level within the first minute of the examination. However, in these cases the pancreas was not contained in the chosen level.

With the chosen contrast dose in the bolus injection technique, a high degree of contrast enhancement is not only substantiated in the spleen and liver, but also regularly seen in the region of the pancreas. The illustration from a patient with acute pancreatitis shows precise delineation of pancreatic tissue from an early exudate in the region of the pancreatic tail. In the early parenchymal phases the amount of contrast concentration in the spleen might be termed as "over-enhancement". In the same phase the vessels of the splenic hilus are well portrayed, just as the intrahepatic branches of the portal vein and enhancement of the gallbladder wall.

The demonstration of the pancreas, with its separation from the splenic vein, mesenteric vein and vessels in the region of the porta hepatis, is to a large part dependent on the choice of slice level for the sequential CT. The bolus technique provides a clear improvement in diagnostic accuracy in the region of the pancreas and in suspected portal venous thrombosis (Fig 4).

After bolus injection of Rayvist 300, compared to Iopromid 300, the behaviour and distribution of contrast agent is virtually the same in the aorta and in the region of the pancreas, with maximum concentration of contrast medium already 22 sec. after the start of injection (Fig 5). Contrast distribution curves show parallel behaviour in the aorta and pancreas from the end of the first minute onward. Within the first minute, if the slice levels are unchanged, a characteristic curve can be demonstrated. In the following 4 minutes the oscillations that arise in the curves may be due to loss of uniform conditions, subject to the table transport and the lack of total consistency in timing of the scans, now obtained at 30 sec. intervals. The course of contrast mediated changes in the liver is identical with both contrast media. After 70 to 80 sec. the density is the same as that in the aorta, and the gradual subsequent decrease in contrast medium parallels that found in the aorta (Fig. 6).

Contrast enhancement occurs earlier in the spleen than in the liver. The peak density reaches a level of approx. 150 Hounsfield units (HU), while a peak of about 110 HU is seen in the parenchymal of the liver. In the region of the upper abdomen, clear overenhancement occurs only in the region of the spleen. The ability to differentiate abnormalities in

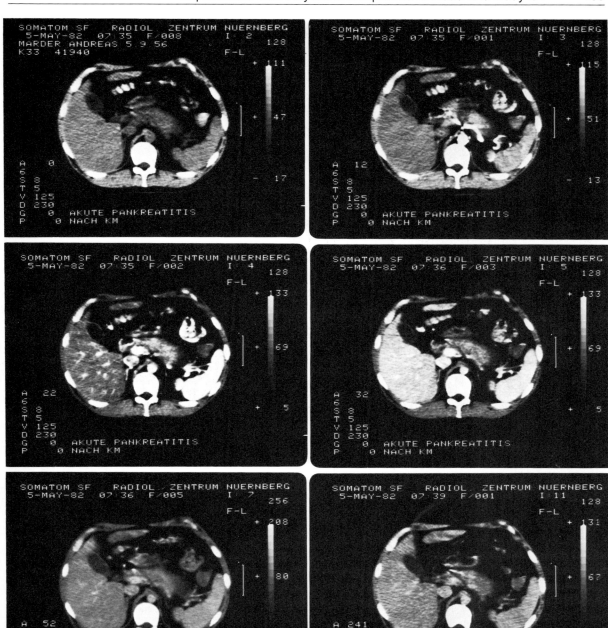

Fig 3 Sequential CT of the upper abdominal organs in 10 sec. intervals in a patient with acute pancreatitis. Emphasis of the intrahepatic branches of the portal vein, enhancement of pancreas, slight exudation in the pancreatic tail

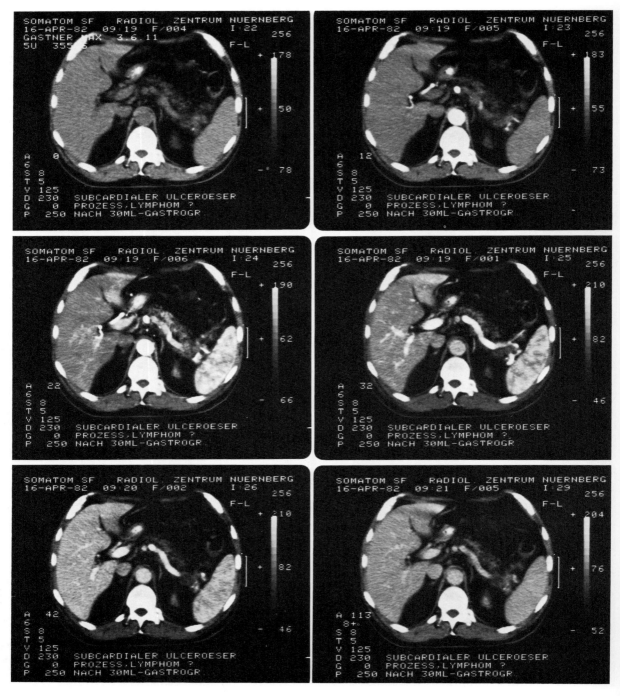

Fig 4 Sequential CT of the upper abdominal organs with clear documentation of the splenic vein. Irregular contrast enhacement in the pancreas, normal contrasting of the intrahepatic vascular structures

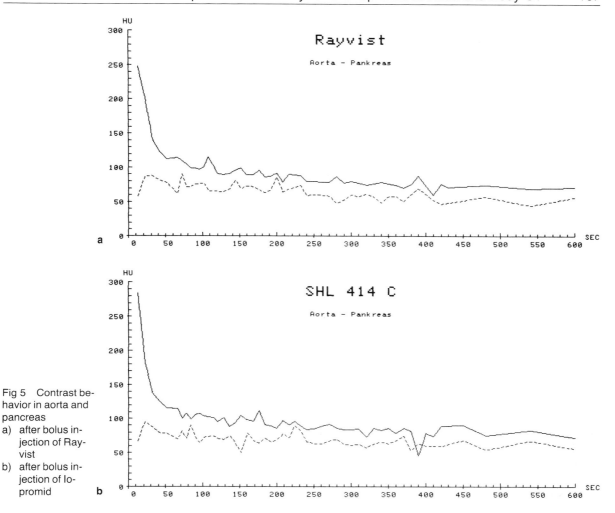

Fig 5 Contrast behavior in aorta and pancreas
a) after bolus injection of Rayvist
b) after bolus injection of Iopromid

the liver is considerably better in sequential CT than in CT after slow contrast media infusion.

The rise in the level of contrast in the coeliac artery occurs within 12 to 14 sec. Contrast values over 150 HU were seen after application of Rayvist, with the simultaneous enhancement of the aorta to 250 HU. After Iopromid injection the highest values measured in the aorta, as well as in the coeliac artery after 12 sec. were higher. The further course, and the gradual decrease in contrast levels were the same with both preparations.

The number of patients we examined with liver metastases was too small to permit us to draw any firm conclusions. It did seem to us, however, that contrast enhancement within liver metastases was quite clear with Rayvist, while after Iopromid enhancement was not as extensive. Therefore, further investigations comparing Iopromid with ionic contrast media in sequential CT should be of special interest with regard to tumor detection.

Analysis of findings in the region of the renal veins shows that 20 to 30 sec. after start of injection there is already prominent appearance of contrast agent in the renal veins, while the aorta and renal arteries are still at the maximum level of enhancement. In this early phase, the density of the renal vein reaches that of the coeliac artery. The following drop in intensity in the renal veins corresponds to that seen in the aorta and the parenchymal organs (Fig 7). The perceptible oscillations in contrast levels may be traced to the difficulties in differentiating precisely renal cortex from medulla. If one doesn't differentiate the behaviour of contrast between renal medulla and cortex, a symmetric drop in the contrast level can be recognized after a maximum between 20 and 30 sec.

Actually, the differential enhancement of cortex and medulla are of special interest in the kidneys. Using regions of interest analysis in 10 patients, it was shown that a two-phase peak was reached after

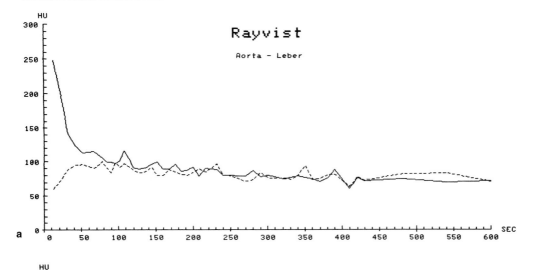
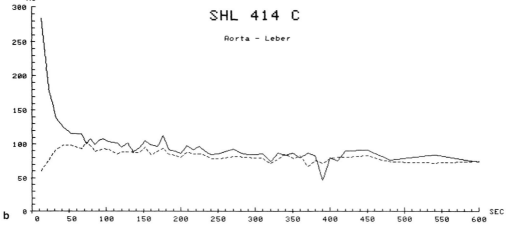

Fig 6 Contrast behaviour of aorta and liver in sequential CT
a) after bolus injection of Rayvist
b) after bolus injection of Iopromid (HU = Hounsfield units)

administration of Rayvist, while this was not seen after Iopromid, but were rather represented by a plateau. The equalization of contrast agent in cortex and medulla occurs earlier after Rayvist than after Iopromid injection (Fig 8). This might promise a better differentiation between cortex and medulla with Iopromid. These results, however, were not seen in all patients.

A comparison of sequential CT of the level of the kidneys (Figs 9 and 10) shows the emphasis of the renal cortex especially well up to 32 sec., and the decreasing differentiation of cortex from medulla as early as 52 sec. with both contrast media. The application of a high contrast medium dose in our study may have favourably influenced the differentiation between cortex and medulla by overenhancement. It remains to be seen whether a smaller contrast medium dose might lead to better differentiation, perhaps for a longer period of time. In order to draw conclusions about the behaviour of the contrast media in the early phases of sequential CT, further studies with narrower scan intervals and larger numbers of patients are needed.

## Discussion

Our investigations of the tolerability and behaviour of contrast agents in the upper abdominal organs and kidneys shows that both Rayvist 300 and Iopromid 300 are well tolerated, and provide essentially the same level of enhancement in the abdominal organs. Substantial contrast media reactions were only observed after the application of Rayvist 300. The prominent enhancement of liver and pancreas within the first 30 sec. after bolus injection compared with drip infusion, is advantageous in the differentiation of anatomic detail from pathologic changes of these two organs. Both contrast media can be used in a similar fashion for this purpose. Both contrast agents are well suited

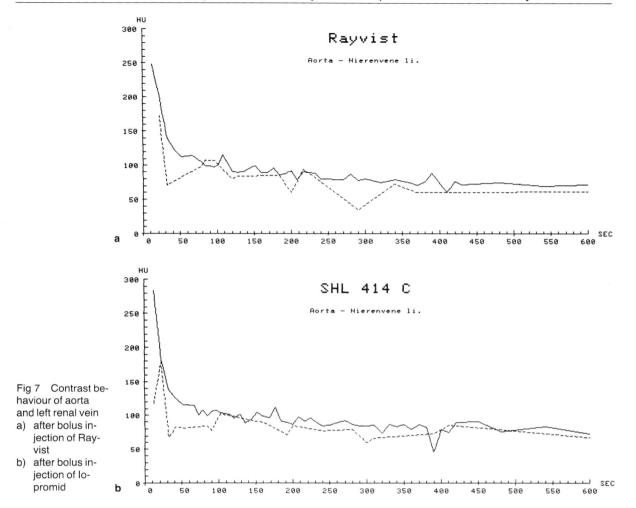

Fig 7 Contrast behaviour of aorta and left renal vein
a) after bolus injection of Rayvist
b) after bolus injection of Iopromid

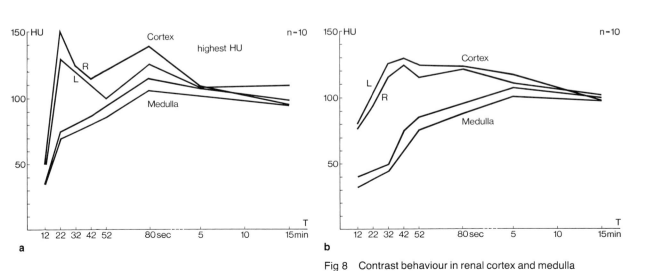

Fig 8 Contrast behaviour in renal cortex and medulla
a) after bolus injection of Rayvist
b) after bolus injection of Iopromid

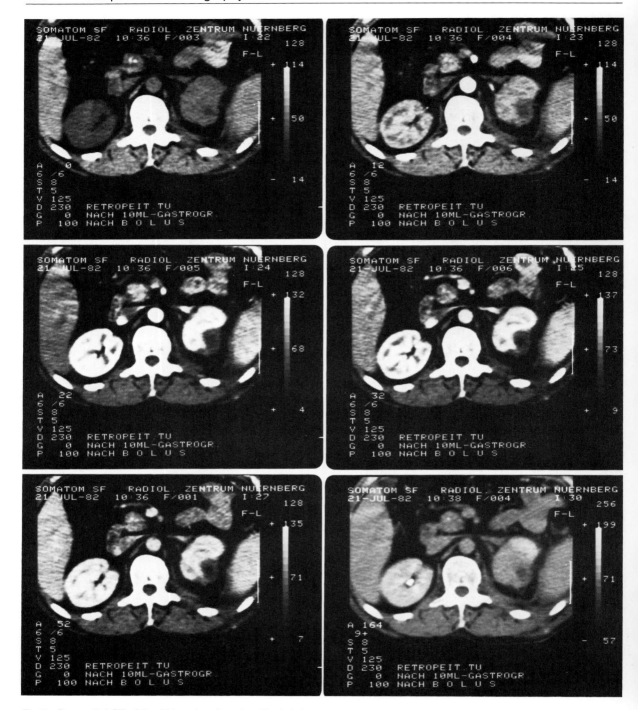

Fig 9 Sequential CT of the kidney in a female with rhabdomyosarcoma after bolus injection of Rayvist

for differentiation of renal cortex and medulla in the early phases of sequential CT. It remains to be established by more extensive studies, whether our initial impression of prolonged transit of Iopromid in the renal cortex proves true.

# Experiences with Rayvist and Iopromid in Head and Body CT

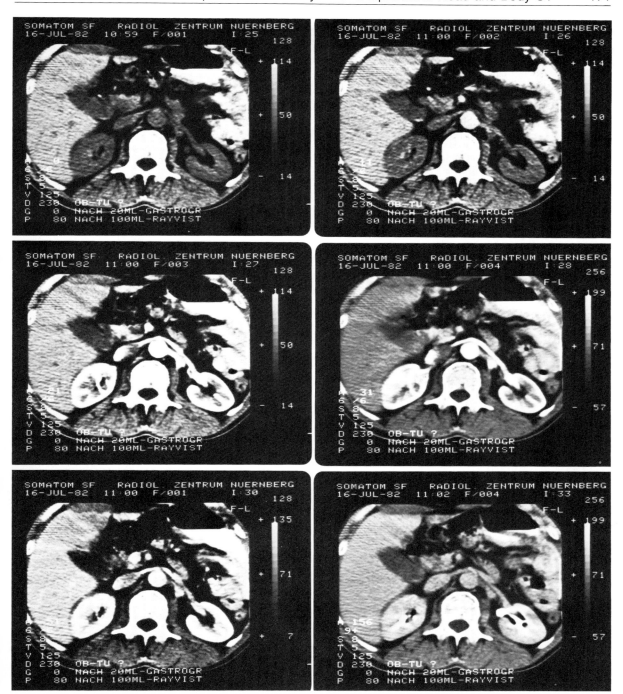

Fig 10 Sequential CT of kidneys and renal veins after bolus injection of Iopromid

## References

1 Baert, A. L., G. Wilms, G. Marchal, P. De Mayer, F. De Somer: Contrast enhancement by bolus technique in the CT examination. Radiologe 20: 279–287, 1980
2 Felix, R., E. Kazner, O. H. Wegener: Contrast Media in Computed Tomography. Excerpta Medica, Amsterdam 1981
3 Fuchs, W. A., P. Vock, M. Haertel: Pharmakokinetik intravasaler Kontrastmittel bei der Computer-Tomographie. Radiologe 19: 90–93, 1979
4 Hübener, K. H., K. J. Klott: "Statisches" und dynamisches Kontrastmittelenhancement der Körperstamm-Computertomographie. Fortschr. Röntgenstr. 133, 4: 347–354, 1980
5 Kirschner, H., A. Kremp, H. Poppe: Vergleich der Häufigkeit von Nebenwirkungen zwischen der zweiphasigen Bolusperfusor- und der einphasigen Bolusinjektion eines Röntgenkontrastmittels in der kranialen Computertomographie. Fortschr. Röntgenstr. 133, 2: 119–124, 1980
6 Kormano, M. J.: Kinetics of contrast media after bolus injection and infusion. In Felix, R., E. Kazner, O. H. Wegener: Contrast Media in Computed Tomography. Excerpta Medica, Amsterdam 1981 (p. 38)
7 Rossi, P.: Contrast Enhancement in CT of the Great Arteries. In Fuchs, W. A.: Contrast Enhancement in Body Computerized Tomography. Thieme, Stuttgart 1981 (p. 45–57)
8 Treugut, H., U. Nyman, J. Hildell: Sequenz-CT: Frühe Dichteveränderungen der gesunden Niere nach Kontrastmittelapplikation. Radiologe 20: 558–562, 1980
9 Wegener, O. H.: Ganzkörper-Computer-Tomographie. Schering-Hausverlag, Berlin

# Subject Index

## A

Adverse reactions, incidence 104, 126, 132, 145, 151, 158, 163
– age distribution 158
Alanine aminopeptidase (AAP) 39
Albuminuria 25, 37
Alkaline phosphatase (AP) 33, 39
Angiography, techniques 94
Arteriography, aortofemoral 78
– cerebral 62, 115
– peripher 50, 57, 62, 102, 107
Arylsulphatase A (ASA) 33

## B

$\beta_2$-microglobulin 43
Blood pressure 71, 79, 122

## C

Calorimetry 108, 117
Chemotoxicity 6, 8
Clotting 18
Complement activation 15, 18, 52
Coronary arteriography 67
Coronary sinus blood, acidosis 70, 72
– electrolytes 70
– osmolality 70, 72

## D

Digital subtraction angiography 125
Dolorimetry 108, 117

## E

EACA epsilonaminocaproic acid 21
ECG 67, 71, 122
Endothelium, damage 52, 137
Enhancement, CT, Iopromide, Ioglicate 167
– – pancreas, liver, kidney 162
Erythrocytes 13, 15, 52

## F

Factor XII a 21, 52
Fibrinolysis 18

## G

Gamma glutamyltranspeptidase (GGT) 32, 39

## H

Hang over effect, pain 57, 112
Heart rate 71, 72, 80, 122
Histamine liberation 14, 15, 52
Hydrogen ionic concentration, coronary blood 72
Hydrophilicity 7, 8
Hypertonicity, side effects 8, 50

## I

Improvement of contrast materials 9
Inotropism 71, 75

## K

Kallikrein 21, 52
Kidney cell-membrane antigen 40

## L

Lactat dehydrogenase (LDH) 32
LD 50  13, 14
Leucin aminopeptidase (LAP) 32
Lidocaine 96
Lysozyme 14

## N

N-acetyl-$\beta$-D-galactosidase (NAG) 31
Nephroangiography 27, 41
Nephrotoxicity 37
Neural tolerance 9, 14, 63, 64

## O

Osmolality 5

## P

Pain, genesis 52
– vascular, arteriography 50, 57, 64, 96, 104, 108, 117
Partition coefficient 6
Pharmacokinetics, Iopromide 85
Physicochemistry, contrast media 2–8, 70, 157, 163
Plasminogen 20
Prophylaxis, CM risks 141
Protein-binding 7
Proteinuria 37, 43

## R

Risk liability, contrast media, endogenous, exogenous factors 130

## S

Shock, causes of, time factor 132
Side effects, see adverse reactions
Surface glycoprotein (SGP) 41

## T

Thrombin 19
Thromboplastin 20
Thymidine 137

## U

Urography 143
– non-ionic contrast media 148, 153

## V

Viscosity 7